Bjørg Marit Andersen

Prevention and Control of Infections in Hospitals

Practice and Theory

Volume II

Springer

Bjørg Marit Andersen
Department of Hospital Infections
Oslo University Hospital
Oslo
Norway

Faculty of Health and Social Science
University of South-Eastern Norway
Oslo
Norway

Original Norwegian edition published by Elefantus Forlag, Moss, 2016

ISBN 978-3-319-99920-3 ISBN 978-3-319-99921-0 (eBook)
https://doi.org/10.1007/978-3-319-99921-0

Library of Congress Control Number: 2018963171

This Springer imprint is published by the registered company Springer Nature Switzerland AG
The registered company address is: Gewerbestrasse 11, 6330 Cham, Switzerland

Preface

Prevention and Control of Infections in Hospitals: Practice and Theory deal with infection control, surveillance and hygienic routines and key topics, both practical and theoretical. The book is adapted to a necessary level of infection prevention to cope with today's emerging and resistant microbes, hygienic challenges and emergency preparedness in practical work. It updates current knowledge about infection protection as basic for selecting routines and guidelines to prevent hospital infections.

Healthcare-associated infection (HAI) is primarily a patient safety issue, causing more than 90% of patient injuries. Leaders at all levels in the healthcare system are responsible for patient safety and infection control, from the director of the hospital to the health minister and government, and this should be warranted by law. Lack of management is associated with overcrowding, understaffing, corridor-beds, poor maintenance of buildings and equipment, inadequate cleaning and basic hygienic measures which often lead to HAIs. Hospital infections may occur in 5–20% or more of hospitalized patients. In Europe, at least 7.5 million patients acquire HAI each year, and more than 147,000 patients die directly or indirectly from HAIs each year in European hospitals.

Hospital infections are detected more often after discharge, due to shorter and shorter stay in hospitals. This may lead to spread of resistant bacteria between healthcare levels and less favourable outcome for the patient with infection. Virus like influenza and norovirus follow the patient and may spread like "fire in dry grass". Entire departments with patients and personnel will be "sick-reported" and must shut down all activity for 2–3 weeks.

The spread of resistant and/or particularly pathogenic, contagious microbes poses a risk to patients, employees, visitors and society as a whole. Dangerous microbes often have a global spread pattern, which requires continuous readiness with effective, limiting measures against epidemics or pandemics.

The book is focused on practical measures against severe hospital infections such as postoperative wound infections; intravascular, blood-borne infections; infections in lower respiratory tract, urinary tract, skin and gastrointestinal tract; and infections in neonates and premature and in other patients with impaired infection defence.

A good hygiene is important to protect patients, visitors and employees against infections. Good hygiene routines, personal infection protection, cleanliness, textile treatment, sterility, disinfection and high professional hygiene standards for patient care increase patient safety and protect the working environment. Daily infection surveillance, infection detection and adequate contraceptive measures and information are required to stop the spread of infection.

The book is intended to be an aid and an optimal standard in practical work to reduce the incidence of serious hospital infections and spread of infection. This increases the quality of patient treatment; patient safety is better taken care of, and infection control becomes a natural part of measures around hospital patients and employees.

Prevention and Control of Infections in Hospitals: Practice and Theory is updated from earlier (1996, 1999, 2003, 2008, 2016) Norwegian handbooks in infection control, lastly published in 2016 (Elefantus forlag, Moss). Each chapter has a practical part and a background information and documentation part.

Thanks to the following colleagues for professional advises and comments:

Infection control nurses, Mette Rasch and Kjersti Hochlin; chief physician, Kjell Olafsen; and professor in medicine, PhD, Inggard Lereim.

In addition, I am grateful to my family, friends and colleagues for friendly assistance and positive support during the writing period. However, my greatest and most enthusiastic fan, my dog, Tito, left forever in May 2018.

Target groups: health professionals; doctors, nurses and other health professionals; students in health-related subjects, hospital leaders and health agencies; and patients and their relatives.

Oslo, Norway
June 2018

Bjørg Marit Andersen

Contents

Part V Respiratory Infections

Part XII Internal Service

Part X

Special Infections: Prevention

Admittance to Hospital

47

Abstract

Multidrug-resistant bacteria constitute a serious global threat—often as a result of dirty conditions treated with overuse of antibiotics. Dangerous microbes are easily transmitted when hygienic measures are inadequate, in the absence of isolation, and by overcrowding and understaffing. Extra costs and human suffering are related to the lack of consistency in the prevention and treatment of infections in the various levels of healthcare: poor and late diagnosis, lack of isolation measures and hygiene and incorrect use of antibacterial agents. Good infection control is linked to good hygiene, prosperity and security and breaks down quickly during disasters and chaos and when large crowds are on the move. Travelling to tropical areas is increasingly causing febrile diseases, by bacteria, viruses or parasites, depending on destination. More and more import-microbes are spread in healthcare and in society as a whole—and among animals by food and contact. Cross-infection occurs internally and between the different levels of healthcare, which can be avoided by good early information, good infectious protection and good disinfection and clearing of environmental contamination. Little by little new or emerging pathogenic microbes are becoming part of the regular human pathogenic flora in most countries and also in Scandinavia. These infections are creating carrier conditions and lead to increased mortality and costs in the healthcare. The following chapter is focused on practical measures to prevent early transmission of infections from patients before and at admittances in hospitals.

Keywords

Imported infections · Admittances in hospital · Pre-examination · Information Isolation · Nosocomial infections · Resistant bacteria · Dangerous virus Infection control · Hygiene · Prevention

B. M. Andersen, *Prevention and Control of Infections in Hospitals*,
https://doi.org/10.1007/978-3-319-99921-0_47

47.1 Purpose

Prevent transmission of multidrug-resistant bacteria and other contagious agents to patients, visitors, staff, equipment and/or environment:

- By pre-examination and information concerning infection—in advance—before admittance.
- By prepared procedures for early infection control [1–3].

47.2 Comprise

All patients to be admitted, examined as outpatient, day-treated or transported in ambulances and healthcare workers inside and outside hospitals—responsible for information of possible infectious patients.

47.3 Responsibility

The hospital's management provides guidelines for advanced information about the patients for early detection and control of import infection, multidrug-resistant agents, other serious infective agents and unknown types of infection, according to the country's infection control act or existing guidelines [1, 2]. The management should also provide resources for isolation and microbiological control of patients with possible infection to protect other patients and personnel.

The department's management implements preventive measures, ensures that employees follow the hospital's routines and reports to the Director in case of lack of resources (personnel, expertise, isolates) for necessary preventive measures.

The leaders of reception, outpatient clinics, day surgery, ambulance transport, emergency services and clinics should ensure that routines are followed and report to the Director regarding non-contraceptive measures that expose patients and personnel to infection.

Doctors and nurses who receive potentially infectious patients for admission or outpatient treatment should ensure satisfactory infection control measures. If relevant, they should inform actual referring doctor and healthcare institution, concerning detection of special infections that should be followed up.

Referring doctor (primary physician) or healthcare institutions who requests admission or outpatient examination/treatment is responsible for informing about possible infection [1, 2].

47.4 Practical Measures

47.4.1 Advanced Information About Infections: Before Admittances

- *Before* admission, day surgery, outpatient clinic, ambulance transport, etc.
- Applies to patient reception, primary care, emergency care, nursing homes and other healthcare institutions.

47.4.1.1 Before/During Admission/Treatment: Pre-Examination

Ask the referring doctor, emergency personnel, patient, etc. questions like: does the patient have:

- Diarrhoea and/or vomiting—now or recently?
- Respiratory infection?
- Influenza?
- Wound infection?
- Been abroad recently?—last year?
- Been in contact with healthcare abroad—last year?
- Previously been infected with MRSA, VRE, ESBL or other resistant bacteria?
- Been exposed to (direct contact with) persons infected/carriers of MRSA or VRE last year?
- Recently been infected with resistant bacteria?

  If yes:

- Treat as possible contagious in a single room/isolate until infection has been clarified (see isolation regimens Chaps. 14–21).

47.4.2 Imported Microbes and Other Microbes That Can Be Spread in Hospitals

47.4.2.1 Information, Advice and Guidance: Contact Infection Control Personnel

1. *Multidrug-resistant bacteria* that cause skin/wound infections, respiratory infections, urinary tract infections, sepsis, gastrointestinal infections, etc.:
   - MRSA (methicillin-resistant *Staphylococcus aureus*) transmitted by contact and air, from infected wounds, hands, equipment and fixtures. All persons present in the room can become carriers if not using PPE, [4] globally a common bacterial infection.
   - MRSA with vancomycin *resistance* (VRSA) or vancomycin *intermediate resistance* (VISA) is unusual today [4].
   - VRE (vancomycin-resistant enterococci) is common in many countries (the United States, Canada, Europe). Particularly *Enterococcus faecium* is resistant against vancomycin. VRE outbreak at several hospitals and nursing homes increases in Norway [5].
   - ESBL (extended-spectrum beta-lactamase-producing). Resistant, gram-negative rod bacteria with ESBL activity are increasing rapidly also in Norway, especially concerning *Escherichia coli*, *Enterobacter cloacae*, *Citrobacter* sp., *Serratia marcescens* and *Klebsiella* sp. [6].
   - Multidrug-resistant, gram-negative bacteria increase. Resistance to carbapenem (CRE), gentamicin, ciprofloxacin, etc., individually or in combinations: *Acinetobacter baumannii*, *Klebsiella oxytoca*, *Pseudomonas* sp., *Pseudomonas aeruginosa*, *Xanthomonas*, *Burkholderia cepacia*, *Stenotrophomonas maltophilia*, etc. [6].

- Penicillin-resistant pneumococci, macrolide-resistant group A streptococci and multidrug-resistant *Haemophilus influenzae* [7, 8].
- Multidrug-resistant, therapy-resistant *Mycobacterium tuberculosis* [9, 10].

2. *Intestinal infections* with bacteria [11]:
   - *Salmonella, Shigella, Campylobacter, Yersinia.*
   - Enteropathogenic *Escherichia coli*, entero-haemorrhagic *E. coli* (EHEC).
   - *Clostridium difficile*—CD (toxin producing and diarrhoea).
   - *Vibrio cholerae* and other vibrions.
3. *Protozoans* that cause intestinal infections [12]:
   - *Giardia lamblia.*
   - Cryptosporidia.
   - Entamoeba *histolytica.*
4. *Viruses* that cause liver infections, blood and/or other infections [13]:
   - Hepatitis A, B, C, D, E and HIV and HTLV.
5. *Viruses* that cause gastrointestinal symptoms [14]:
   - Norovirus, rotavirus, sapovirus, etc.
6. *Viruses* which cause respiratory symptoms [15]:
   - Influenza virus, parainfluenza virus, metapneumovirus, bocaviruses, enteroviruses, RSV, adenovirus.
7. *Fungus infections*—invasive [16].

47.4.3 Definitions and Short Versions of Measures

1. Imported infection

Patients from abroad infected/carriers with resistant and/or virulent microbes, more frequently occurring abroad than in actual country:

- Directly in isolation if admitted—until known infection status (sampling and control). Use of personal protective equipment (PPE).
- Infection prevention measures for outpatient treatment.
- In case of negative tests—no more measures (no testing of personnel etc.)
- By positive tests—continued isolation, treatment and information.
  - Information concerning infection to the patient's next and possibly previous treatment unit.
  - If detecting MRSA, recommend testing of personnel who have had *unprotected* (without using PPE), direct contact with the patient. *See MRSA for further action, Chap. 49.*

2. Known infection

Patient admitted with a known infection such as MRSA, VRE, other multidrug-resistant bacteria (ESBL, CRE, TBC, CD), etc. For MRSA, this always applies (previously infected with MRSA,—ever).

- Directly in isolation if admitted. Check infection status.
- Infection prevention measures for outpatient treatment. Check infection status.
- In case of negative tests—no more measures.
- For negative tests in previous MRSA-positive patients, See MRSA for further action, Chap. 49.
- For positive tests—continued isolation and information to the patient and to the earlier and next treatment unit. *See Chap. 49 for further action.*

3. Unknown infection, detected randomly in clinical samples or by new information

In the event of unexpected discovery of resistant or special microbes and the patient has not been isolated:

- Directly in isolation if admitted.
- Infection prevention measures for outpatient treatment.
- Disinfection of relevant rooms and surfaces exposed to the infected patients.
- Infection control measures concerning exposed patients and personnel.
- Possible infection tracing (testing) and other measures, depending on the agent.
- Information to the patient and to previous and next treatment units.
- For detected MRSA and other special agents, *see the relevant chapter.*

NB! The isolation regime should not prevent necessary diagnostics and treatment!

47.4.4 Implementation of Measures

1. Preliminary assessment of infection risk:
   - *First contact*: Ask if the patient has been treated abroad or been a carrier/infected with resistant bacteria or other infectious agents. Risk of infection is addressed by telephone (postdoctor) or outpatient *before* admission/readmission.
   - In case of elective treatment, consider postponement until infection is resolved, possibly sanitized.
   - *In case of suspected highly infectious, severe import disease or other serious contagious disease (viral haemorrhagic fever, therapy-resistant pulmonary tuberculosis, diphtheria, pest,* etc.*)*, contact infection control personnel. Such patients should directly be in strict isolation, not through reception. (See chapters on strict isolation, highly infectious and serious import disease—PPE, bioterrorism).
2. Outpatient assessment first—if possible:
   - Determine the risk of infection and take samples.
   - Minimal equipment available in the room so that it can easily be washed afterwards.

- Staff wears surgical mask/cap, gloves and gown at all examinations and treatments.
- The room is disinfected and washed afterwards; inform cleaning staff!
- Responsible physician provides microbial sampling of the patient.

3. Admission in hospital and ward and suspected imported or other known infection: *isolation*
   - The ward/physician in charge provides isolation.
   - Not via patient reception but directly to current isolate.
   - Personnel who follow the patient to the hospital should not enter the ward. Exceptions are immediate help or when using PPE. If personnel accompany the patient from institutions abroad, see measures for healthcare professionals, Chap. 48.
   - Personnel/companions who have been MRSA-positive, have active tuberculosis infection, are infected with known resistant microbes, or have recently had symptoms of gastrointestinal infection, etc. should not enter the ward without agreement with the ward coordinator.
   - If *suspected* highly infectious, *severe import illness*, see point 1.
4. Isolate for imported infection, possible pulmonary tuberculosis or known MRSA—*see isolation routines, Chaps. 14–21*. Always wear gown, gloves and surgical mask/cap when receiving the patient! The following isolate types may be used for human pathogenic infectious agents:
   - *Isolate for air-/droplet-borne infections with negative air pressure.* In case of suspected pulmonary tuberculosis and other dangerous airborne agents, use respiratory protection (P3 mask) instead of surgical mask.
   - *Isolate for mainly contact-borne infections.* In case of suspected pulmonary tuberculosis, use respiratory protection (P3 mask), and transfer patient as soon as possible to isolate with negative air pressure.
   - *Single-patient room with anteroom and separate toilet/shower*—so that the patient is not using common corridor, etc. with other patients is an emergency solution. In case of suspected pulmonary tuberculosis, use respiratory protection (P3 mask) and transfer patient as soon as possible to negative air pressure isolation.
   - *Single-patient room without anteroom and/or without a separate toilet/shower* is a short-term emergency solution, *but should not be used in suspected pulmonary tuberculosis*. The patient should not enter the common hallway and must therefore use the mobile toilet seat in the room.
   - The *isolation* should continue until the microbiological control is negative.
   - Further *isolation* level (contact/air droplet) is determined when the infectious agent is known.
5. Immediate-help patient:
   - The *isolation* regime should not prevent necessary diagnostics and treatment.
   - Other *patients* and personnel should not be exposed to infection.

6. Treatment, transport, operation and other activities *outside* of the isolate—*see isolation routines*:
   - Inform relevant departments that had been or should be in contact with the patient.
   - Avoid unnecessary transport, examination and treatment of the patient before a negative test response exists.
   - Put on PPE before entering the patients' room.
   - Transport (if needed) the patient in a clean, new bed with clean clothes and clean bandages. The patient uses surgical mask (optionally respiratory protection) if respiratory symptoms are present.
   - Disinfect and wash locally at the places the patient has been. Inform cleaning staff!
   - If *suspected* of high-risk infection (viral haemorrhagic fever or pulmonary tuberculosis, etc.) contact infection control personnel immediately.
   - See the *operation* department's procedures for surgical treatment of patients with infections.
7. Procedure for test sampling:
   - Wear *gloves*, surgical mask/cap and gown with cuffs, and follow routines for taking on and off the PPE.
   - Rapid *tests*, such as MRSA and flu, are used for rapid clearance of infection status and to reduce isolation time; answer after about 2 h.

7(a) *Clinical samples*

Samples from wounds/pus/tissue/blood/catheters and other relevant infectious sites. Fill out the referral and inform about "*import* infection"/resistant microbes so that the laboratory can check the profile of resistance.

- Use ordinary sterile pencil that is placed in transport medium.
- Wet the pencil in sterile water before each sampling.
- Virus testing—follow routines; use virus transport medium.
- Rapid transport to the laboratory.
- Inform the laboratory of the need for quick response and if many tests will be done (infection tracing among other patients).

7(b) *Colonization or carrier state (import, MRSA, VRE, ESBL, CRE or other microbes).*

MRSA detection usually consists of four brush samples that can also be used for other bacteria:

- Sterile pencil in transport medium.
- Wet the pencil in sterile water before each sampling:
- One nose sample (front part of the nose floor/and internal walls, both nostrils—roll around three times in each nostrils).

- One throat sample (over the soft palate and tonsils three times).
- One from both wrists and hands ("wash" both hands and wrists).
- One from the perineum (stretches the area between the urethra and rectal openings three times).
- One from wounds/eczema/rash/scars, etc.

Record clinical information and ask for resistance profile.

7(c) *Other microbes*
- Wound/pus/expectorated specimens and samples from other relevant infection sites.
- VRE: perirectal/rectal samples.
- Imported intestinal infections or occurring in the actual country.
  - Faeces samples, possibly samples from vomiting, are sent for microbiological examination (bacteria, Clostridium difficile—toxins, viruses, parasites).
- *Mycobacterium tuberculosis*—expectorate samples for microscopy, rapid test and cultivation on suspicion of pulmonary tuberculosis.

8. Microbiological department
   - Remember clinical information and ask for resistance pattern.
   - In case of infection tracing, contact the microbiologist for the extent, shipment, rapid tests (MRSA, influenza, other respiratory tract infection, etc.) and rapid response procedures (by telephone).

9. Measures if detected infection
   - *See routines for isolation of MRSA and other resistant bacteria, tuberculosis, gastrointestinal infections, respiratory tract infections,* etc.
   - *Infection exposure?* Patient with proven infection/carrier state—*not isolated* from admission on—and with defined risk of transmission to the environment, personnel and other patients.
     - Infection tracing and eventually microbial screening of exposed patients and personnel (MRSA, tbc, etc.).
     - Exposed patients who have been in the same room as the infectious patients are isolated in a separate room until infection status has been clarified (norovirus, MRSA, VRE, *C difficile*, etc.).
     - Disinfection and washing are carried out in all rooms where the infectious patient has stayed.
     - Other measures are followed up by the department's management in consultation with hygiene nurses and according to proven agents and isolation routines.
10. Isolation is lifted
    - See isolation routines and chapters of special microbes.

11. Information and registering of critical infections
    - Patients with detected *MRSA or other resistant bacteria* may periodically be carriers/infected for one or more years (especially MRSA, resistant enterococci and gram-negative rod bacteria in the intestine).
    - Patients with proven *tuberculosis* may experience relapse if treatment is not followed up/completed and control fails.
    - The patient is advised to inform—about infective status—health professionals at the next contact or hospitalization/healthcare/primary care service.
    - Information and registration in the journal, by "flagging out" important information and good, written information to the next and possible previous treatment.
12. Follow-up and treatment of carrier status/infection

It may take some time for the patient to get rid of the infection/carrier status, and a few will be carriers. Continuous environmental sanitation reduces microbial load and risk of reinfection.

The carrier status is less important for the patient's own health if in a general good condition but can affect disease progression in disease and cause infection risk to personnel and exposed patients if no effective preventive measures are taken.

- *MRSA (see separate Chap. 49)* is the only *carrier state* that is practically followed up, cleared and controlled in Norway and in some other countries in Europe. Follow up for at least 12 months after the first three test sets are negative, or according to national guidelines.
- *Other microbes.* VRE and ESBL are followed up and checked, but are not usually cleared for infection. It is recommended that multidrug-resistant gram-negative rod bacteria should be followed up as MRSA, with the exception of clearing. Many get rid of their carrier status after wound healing and completed treatment.
- *Tuberculosis.* Exposure to tuberculosis and infective status are followed up, treated and controlled according to national guidelines.

13. Marking of the journal, possibly "flagging out" of the infectious agent

47.5 Background Information

Multidrug-resistant bacteria are increasing problems [17]. Prevalence of MRSA increases both in- and outside hospitals in Norway and has also been introduced in food production [4, 17–24]. There is increasing tendency to find resistant, gram-negative rods with extended beta-lactamase resistance: ESBL and enterococci with enhanced resistance to vancomycin and similar agents, VRE [5, 6, 17, 25].

Multidrug resistance is associated with overuse of antibiotics and is easily transmitted when hygienic measures are inadequate, in the absence of isolation, and by overcrowding and understaffing [18–30]. Unusual, multidrug-resistant/super-resistant *Acinetobacter baumannii, Klebsiella oxytoca, Pseudomonas aeruginosa, Burkholderia cepacia* and *Stenotrophomonas maltophilia* with infectious resistance genes (like New Delhi metallo-beta-lactamase 1, NDM-1) that spread to almost all types of gram-negative bacteria pose a serious global threat [6, 31–38]. From the 1990s on, and especially since the 2000s, resistant gram-negative bacteria have become a noticeable problem, also in Norway [6, 17, 39–41].

47.5.1 Import Increases

Good infection control is linked to good hygiene, prosperity and security and breaks down quickly during disasters and chaos and when large crowds are on the move [42].

Gastrointestinal infections often occur during international travel. Among 25,900 travellers examined after returning home, almost 30% had an infectious gastrointestinal disease, most commonly detected in women, younger travellers and regular tourists [43]. Among the clinically significant infectious agents were parasites, 65%; bacteria, 31%; and virus 3% [43].

Travelling to tropical areas is increasingly causing febrile diseases, by bacteria, viruses or parasites, depending on the destination [44]. Among 42,200 sick travellers studied in the period 2000–2010 came 26% from sub-Saharan Africa, 17% from Southeast Asia, 15% from South Central Asia and 10% from South America [45]. Intestinal infections and dengue fever increased, with clusters of malaria in Africa in 2000 and 2007, dengue fever in Thailand in 2002 and India in 2003 and salmonella infections in Nepal in 2009 [45].

In 2010, international travel activity was estimated at almost a billion tourists with a strong increase to visit developing countries [45]. More than half of those travelling to developing countries on vacation get sick, and 8–10% of these seek medical treatment during or after the trip [45].

The most serious infectious diseases are rarely imported to Norway, but an increase is recorded, especially for intestinal microbes [11, 46, 47].

47.5.2 Expenses

More and more import microbes are spread in healthcare and in the society as a whole—and among animals by food and contact. And little by little, they are becoming part of the regular human pathogenic flora in most countries and also in Scandinavia. These infections may be invalidating; they are creating carrier conditions and lead to increased mortality.

Costs—human and resources—are related to the lack of consistency in the prevention and treatment of infections in the various levels of healthcare: poor and late diagnosis, lack of isolation measures and hygiene and incorrect use of antibacterial agents [20, 24–32, 36–38, 48–51]. Cross-infection occurs internally in and between the different levels of healthcare, which can be avoided by good information, good infectious protection and good disinfection and clearing of environmental contamination [33–39, 41, 52–59].

Good isolation measures and routines for screening and information may effectively reduce costs in all levels of healthcare, especially associated to reduce length of stay at intensive departments and fewer problems with transmission of infected patients to long-term institutions without isolates and non-competent personnel [21–25, 49–51].

References

1. Regulations on infectious diseases in health institutions – hospital infections. Ministry of Social Affairs and Health 5 July 1996, § 4-7 and § 7-11 in law of 5 Aug 1994, Communicable Disease Control Act No. 55 on protection against communicable diseases. Norwegian Board of Health, Oslo. 1996.
2. Advice for the application of the Infection Protection Act § 3-3 pre-examination of patients – infectious diseases. IK-28/96. Norwegian Board of Health, Oslo. 1996.
3. Andersen BM. Prevention of import-infection and unknown infection. In: Handbook in hygiene and infection control for hospitals. Oslo: Ullevål University Hospital; 2008. p. 406–15.
4. Andersen BM. MRSA. Handbook in hygiene and infection control for hospitals. Part 1: Microbiology and infection protection. Fagbokforlaget. 2014. p. 39–57.
5. Andersen BM. Enterococci. Handbook in hygiene and infection control for hospitals. Part 1: Microbiology and infection protection. Fagbokforlaget. 2014. p. 59–64.
6. Andersen BM. Gramnegative rod bacteria in the intestine and/or environment. Handbook in hygiene and infection control for hospitals. Part 1: Microbiology and infection protection. Fagbokforlaget. 2014. p. 85–92.
7. Andersen BM. Streptococci and pneumococci. Handbook in hygiene and infection control for hospitals. Part 1: Microbiology and infection protection. Fagbokforlaget. 2014. p. 65–70 and 71–8.
8. Andersen BM. Haemophilus influenzae. Handbook for hygiene and infection control for hospitals. Part 1: Microbiology and infection protection. Fagbokforlaget. 2014. p. 83–5.
9. Andersen BM. Mycobacteria. Handbook for hygiene and infection control for hospitals. Part 1: Microbiology and infection protection. Fagbokforlaget. 2014. p. 135–43.
10. Norwegian Board of Health. Tuberculosis guideline. 07/04/2010.
11. Andersen BM. Gastrointestinal and intestinal bacteria. Handbook in hygiene and infection control for hospitals. Part 1: Microbiology and infection protection. Fagbokforlaget. 2014. p. 95–106.
12. Andersen BM. Tarmpatogenic protozoa. Handbook in hygiene and infection control for hospitals. Part 1: Microbiology and infection protection. Fagbokforlaget. 2014. p. 356–63.
13. Andersen BM. Hepatitis and other blood borne infections. Handbook in hygiene and infection control for hospitals. Part 1: Microbiology and infection protection. Fagbokforlaget. 2014. p. 167–206.
14. Andersen BM. Gastrointestinal virus infections. Handbook in hygiene and infection control for hospitals. Part 1: Microbiology and infection protection. Fagbokforlaget. 2014. p. 248–54.
15. Andersen BM. Influenza and other respiratory tract virus infections. Handbook in hygiene and infection control for hospitals. Part 1: Microbiology and infection protection. Fagbokforlaget. 2014. p. 206–47.
16. Andersen BM. Fungi-human pathogenic. Handbook in hygiene and infection control for hospitals. Part 1: Microbiology and infection protection. Fagbokforlaget. 2014. p. 393–400.
17. NORM/NORM-VET 2011–2016, yearly reports. Norwegian Veterinary Institute, Norwegian Institute of Public Health.

18. Andersen BM, Bergh K, Steinbakk M, Syversen G, Magnes B, Dalen H, Bruun JN. A Norwegian nosocomial outbreak of methicillin-resistant *Staphylococcus aureus* resistant to fusidic acid and susceptible to other anti-staphylococcal agents. J Hosp Infect. 1999;41:123–32.
19. Andersen BM, Syversen G. Methicillin- resistant *Staphylococcus aureus* in Oslo in 2000. Tidsskr Nor Legeforen. 2001;121:1844–7.
20. Andersen BM, Lindemann R, Bergh K, Nesheim BI, Syversen G, Solheim N, Laugerud F. Spread of methicillin-resistant *Staphylococcus aureus* in a neonatal intensive unit associated with understaffing, overcrowding and mixing of patients. J Hosp Infect. 2002;1:1–7.
21. Andersen BM, Rasch M, Syversen G. Is an increase of MRSA in Oslo, Norway, associated with changed infection control policy? J Infect. 2007;55:531–8.
22. Sie I, Thorstad M, Andersen BM. Infection control and methicillin-resistant *Staphylococcus aureus* in nursing homes in Oslo. J Hosp Infect. 2008;70:235–40.
23. Andersen BM, Tollefsen T, Seljordslia B, Hochlin K, Syversen G, Jonassen Ø, Rasch M. Rapid MRSA test in exposed persons: costs and savings in hospitals. J Infect. 2010;60:293–9.
24. Thorstad M, Sie I, Andersen BM. MRSA: a challenge to Norwegian Nursing Home Personnel. Interdiscip Perspect Infect Dis. 2011;2011:197683., 6p. https://doi.org/10.1155/2011/197683.
25. Andersen BM, Seljordslia B, Hochlin K, Rasch M, Syversen G. A predicted outbreak in an overcrowded, administratively neglected and run-down haemodialysis unit as an offer of «New Public Management» in Norwegian hospitals. J Hosp Admin. 2013;2:15–24.
26. Eveillard M, Schmit JL, Eb F. Antimicrobial use prior to the acquisition of multiresistant bacteria. Infect Control Hosp Epidemiol. 2002;23:155–8.
27. Saulnier FF, Hubert H, Onimus TM, et al. Assessing excess nurse workload generated by multiresistant nosocomial bacteria in intensive care. Infect Control Hosp Epidemiol. 2001;22:273–8.
28. The Brooklyn Antibiotic Resistance Task Force. The cost of antibiotic resistance: effect of resistance among *Staphylococcus aureus*, *Klebsiella pneumoniae*, *Acinetobacter baumannii*, and *Pseudomonas aeruginosa* on length of hospital stay. Infect Control Hosp Epidemiol. 2002;23:106–8.
29. Montecalvo MA, Jarvis WR, Uman J, et al. Costs and savings associated with infection control measures that reduce transmission of vancomycin-resistant enterococci in an endemic setting. Infect Control Hosp Epidemiol. 2001;22:437–42.
30. Sievert DM, Boulton ML, Stoltman G, Johnson D, et al. *Staphylococcus aureus* resistant to vancomycin - United States, 2002. MMWR. 2002;51:565–7.
31. Koeleman JGM, van der Bijl MW, Stoof J, Vanderbroucke-Grauls CMJE, Savelkoul PHM. Antibiotic resistance is a major risk factor for epidemic behaviour of *Acinetobacter baumannii*. Infect Control Hosp Epidemiol. 2001;22:284–8.
32. Mahgoub S, Ahmed J, Glatt AE. Completely resistant *Acinetobacter baumannii* strains. Infect Control Hosp Epidemiol. 2002;23:477–9.
33. Paavilainen T, Alanen M, Makela M, Routamaa M, Jarvinen H, Houvinen P, et al. Infrequent isolation of multiresistant *Acinetobacter baumannii* from the staff tending a colonized patient with severe burns. Infect Control Hosp Epidemiol. 2001;22:388–91.
34. Pitten FA, Panzig B, Schrøder G, Tietze K, Kramer A. Transmission of a multiresistant *Pseudomonas aeruginosa* strain at a German university hospital. J Hosp Infect. 2001;47:125–30.
35. Assadian O, Berger A, Aspøck C, Mustafa S, Kohlhauser C, Hirschl AM. Nosocomial outbreak of *Serratia marcescens* in a neonatal intensive care unit. Infect Control Hosp Epidemiol. 2002;23:457–61.
36. Munoz-Price LS. Carbapenem-resistant *Enterobacteriaceae*, long-term acute care hospitals, and our distortions of reality. Infect Control Hosp Epidemiol. 2013;34:829–33.
37. Lewis JC, Bishop M, Heon B, et al. Admission surveillance for carbapenemase-producing *Enterobacteriaceae* at a long-term acute care hospital. Infect Control Hosp Epidemiol. 2013;34:832–4.
38. Willemsen I, Nelson J, Hendriks Y, et al. Extensive dissemination of extended sprectrum beta-lactamase-producing *Enterobacteriaceae* in a Dutch nursing home. Infect Control Hosp Epidemiol. 2015;36:394–400.

39. Olafsen K, Hotvedt R, Andersen BM, Almdahl SM, Sørlie D. Nosocomial infection with resistant *Enterobacter cloacae*. Tidsskr Nor Legeforen. 1989;109:332–6.
40. Andersen BM. Concerned about development of resistant Gram-negative rod bacteria. Dagens Medisin, 16 Aug 2001.
41. Bukholm G, Tannæs T, Kjelsberg ABB, Smith-Erichsen N. An outbreak of multidrug-resistant *Pseudomonas aeruginosa* associated with increased risk of patient death in an intensive care unit. Infect Control Hosp Epidemiol. 2002;23:441–6.
42. Uckay I, Sax H, Harbarth S, Bernard L, Pittet D. Multi-resistant infections in repatriated patients after natural disaster: lessons learned from the 2004 tsunami for hospital infection control. J Hosp Infect. 2008;68:1–8.
43. Swaminathan A, Torresi J, Schlagenhauf P, et al. A global study of pathogens and host risk factors associated with infectious gastrointestinal disease in returned international travelers. J Infect. 2009;59:19–27.
44. Johnston V, Stockley JM, Dockrell D, et al. Fever in return travellers presenting in the United Kingdom: recommendations for investigation and initial management. J Infect. 2009;59:1–18.
45. Leder K, Torresi J, Brownstein JS, et al. Travel-related illness trends and clusters, 2000–2010. Emerg Infect Dis. 2013;19:1049–73.
46. Blystad H, Nilsen Ø, Løvberg AB. Imported infections to Norway 2001. MSIS. 2002;30:9.
47. Bruun JN. Tourism, climate change and diagnostics. Tidsskr Nor Legeforen. 2012;132:670.
48. Skov Simonsen G, Andersen BM, Digranes A, Harthug S, Jakobsen T, Langeland N, et al. Low fecal carriage rate of vancomycin resistant enterococci in Norwegian hospital patients. Scand J Infect Dis. 1998;30:465–8.
49. Mayhall CG. Control of vancomycin-resistant enterococci: it is important, it is possible, and it is cost-effective. Infect Control Hosp Epidemiol. 2002;23:420–3.
50. Srinivasan A, Song X, Ross T, Merz W, Brower R, Perl TM. A prospective study to determine whether gowns in addition to gloves reduce nosocomial transmission or vancomycin-resistant enterococci in an intensive care unit. Infect Control Hosp Epidemiol. 2002;23:424–8.
51. Muto CA, Giannetta ET, Durbin LJ, Simonton BM, Farr BM. Cost-effectiveness of perirectal surveillance cultures for controlling vancomycin-resistant *Enterococcus*. Infect Control Hosp Epidemiol. 2002;23:429–35.
52. Weist K, Pollege K, Schulz I, Ruden H, Gastmeier P. How many nosocomial infections are associated with cross-transmission? A prospective cohort study in a surgical intensive care unit. Infect Control Hosp Epidemiol. 2002;23:127–32.
53. D'Agata EMC, Thayer V, Schaffner W. An outbreak of *Acinetobacter baumannii*: the importance of cross-transmission. Infect Control Hosp Epidemiol. 2000;21:588–91.
54. Eveillard M, Quenon JL, Rufat P, Mangeol A, Fauvelle F. Association between hospital-acquired infections and patient transfers. Infect Control Hosp Epidemiol. 2001;22:693–6.
55. Levin AS, Gobara S, Mendes C, Cursino R, Sinto S. Environmental contamination by multidrug-resistant *Acinetobacter baumannii* in an intensive care unit. Infect Control Hosp Epidemiol. 2001;22:717–20.
56. Shiomori T, Miyamoto H, Makishima K, et al. Evaluation of bedmaking-related airborne and surface methicillin-resistant *Staphylococcus aureus* contamination. J Hosp Infect. 2002;50:30–5.
57. Trautmann M, Michalsky T, Wiedeck H, Radosavljevic V, Ruhnke M. Tap water colonization with *Pseudomonas aeruginosa* in a surgical intensive care unit (ICU) and relation to pseudomonas infections of ICU patients. Infect Control Hosp Epidemiol. 2001;22:49–52.
58. Ministry of Social Affairs and Health, Norway Regulation on tuberculosis control, 2001, 2002.
59. Byers KE, Anglim AM, Anneski CJ, Farr BM. Duration of colonization with vancomycin-resistant *Enterococcus*. Infect Control Hosp Epidemiol. 2002;23:207–11.

Healthcare Professionals 48

Abstract

Healthcare professionals may become sick or infected with human pathogenic microbes during travel, work and stay in other countries (imported infection) and at home. In some cases, the infection occurs nosocomial by direct or indirect work with infected patients, employees or the environment. Personnel can therefore be "sources, carriers and victims" of infection with a variety of different microbes, including MRSA. Most infections and carrier states among healthcare personnel are preventable and subclinical and may cause large outbreaks in hospitals and other healthcare institutions.

The following chapter is focused on practical measures to detect and prevent transmission of infections from healthcare personnel before and during work in healthcare institutions.

Keywords

Imported infections · Work in hospital · Pre-examination · Information Nosocomial infections · Resistant bacteria · Dangerous virus · Infection control Hygiene · Prevention

48.1 Purpose

Control of personnel after contact with healthcare abroad or after work in war areas, refugee camps or otherwise exposed to particularly infectious microbes:

- By pre-examination and information—in advance.
- By preparing procedures for early infection control.

B. M. Andersen, *Prevention and Control of Infections in Hospitals*,
https://doi.org/10.1007/978-3-319-99921-0_48

48.2 Comprise

- All personnel, including students, temporary workers, visitors, etc., after contact with healthcare abroad or after work in war areas, refugee camps or otherwise exposed to particularly infectious microbes at other departments, healthcare institutions or other known infectious contacts.
- All personnel that has direct or indirect contact with patients, examination, treatment and care, textiles, equipment, cleaning, transportation, handling food, etc.
- Check for blood-borne virus infection (see also section on employees with infectious/carrier status).

48.3 Responsibility

The National Board of Health decides issues concerning preliminary examination of workers after possible exposure to antibiotic-resistant bacteria [1–9]. Practice today, for instance, in Norway, is the examination of MRSA and tuberculosis [1–9].

The hospital's management provides a control system for employment via agency and other offering personnel to the hospital and for students, temporary workers and other visitors—at the resource—and recruitment centre, corporate health service centre or otherwise.

The department management checks when recruiting/reinstating the position. This applies to all employees, temporary staff, assistants or students and visitors.

The personnel are required to provide information about exposure/illness prior to entry/reinstatement of the work and to perform current routine examinations (including students, guests, etc.).

48.4 Practical Measures

Requirement for microbial testing after healthcare contact abroad.

These routines may vary between countries. In Norway it is required testing after international stays in connection with *healthcare* or *being a patient* [1]. Only the county governor can exempt for testing [1]. All personnel, including temporary staff, short-term employees and hospitals, are tested prior to work at hospitals and at other healthcare institutions following healthcare or as a patient abroad—or in areas at home and abroad where multidrug resistance is a problem. This applies especially to the *last 12 months before employment* and *always* if previously been MRSA-positive.

1. The recruitment centre/department management verifies that documents relating to infection exposure are understood and signed by employee, student, guest, etc.
2. The head of department asks the employee to contact the hospital's medical officer/general practitioner for the relevant microbial tests *before* work.

3. Await test result (2–4 days for MRSA), or use quickest (approximately 2 h). Avoid clinical work during this period.
4. In case of *suspicion* of positive test answers, the microbiological laboratory contacts the hospital's medical officer/general practitioner and infection control staff.
5. The medical officer/general practitioner contacts eventually the carrier personnel, and the infection control staff contacts the head of the department if the employee is at work.
6. MRSA testing during the last 14 days before starting work at the hospital is approved, also if satisfactory testing has been carried out abroad. The test results must be documented in writing.
7. The medical officer/general practitioner will provide further follow-up on suspicion of tuberculosis or other specific infections/carriers.

48.4.1 Sampling/Treatment/Post-Control in MRSA Suspicion

See Chap. 49 on MRSA infection detection and control.

48.4.2 Suspected Tuberculosis

See Chap. 56 on tuberculosis and tuberculosis control.

48.4.3 Suspected Gastrointestinal Infections

See Chaps. 52–54 on gastrointestinal infection and norovirus.

48.5 Background Information

Healthcare professionals may become sick or infected with human pathogenic microbes during travel, work and stay in other countries (imported infection) and at home [10–13]. In some cases, the infection occurs nosocomial by direct or indirect work with infected patients, employees or the environment. The personnel can therefore be "sources, carriers and victims" of infection with a variety of different microbes, including MRSA [10–13].

References

1. Norwegian Board of Health. Regulation on pre-examination of workers in healthcare-antibiotic resistant bacteria IK-36/1996.

2. Norwegian Board of Health. Advice for the application of the Infection Act § 3-3 pre-examination of patients – infectious diseases. IK-28/96. Oslo: Norwegian Board of Health; 1996.
3. Regulations on infectious diseases in health institutions – hospital infections. Ministry of Social Affairs and Health 5 July 1996 pursuant to section 4-7 and § 7-11 in law August 5, 1994 Act no. 55 on protection against communicable diseases. Norway.
4. Andersen BM. Personnel exposed to infection. In: Handbook in hygiene and infectious diseases for hospitals. Oslo: Ullevål University Hospital; 2008. p. 416–21.
5. National guideline for prevention of MRSA in health care; MRSA guide. The Norwegian Institute of Public Health and the Directorate for Health and Social Affairs. 2004, 2008.
6. Andersen BM. MRSA. Handbook in hygiene and infection control for hospitals. Part 1: Microbiology and infection protection. Fagbokforlaget. 2014. p. 39–57.
7. Ministry of Social Affairs and Health. Regulation on tuberculosis control, 2001, 2002.
8. Norwegian Board of Health. Tuberculosis guideline. 07/04/2010.
9. Andersen BM. Mycobacteria. Handbook in hygiene and infection control for hospitals. Part 1: Microbiology and infection protection. Fagbokforlaget. 2014. p. 135–43.
10. Starke JR, Jackson MA. When the health care worker is sick. Premium non nocere. JAMA Pediatr. 2015;169:809–10.
11. Wang JT, Chang SC, Ko WJ, Chang YY, Chen ML, Pan HJ, Luh KT. A hospital-acquired outbreak of methicillin-resistant *Staphylococcus aureus* infection initiated by a surgeon carrier. J Hosp Infect. 2001;47:104–9.
12. Ben-David D, Mermel LA, Parenteau S. Methicillin-resistant *Staphylococcus aureus* transmission: the possible importance of unrecognized health care worker carriage. Am J Infect Control. 2008;36:93–7.
13. Albrich WC, Harbarth S. Healthcare workers: source, vector or victim of MRSA? Infect Lancet. 2008;8:289–301.

49 MRSA Prevention

Abstract

Methicillin-resistant *Staphylococcus aureus* (MRSA) is a serious and increasing global problem. MRSA infection is linked to patients from abroad (imported infection), war injuries, high antibiotic consumption, lack of environmental hygiene and infection control, understaffing, overcrowding and absence of isolation procedures. MRSA is a *S. aureus* bacterium that has developed resistance to several good antibiotics and that may harbour special dangerous virulence genes. *S. aureus* is causing infections in two out of seven billion peoples in the world each year, and 10–50% of the most serious types are caused by MRSA. MRSA is causing one of the largest infectious diseases in the world with a rather high death rate. It is easily spread by contact, droplets, air, equipment and dust and may survive in dry state outside the body for up to 1 year.

Everyone should be protected against infection with MRSA since it is a highly preventable infectious disease. In countries with strict infection control, like in Scandinavia, high standards (like "Ullevål standard") have been used with rather good experiences. Still, the infections are increasing because of a high mobility in the population and spread of MRSA in the environment, in the community and among animals and via food chains. Healthcare professionals may become infected with MRSA and may be the "source, carriers and victims of infection". Carrier states are preventable, subclinical and may cause large outbreaks in hospitals and other healthcare institutions. The following chapter is focused on practical measures to detect and prevent transmission of MRSA in healthcare institutions.

Keywords

MRSA in and outside hospitals · Imported from abroad · CA-MRSA · HA-MRSA Resistance genes *Mec*A, *Mec*B, *Mec*C · Admission to hospital · Pre-examination Information · Screening · Testing · Isolation · PPE · Sanitation · Decontamination Eradication · Nosocomial infections · Infection control · Hygiene · Prevention

B. M. Andersen, *Prevention and Control of Infections in Hospitals*,
https://doi.org/10.1007/978-3-319-99921-0_49

49.1 Purpose

Prevent the introduction and spread of MRSA in the hospital by information, testing and isolation of suspected MRSA-infected persons.

Control of personnel and patients after contact with healthcare abroad or after work in war areas and refugee camps or otherwise exposed to MRSA—or earlier tested as MRSA positive—at home or abroad.

- By pre-examination and information—in advance.
- By implemented procedures for early infection control.

49.2 Comprise

Close contact of MRSA-infected patient or personnel, patients in the same room and others who have been in direct contact with the source of infection without personal protective equipment (PPE).

Environmental contamination: patient room, toilet/bathroom, ward office, living room, disinfection room (cleaning room), etc.

Outbreak: one single case (or more) of MRSA if the infection/colonization has occurred after admission and is not known positive on or beforehand or not previously exposed to known infection.

49.3 Responsibility

The hospital's management provides routines and guidelines regarding MRSA and of infection detection and control [1–12].

The department management implements routines, following up outbreaks in collaboration with the infection control unit, provides for testing after possible exposure and contacts the Director at increased risk of infection for patients and personnel.

Personnel follow routines and measures.

49.4 Practical Measures

All patients, visitors and personnel should be protected against infection with MRSA which is a highly preventable disease [1–24].

49.4.1 Coordination of Outbreaks of MRSA

Infection control personnel coordinate infection control measures, give hygienic advices, guidance and information during outbreaks and inform the Director of larger outbreaks, extensive use of resources and possible deaths in connection with MRSA.

49.4.1.1 Department/Ward Manager—Where the Problem Occur—Coordinates

- Preventive measures (patient isolation, testing of contacts, use of PPE, disinfection, etc.).
- Information to exposed personnel to not work elsewhere because of risk of transmission (extras, etc.).
- Establish overview of patients/employees/environment that have been exposed (direct contact).
- "Flagging out" MRSA into patient journal—critical information.
- Information to other departments/personnel exposed to the infection.
- Follow-up of MRSA-infected persons in cooperation with the hospital's medical officer (personnel) and the infection control unit.

The MRSA responsible physician of the ward requests samples from patients and personnel and informs the microbiological department of the number of samples in case of outbreaks. Employees with proven MRSA are referred to the medical officer/infection control doctor/general practitioner for possible disinfection and follow-up. Test responses (from staff) are administered in hospital archives.

49.4.2 Pre-Examination: Before Entering Hospital

Preliminary examinations of patients and personnel should be conducted *prior to* hospitalization.

49.4.2.1 Patients

- Presurvey (telephone, formal letter and information to the patient, etc.): was there any contact with healthcare abroad or exposure to resistant bacteria? Determine infection risks by telephone (referring doctor) or outpatient for elective patients and for immediate help.
- The preliminary examination can be carried out with the GP. The patient receives information from the hospital and is asked to contact the GP if exposed to MRSA infection for the past 12 months or earlier, or MRSA infected—if ever. The patient is tested at the GP in the same way as in the hospital.
- *Critical information.* Check if the patient's journal is flagged out under critical information.

49.4.2.2 Personnel (Including Temporary Staff, Guest Visitors, Students)

- Possible exposure (last 12 months), or previously infected with MRSA; tested prior to employment/re-entry, etc. at the hospital.
- The preliminary examination can be carried out by own GP.
- Personnel from healthcare abroad can be pretested abroad 14 days prior to arrival at the hospital. The test result is brought and delivered to the department manager. Patient is tested in the same way as in the hospital.
- Personnel with chronic wounds or eczema should not work with MRSA patients.
- Exposed personnel, pre-examined before employment, should not work in the healthcare system before a test response is available.

49.4.3 Testing/Screening of Patients and Personnel Suspected of MRSA

49.4.3.1 Ullevål—Standard for Detection, Isolation and Follow-Up on Suspicion of MRSA (Tables 49.1 and 49.2)

Table 49.1 Who should be MRSA screened?

Ask patient/personnel	If yes
Import? Have you been in contact with healthcare abroad for the last 12 months?[a]	• Directly take the patient in an isolated/single room and conduct the test (outpatient or inpatient); isolate the patient until the test result is completed • PPE: Surgical mask/cap, gloves, gown for the one who is testing/entering the room • *Patient:* Isolated until test results are clear • *Personnel:* Should not work with patients before the test result is complete
Earlier MRSA positive? Have you ever been infected with MRSA? (no matter how far back in time)	• As above
MRSA exposed last 12 months? Have you been in contact with people infected with MRSA infection in nursing homes, home care, primary healthcare, hospitals, etc. during the past 12 months?[b]	• As above

[a]Examined/treated/worked at hospital, outpatient clinic, primary care, nursing home, abroad, etc. exceptions are the consultation, prescription or attestation of a doctor
[b]Except for protected contact with MRSA (use of PPE and patient isolated)

Table 49.2 Testing for MRSA

Test sampling equipment	• Sterile pencils and transport medium (from microbiological department) • Sterile water/saline. The pencil is always wetted before sampling
Sample locations (anatomical)	• Nose—inside, outer part of inside • Throat—tonsils and soft palate • Hands and wrists • Perineum—between the urethral opening and rectum • Wounds, eczema, scarring, catheter and drainage • A common test kit for patients and personnel: nose, throat, hands, perineum
Remisse	• Information per test kit (nose, throat, hands, perineum, event elsewhere) from a patient/person • Record the name, date and test mark of the referral and the samples • Note remarks of MRSA (import, exposed, etc.)
Sample vials and test answers	• A test kit (per patient) is bundled together • Test kit and referral will be delivered to the microbiological department directly and as soon as possible • Go and get test answers or use telephone—with the post it is taking time

49.4.3.2 Procedure Description: Equal to Patients and Personnel

- Nose—both nostrils: wet the pencil. Roll the pencil three times around inside each nostrils—outermost.
- Throat: wet the pencil. Roll the pencil over tonsils and soft palate region three times.
- Hands and wrists: wet the pencil. Roll the pencil on both sides of the palm, between fingers, over fingertips and around wrist.
- Perineum: wet the pencil. Roll the pencil between the urethra opening and rectal opening three times back and forth. Employees take the sample themselves.
- Wounds/scars/eczema/skin lesions: wet the pencil. Roll the pencil over areas with wounds, eczema, etc.
- All types of catheter: wet the pencil. Roll the pencil and wipe it well around the insertion site/catheter/drain, etc. Take eventually, in addition, urine test, tracheal secret, drain secret, etc.

49.4.3.3 Testing of Staff at Outbreaks

- The department manager or delegated staff is responsible for screening of exposed personnel.
- In case of major outbreaks, a list of exposed patients and personnel is made, and the number of persons to be tested for microbiological laboratory is reported.
- Non-medical personnel (cleaning, technical or other service personnel) address the occupational health services or other defined units by appointment.

49.4.3.4 Important!

- Personnel in close contact with MRSA patient, equipment/bed, etc. are tested. During the period of the test (3–5 days), the personnel are using surgical mask/cap, gown and gloves for all patient care in the actual ward with outbreak. In rooms with more patient beds/cohort, change gloves between each patient.
- Personnel, temporary workers, students, etc. should not work elsewhere while infection tracing is in progress before the results are available (event sickness reports). Exposed personnel can still work in the particular ward, while infection tracing is in progress, but should use PPE; see above.

49.4.3.5 Interpretation of Test Answers

MRSA Test Negative: Previously Not Detected MRSA Positive and All Samples Taken Now Are Negative

- Patients/personnel are declared free of infection after a complete set of tests (nose, throat, hands, perineum and clinical samples).
- Prerequisite: MRSA testing is done properly, and the patient is not recently on antibiotics (last 14 days) or disinfection (last 10 days).

MRSA Test Positive

- Isolation of this patient is continued. In case of isolation measures started from the day of admission, infection tracing (testing of other patients, personnel, etc.) is unnecessary.
- In case of occasional discovery, the patient is isolated, and a number of preventive measures are taken (see below).
- Personnel who are diagnosed as MRSA positive should avail sick leave and submit an information concerning accident statement (infected on job), and adequate protection measures are taken for any close contacts and for the contaminated environment (see later).
- Check the findings of MRSA (repeat sample from nose, throat, hands, perineum, etc.) before taking disinfection measures to verify findings and map the infection sites.
- Written information on infection and disinfection measures.

49.4.4 Patients with Known MRSA at Admission/Outpatient Clinic

- The patient is isolated throughout the stay!
- Inform the patient about infection prevention measures.
- Always isolate—no matter how far back MRSA was detected.
- The department/responsible physician provides suitable isolation room and agrees with this before admission/outpatient clinic.

- Isolation for airborne infections with negative air pressure is recommended, especially if having respiratory symptoms, respiratory treatment and widespread skin ulcers.
- Contact isolation with separate toilet/shower/decontaminator can be used.
- Single room with anteroom and separate toilet/shower, attached room (not in common hallway), is a short-term emergency solution.
- The staff use surgical mask/gloves/cap/gown and follow routines for the removal and disposal of PPE.
- Check if the journal is flagged out under critical information.
- Examination and treatment at other units, etc. are carried out by appointment and with protective measures (patient in a clean bed, clean clothes and with a mask if coughing—to the actual unit).

49.4.5 Suspected MRSA–Not Been Isolated in the Ward

The patient or relatives may, for example, after a few days tell about contact with healthcare abroad or exposed to MRSA otherwise.

- Isolation due to MRSA status is clarified. MRSA is tested; rapid test + cultivation are recommended. Fastest possible clarification regarding infection status.
- *Await MRSA testing* of exposed patients and personnel until results from the index patient are available.
- Inform the patient about infection prevention measures.
- Treat MRSA infection until test results are negative.
- Hand hygiene and personal hygiene should be done.
- Patients in contact with the actual suspected patient are registered and isolated in their own room.
- Personnel with direct contact with the patient are registered.
- Disinfection and washing of important common rooms such as X-ray rooms, operating rooms, etc. where the index patient has been treated—contact infection control personnel for advices.
- The staff wear surgical masks/cap/gloves and gown when entering the room of index patient/exposed patients and follow the procedures for the removal and disposal of PPE afterwards.
- Examination and treatment by other units, etc. are carried out by appointment and with preventive measures (patient in a clean bed, clean clothes and with a surgical mask if coughing—to the unit responsible for examination/treatment).
- If the test result of the index patient is negative, the patient is considered to be not MRSA-infected if the samples are taken in a proper manner.
- No testing of patients or personnel if the patient's test result is negative.

49.4.6 Unexpected Discovery of Inpatient Patient with MRSA

Example: MRSA detected in clinical samples of a patient after some days in the ward. The patient has been in a four-bed room with other patients, used common living rooms and toilets and been on other units for X-ray, etc. Most nurses on the ward have been caring for this patient.

49.4.6.1 Isolation

The ward/physician in charge provides for isolation of the MRSA patient who is isolated throughout the stay and informed about infection control measures.

49.4.6.2 Personal Protective Equipment (PPE)

- Surgical mask put on outside the cap, gloves with long cuff and single-use gown. Check that the staff can use PPE—donning and doffing.
- PPE is used for the care of all patients in the ward until the test result is available—to prevent spread of infection.

49.4.6.3 Hand Hygiene

- Tighten up general personal hygiene and hand hygiene.
- Check hand disinfectant and procedures for hand disinfection.

49.4.6.4 Exposed Patients

- Patients on the same room may often be colonized or infected. Inform by writing about infection prevention measures.
- Exposed patients are transferred to a clean bed with clean clothes (the unclean is treated as infectious) and returned to the patient room after disinfection of the room has been completed (takes about 1–2 h)—or to another clean room—and isolated. They are MRSA tested and isolated until test results are negative.
- Cohort isolation (same room) may be used during large outbreaks (but should be avoided).
- Until test results are negative, patients are treated as MRSA positive in examination, treatment, care and transportation.
- Avoid relocation of MRSA-exposed patients to other wards or to nursing homes, home nursing, etc.
- Message is sent to departments and institutions that have received exposed patients before the current case was detected. They are isolated and tested where they are located.
- If necessary, transfer to other departments/hospitals/health institutions *before negative test response is available*; notify exposure to MRSA *prior* to transmission.

49.4.6.5 Exposed Personnel

- Tighten up general personal hygiene and hand hygiene.
- Register, test and use PPE for care of patients until the infection situation has been resolved.

- Inform about protective measures—written.
- Do not work elsewhere, at other departments/health institutions, before test results are present; contact infection control personnel if there are questions.
  - Exception: in special circumstances, be careful. Change clothes (gown) and disinfect hands when leaving the outbreak ward. At work elsewhere: clean gown, surgical mask/cap and gloves. This is carried out until infection status is clarified.

49.4.6.6 Visitors/Relatives

- Inform about infection prevention measures.
- Must follow isolation routines, hand hygiene, etc.
- Do not stay anywhere else in the ward (direct to and from).
- Close relatives (direct contact) are recommended to undergo MRSA testing at their own GP.

49.4.6.7 Disinfection and Cleaning of Exposed Rooms and Equipment

- Personnel in charge provide rapid disinfection and cleaning of contaminated rooms and objects (see contamination/room disinfection) in cooperation with cleaning and hygiene staff.
- The same procedures are done elsewhere in the hospital where the MRSA patient has been treated/examined.
- During disinfection, the room is emptied—the patient is moved to another room.
  - Exception: If the condition of the MRSA patient is such that he cannot be moved to isolation immediately (for instance, ICU patient), contact infection control personnel for advices. If there is shortage of rooms, a local disinfection around the patient may be done—as an exception. Then other patients on the same room may be moved to a new, clean bed with clean bedding/equipment and still considered to be exposed to MRSA infection.
- If there are problems with disinfection of rooms due to a lot of single-use or other equipment, fixtures, etc., assess decontamination by dry hydrogen peroxide gas—contact infection control staff.

49.4.6.8 Flagging-Out Journal

- Check if the patient's journal is flagged out under critical information.
- Flagging-out mark should not be removed even if the patient is disinfected!

49.4.6.9 Message Information

- Manager in charge at the relevant ward reports the MRSA result to other units/wards/departments that have been in direct, unprotected contact with the patient (X-ray, surgeons, anaesthesia, porters, bioengineers, transport staff, ambulance, etc.) and to other hospitals, nursing homes, home care services, etc. (see more later).

49.4.6.10 Screening of Whom?

- Close contacts and patients who have been in the same room (not necessary if the index patient has been isolated from hospitalization due to other infections).
- Other patients exposed due to local conditions (open units, e.g. intensive), less good hygienic conditions, use of common exposed personnel, common service space over time, etc. Ask for specific additional MRSA examination when sending microbial samples. Contact infection control personnel for advice.
- Exposed personnel: direct contact with the patient or patient's room/equipment or other patients in the same room.
- NB! Inform the microbiological department about the number of people to be tested!
- Infection control personnel provide advice on the extent of testing.

49.4.7 Unexpected Findings of MRSA in Several Inpatient Patients

If there is detected spread of infection among several patients or personnel, it may be necessary to repeat MRSA screening, disinfection of rooms, isolation and closing the ward for new intake until the situation is under control.

- If another patient in the same room as the MRSA patient (index) is detected of infection, have new control measures of patients in the same room and actual personnel and decontamination on actual rooms (measures as above).
- If one or more patients in *other* patient rooms (in addition to the index room) are infected, the entire ward (patients and personnel) may have been exposed and are tested. Evaluate stop for new intake (measures as above).
- If MRSA is detected in one or more personnel at the department, all (patients and personnel) are tested; stop for intake (measures as above).
- If MRSA is detected in personnel from other wards (been in contact with the outbreak ward), these contacts are followed up with measures in cooperation with infection control personnel (measures as above).
- Always check the findings of a positive MRSA result.

49.4.8 Unexpected Discovery of MRSA in a Healthcare Worker

- MRSA detected in one or more personnel at the department: test all (patients and personnel) and stop for intake (measures as above).
- Personnel with proven MRSA are on sick leave and followed up/treated by the GP or other doctors in collaboration with infection control personnel.
- MRSA is registered as occupational disease, and injury claim form is completed.

- In case of detected MRSA: no patient-related work as long as the person is infected/carrier.
- Infection tracing in the family of healthcare professionals with proven MRSA infection varies. It is most often required to remove carrier status. In case of recidiv of carrier status, and if others in the family are working in the healthcare system or are to be treated by the healthcare service, infection tracing and sanitation are especially important to be carried out.
- MRSA disappears in 10–40% of infected healthcare professionals within 14 days to 3 months and most within 12 months after adequate sanitation. Prolonged carrier status is less likely after adequate sanitation, with the exception of wounds/eczema. Best chance of successful treatment if it starts immediately.
- Personnel with chronic wounds or eczema should not work with MRSA patients because they are more vulnerable to become long-term carriers.
- Check the findings of MRSA before any treatment (nose, throat, hand-wrist, perineum, eczema, ulcers, scars, etc.).

49.4.9 Follow-Up of MRSA-Infected Person

Infected healthcare personnel should be followed up quickly and efficiently; they should be taken care of and come back to work as quickly as possible.

49.4.9.1 Follow-Up of MRSA Tests Concerning Infected Person: Patient or Personnel

- In the case of detected MRSA, three consecutive test sets taken at 3 days intervals must be negative before the person is defined as “low MRSA risk”. It is assumed that the sampling will start at least 10 days after completion of the sanitation/disinfection and at least 14 days after the end of the use of antibacterial agents.
- Then follow up for 12 months with frequent testing at the start—for instance, every week—and later on testing after 3, 6, 9 and 12 months. Each time three sets of tests are taken at 3 days intervals. After at least 15 consecutive negative test sets/(0, 3, 6, 9, 12 months) during 1 year and no positive findings in between, there is less chance of permanent MRSA status.
- In the event of residiv, a new sanitation period and follow-up over 1 year until the patient/personnel has been continuously negative for 1 year (*see sanitation*).
- Personnel are on sick leave and followed up by the GP (or infection control doctor in the community)—in cooperation with infection control personnel at the hospital.
- All expenditure on tracing of infections, sanitation and other treatment of MRSA-positive cases and exposed environment should be charged to the current institution/primary healthcare.

49.4.9.2 Patient

- Control samples from the nose, throat, hands, perineum, wounds, eczema, scars, catheters, drainages, secretions, pus, etc.
- Sanitation started early if not quickly negative (see sanitation).
- Considered as "low MRSA risk" if three consecutive test sets taken with 3-day intervals are negative at least 10 days after completion of sanitation and at least 14 days after the end of the antibiotic cure.
- Considered possible MRSA positive when readmitted/any contact with the healthcare, and the journal is "flagged out" under critical information.
- Sanitation and follow-up are carried out at different healthcare levels where the infected patient stays; at hospitals, nursing homes, home nursing and at home, in collaboration with the GP and in consultation with infection control personnel.
- If there's a need for use of systemic antibacterial treatment, contact specialist in infection medicine.
- Reported as hospital-associated/healthcare-associated infection if encountered after contact with healthcare in and outside the country.

49.4.9.3 Personnel in Healthcare Institutions

- Sick leave when detected—not at work before MRSA negative and informed about further action.
- Mapped, reported, sanitation and followed-up as above.
- Considered as MRSA negative after 1 year with only negative control samples taken at certain intervals.
- Re-entry into work is planned as early as possible (see below).
- Carrier state and infection must be reported as occupational injury.

49.4.10 Sanitation for Patient and Personnel to Get Rid of MRSA Contamination

Sanitation is a combination of whole-body disinfection and effective disinfection and cleaning of the environment, equipment, textiles, etc. While the sanitation period is ongoing, the person is nearly not infectious, because of the daily effect of the disinfectant used. Written information is always included in sanitation measures. Contact infection control personnel for advice and guidance.

49.4.10.1 Sanitation Steps: Short Version

- Mapping MRSA status and requesting complete resistance form from microbiological laboratory, including mupirocin resistance.
- Patients and relatives are informed of the treatment.

- All sanitation take place at the same time; if more people live together, all of them are treated regardless of MRSA status (exceptions—contact infection control personnel).
- Disinfection, cleaning and environmental treatment to avoid recontamination from own environment: disinfect switches, door handles and other common touch points three times a day.
- Disinfect whole body and hair × 1 per day (hibiscrub/stellisept/other recommended disinfectant) for 10–14 days. Soap in twice for 2 minutes each time with the disinfectant. Rinse off the disinfectant soap thoroughly afterwards–otherwise skin problems! *The disinfectant must be tolerated by the skin!*
- Switch to clean personal clothing and bedding—after each whole body's disinfection. The used laundry is washed at a temperature above 65 °C. (Eventually, textiles that does not withstand high temperature is washed 2× at 45 °C.)
- Disinfect the nasal cavity with Bactroban nasal (mupirocin) 3× per day for 10 days. Disinfect so much that the taste is felt in the throat.
- If mupirocin resistance is detected, use Naseptin® which contains 0.1% chlorhexidine and 0.5% neomycin/or other recommended disinfectants.
- Disinfect mouth with chlorhexidine mouthwash 3× per day for 10–14 days.
- Disinfect toothbrush, glass, toothpaste, denture, comb, etc. 2× per day for 10–14 days.
- Avoid using jewellery, piercing, makeup, lipstick, creams, etc. that may easily be contaminated.
- Hand hygiene with 70% alcohol-chlorhexidine with glycerol: 10–20 times per day, optionally using alcohol wipes.

49.4.10.2 Special Problems

- *Surface wounds/eczema:* The disinfectant (hibiscrub/stellisept) is usually tolerated on superficial wounds; possibly use diluted alcoholic-chlorhexidine 3–4 times a day—or chlorhexidine aqueous disinfectant (Note chlorhexidine—not in the ear!).
- *Alternatively by wound*: Chlorhexidine liniment/rinsing fluid for wounds/mucous membranes, Bactroban ointment 3×/day, Bacimycin wound powder/ointment, not fucidin.
- *Eczema:* Contact a skin specialist if widespread, superficial wounds/eczema.
- *Carrying MRSA in the throat*, etc. Contact specialist in infection medicine for assessment of antibacterial agent for systemic therapy in addition to sanitation. Current agents may be minocycline, trimethoprim-sulpha and linezolid—after resistance pattern.
- *Mupirocin resistance:* use Naseptin® containing 0.1% chlorhexidine and 0.5% neomycin or other recommended medicament.
- *Ointments and other skin care products*—Contact infection control personnel. A variety of skin ointments can inactivate chlorhexidine.

49.4.10.3 Sanitation Kit

- Sanitation kits for treatment of MRSA carrier state may be pre-packaged as cleaning kits—every set for 5 days of treatment.
- Contents may be disposable bed sets and towels, disposable vials and other personal hygiene equipment.

49.4.10.4 From the Pharmacy

- Disinfectants like hibiscrub/stellisept/hand disinfectants/mouth disinfectant, etc.
- Mupirocin ointments, bactroban, etc. after prescription by the responsible physician (Table 49.3).

49.4.11 Information and Registration

- Inform patient or relatives that MRSA may be present on the body periodically in 40–60% of the cases a time following infection (12 months or more), if the patient is not being sanitized. It may also disappear spontaneously. The infection is usually not dangerous for healthy people.
- The patient should inform about MRSA infection/carrier state to actual treating healthcare providers.
- Journal tagged and flagged out under critical information.
- The patient is monitored for MRSA carrier state in new contact with healthcare.
- In the United States, influenza vaccination is recommended in former or current MRSA-infected people to prevent serious respiratory infections and the spread of infection with MRSA.

49.4.12 Administrative Measures and Cancelling Restrictions

- MRSA patients and carriers are out of the hospital system/or isolated.
- Disinfection and cleaning are completed.
- Personal and general hygiene must be tightened up.

Table 49.3 Scheme for sanitation of MRSA in patients or personnel

NB. No investigation or treatment is postponed due to suspicion of MRSA
• Mapping MRSA prevalence on the body before sanitation—with one or more sets of tests • Ask for complete resistance pattern from the microbiological department, including mupirocin • Patients and relatives are informed of the treatment • All sanitation should be carried out at the same time, possibly with the addition of antibacterial treatment • Disinfection and cleaning—daily—are important in the process to avoid recontamination from own environment • Follow-up with control tests starting 10 days after completion of sanitation and 14 days after antibiotic treatment

(continued)

Table 49.3 (continued)

<table>
<tr><td>Sanitation measures for 10–14 days
Contact infection control nurse for advice and guidance
1. Disinfect whole body and hair once per day for 10–14 days
• Soap in twice for 2 min with the disinfectant, with thorough rinse between the washes afterwards
• The disinfectant (chlorhexidine, stellisept or another) must be tolerated!
• Switch to clean personal clothing and bedding—after each body's disinfection
• The laundry must withstand washing, 65–85 °C
2. Disinfect the nasal cavity (mupirocin) 3× per day for 10–14 days
3. Disinfect mouth with chlorhexidine mouthwash 3× per day for 10–14 days
4. Disinfect the toothbrush, denture, prosthesis 2× for 10–14 days: Wash at temp >65 °C or chlorhexidine alcohol (70% alcohol, 5 mg/ml chlorhexidine)
New glass/disposable cup for every mouth care
Do not contaminate the toothpaste (or small portions in single cups)
5. Disinfect all patient-related equipment (comb, jewellery, watch, glasses, etc.) and remove makeup
6. Hand hygiene with chlorhexidine alcohol (70% alcohol, 5 mg/ml chlorhexidine) or alcohol-based agents added glycerol, 10–20 times per day; in an event, use alcohol wipes
7. Wipe (alcohol wipes) surfaces, switches and common touch points 3× for 10 days
8. Ointments and other skin care products—Contact infection control nurse for advice</td>
<td>Steps at the same time
1. Soap in with disinfectant once for 10–14 days
• Twice for 2 min each with rinsing between
• Wash over the soap container surface with the disinfectant. Use disposable washcloth
• Remember hair, ears, genitalia, between toes
• Rinse off the disinfectant thoroughly afterwards—otherwise skin problems
• Rinse the shower cubicle walls with warm water. Step out on a clean towel or in an area that is disinfected with alcohol and wipe yourself with another clean towel
• Both towels are placed in yellow plastic bag for contaminated textiles after use
2. Disinfection of the nasal cavity: Bactroban/mupirocin 3× for 10–14 days
• Disinfect hands and outside of the ointment box with hand disinfectant
• Take ointment on a clean Q-tip and smear well in each nasal cavity or use disposable gloves for the procedure
3. Disinfect the mouth: Chlorhexidine mouthwash 3× for 10–14 days
• Disinfect the hands and outside of the bottle/cup
• New cup for every rinse
• Rinse your mouth well, put your head back and "gurgle" mouth rinse in your throat for 2–3 min. Do not swallow
4. Brush your teeth, dentures, prosthesis 2× for 10–14 days and disinfect the equipment—see point 4, left</td></tr>
<tr><td colspan="2">Special problems
• Surface wounds/eczema: body disinfectants (hibiscrub/stellisept/alcohol) are usually tolerated in superficial wounds or chlorhexidine 0.5–1 mg/ml in aqueous solution 3–4×/day (note chlorhexidine—not in the ear and has short durability after opened: 1 week). Optionally mupirocin ointment (should generally be avoided)
• Alternatively when wound: Chlorhexidine liniment/rinsing liquid to wounds/mucous membranes, Bactroban ointment 3×/day, Bacimycin wound powder/ointment, but do not use fucidin ointment. Request resistance pattern of the MRSA strain
• By mupirocin resistance, use Naseptin® containing 0.1% chlorhexidine and 0.5% neomycin
• Eczema: Contact dermatologist if there is widespread superficial wounds/eczema
• Carrier state in throat, etc. contact specialist in infection medicine for selecting antibacterial agent for systemic therapy if failure of the sanitation
• Infection with fever. Contact specialist in infection medicine</td></tr>
</table>

Source for Ullevål standard: Refs. 13–24

- Initial control of exposed personnel is mostly carried out, and no new infected persons are found.
- Activity is normalized after consulting with infection control personnel.

49.4.13 Discharge to Community Health Centres, Primary Health

Responsibility: management by relevant department in collaboration with infection control/hygiene nurse.

- When transferring to other health institutions, nursing homes and home care, notify MRSA infection in the actual ward, even if the patient has negative samples at discharge.
- Follow-up and sanitation can take place outside the hospital in consultation with the family doctor/responsible institution/infection control (see earlier).
- Good discharge procedures and information about MRSA control and infection control procedures to patients, relatives and receiving health unit *before* the patient is discharged.
- Good monitoring by nursing/retirement home/condominiums/home care, preventing the spread of infection.
- MSA patients in institutions, in home care or special living units must get patient-responsible doctor and nurse who follow up with the controls and treatment until the MRSA patient is negative in consecutive samples for 1 year after the last positive sample.

49.4.14 Outpatient Treatment and Examination When MRSA Is Infected

- Planned at the end of the day, prepared well.
- Clear away equipment, etc.—not fabric chairs or a lot of equipment.
- Use personal infection control equipment (gloves, face mask/hood, infection coat).
- Take the patient directly into the office—not in the waiting room.
- Let the patient sit on a chair or on an examining table—and do not touch the stuff in the room.
- Calm examination and treatment—have all the necessary equipment available—do not leave the room with PPE on.
- Afterwards disinfect relevant surfaces and contact points—including floors that the patient has been in direct contact with using disinfectant—alcohol, chloramine, chloricide, peracet acid, etc.
- Remove the PPE without contaminating hands, own clothes or the environment—and treat it as infectious waste.

49.4.15 Notification Responsibilities

- Microbiological laboratory reports telephonic identified/suspected MRSA to department/ward and infection control personnel.
- Department manager (event in charge) contacts infection control personnel and other departments where patients have been and sends nominative message.
- Nursing homes, home care and primary health service in general are notified if infected patient/employee has been in contact with these.
- Employees are obliged to inform about exposure to MRSA.
- Infection control doctor reports to the Director, National Institute of Public Health, the County and the State Board of Health during major outbreaks of MRSA. The Director is also notified by fatalities due to MRSA and/or particularly costly measures.

49.5 Background Information

MRSA is an increasing problem in healthcare worldwide and also in Scandinavia, including Norway [15, 18]. The largest hospital outbreak of MRSA in Norway occurred at the Regional Hospital of Trondheim during 1970–1974 with 144 cases, 48 (31.6%) deaths (direct or indirect), 15 infected employee (13 nurses/assistants, one physiotherapist, one physician) and did not end before a separate isolation ward was established [15, 25]. The index case was a 59-year-old woman with postoperative wound infection (never been outside Norway), treated with cephalothin and ampicillin. The highly virulent strains of MRSA were found in environmental samples from air in several patient rooms, equipment, bed-lining, dust on floors under the beds and in the beds, etc. [25]. The entire hospital was nearly paralyzed during the endemic—because of lack of isolation units and qualified personnel, difficulties concerning information, disagreement concerning infection control and more or less follow-up of doctors that did not believe in the effect of infection control measures [15, 25]. The same problems are still present in many hospitals, also in Norway.

- *MRSA* is unusually robust with long survival in dry state in the environment—up to 10 months, and with ability to spread to animals and grazing land and to nutrients as food and drink [18, 24, 26].
- *MRSA* is resistant to all penicillins, cephalosporins and carbapenems; all types of beta-lactam antibiotics have resistance genes *Mec*A and/or *Mec*C and is often resistant to other good staphylococcal medicaments, especially import strains.
- *HA-MRSA (hospital-associated MRSA)* is nosocomial, often more antibiotic resistant than MRSA occurring outside healthcare: CA-MRSA [18, 24].
- *HACO-MRSA (hospital-associated community-onset MRSA)* is increasing in the United States and Europe where MRSA infection is discovered first after a few months after hospitalization. This is due to ever-shorter hospital stay.

- *CA-MRSA (community-associated MRSA)*—outside health institutions, often in young, healthy people—with no previous contact with the healthcare system [18, 24, 27]. Serious abscesses in the skin and other acute infections are associated with CA-MRSA. The MRSA is sensitive to other staphylococcal medicaments but may produce dangerous toxins that PVL (Panton-Valentine Leukocidin) and is associated with greater virulence than HA-MRSA [18, 28].
- *LA-MRSA (livestock-associated MRSA)* is a new type of MRSA (first occurring in Denmark, Netherland and USA) transmitted by a high production of animals, especially of pigs, and also found in bulk milk and other foodstuffs [18, 24, 26, 29].
- *Mixing of MRSA types:* MRSA transmission happens very fast. In hospitals today, there are both CA-MRSA and LA-MRSA—types, in addition to HA-MRSA, and vice versa [18, 24, 30]. In the United States, type USA300 is spread both outside and within the healthcare system [31].
- *VRSA* is vancomycin resistant (VRSA) or vancomycin intermediate resistant (VISA)—MRSA which are selected by the high prevalence of MRSA and VRE, combined with the use of vancomycin [32–34].
- *MRSA tracing*: sampling of close contacts of the MRSA case and/or the environment surrounding the source of infection. Typing of MRSA-genotyping (PFGE, sequencing of the entire genome etc.) show similarity between bacteria which indicates the pathways of infection and sources [18, 19, 21–23, 35, 36].
- *Mupirocin*– disinfectant of skin and mucous membranes and is used in ointments to kill MRSA during decontamination of MRSA [37].

49.5.1 Incidence, Cost and Mortality

Occurrence varies from 40–60% of *Staphylococcus aureus* in Southern Europe to 1–4% in Norway, Sweden, Finland and Denmark (Fig. 49.1) [38].

In the United States, the percentage of MRSA among *S. aureus* isolates was 55% from cases with catheter septicaemia, 60% from UVI catheters, ca 50% from VAP cases and 44% from postoperative wounds [12]. MRSA-type USA300 is spreading, and serious nosocomial pneumonia cases increase [31, 39]. Carrier state of MRSA in the population is high. In routine samples from 250 pregnant women in the United States, MRSA were detected in 10.4% of recto-vaginal swabs. Carrier state in pregnant women can lead to complications around birth and in the child [40].

From 2002 to 2009, MRSA increased significantly at Veterans Affairs Healthcare System (a large healthcare chain in the United States) at hospitals 14%, nursing homes 10% and outpatient clinics 37% [41]. Hospitals in the chain had during this period 44,668 MRSA-infected patients! Despite the increase in MRSA—cases, the clinical outcomes were better [41].

The risk of spread of MRSA is great in nursing homes, home care, day care, schools and among families of infected healthcare professionals. MRSA among pet, pig herds, in grazing land, recreation areas, foods, bulk milk, meat, etc. promotes the spread in the environment and in the population [18, 24, 26].

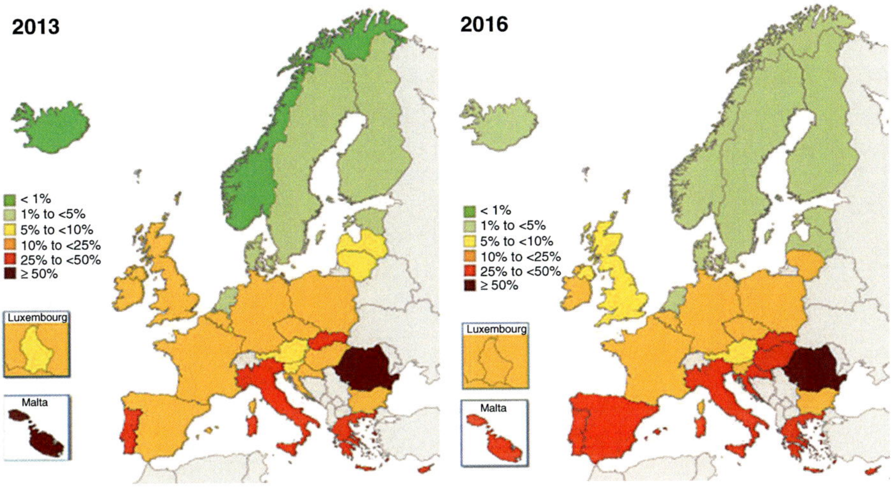

Fig. 49.1 Percentage (%) of invasive isolates resistant to methicillin (MRSA), by country, EU/EEA countries, 2013 and 2016. Source: ECDC, 2013, 2017 [38]

Attack rate of infection after colonization in hospitals is 26–33% and may even be almost 50% in infants [12, 18]. Attack rate of CA-MRSA can be up to 100% [18]. Certain epidemic clones, USA300 and USA400 is easily transmitted and harder to get rid of than others [12, 18].

In Norway, MRSA increased to 1867 cases in 2014, hence 832 with infections and 1035 carriers (Fig. 49.2, source: MSIS). MRSA has been out of control, with outbreaks in pig herds, much like in Denmark, but is now followed up by the Norwegian Veterinary Institute [18, 24].

Costs associated with MRSA infections are dependent on active infection control that prevent transmission of infections in hospitals. Good isolation measures and procedures for screening and decontamination is cost-efficient and leads to control [12, 18–24, 42–45]. There is less spread if the infected patient is diagnosed quickly [18, 23, 24, 46, 47]. Costs are associated with extra length of stay at the ICU, up to 20 extra days, and are significantly higher than for other infectious agents [12, 18].

At Ullevål University Hospital (UUH), one patient with MRSA was costing in 1997 526,000 NKr (ca. 75,150 USD), including extended length, transmission of MRSA to a hospital employee, screening tests, disinfection, sanitation and antibacterial treatment [19]. An outbreak of MRSA in the same hospital's neonatal intensive department in 1999 resulted in additional costs of 375, 000 NKr (53,600 USD) per MRSA positive patient, including isolation costs, disinfection, screening and extra days in hospital—a total of ca. three million NKr (ca. 429,000 USD) [21].

A rapid MRSA test within 2 h, combined with regular cultivation, may save huge costs for patients and personnel exposed to MRSA or suspected to be MRSA infected [23]. A rapid MRSA test is saving isolation measures, and exposed personnel can go directly to work without being on sick leave while waiting for the test result [23].

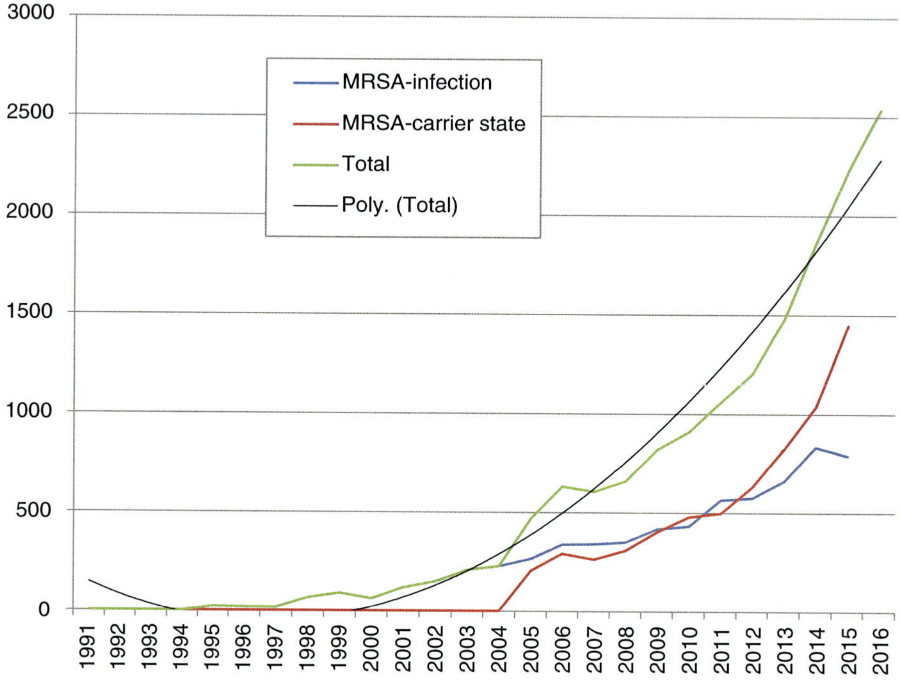

Fig. 49.2 Development of MRSA cases in Norway; 1991–2016 (source: MSIS, National Public Health)

Active screening and isolation is significantly cheaper for the healthcare than uncontrolled transmission of MRSA which can result in serious infection and death and lead to "hopeless" endemic conditions and even more antibacterial resistance problems!

Mortality among people over 65 years of MRSA bacteraemia is found to be ca. 36%, compared with 12% below 65 [15, 18, 48]. Among ca. 3400 cases of *S. aureus* bacteraemia in Europe and the United States (2006–2011), more than 20% of cases were caused by MRSA as an independent risk factor for death [49]. Survival period after MRSA bacteraemia was 14 months, compared to 54 months after MSSA (methicillin-sensitive *S aureus*) bacteraemia [50]. Mortality associated with MRSA bacteraemia is evaluated to be more than three times higher than that of MSSA bacteraemia [12, 18].

49.5.2 Isolation and Testing Prevents the Spread of Infection

The presence of MRSA at hospital admission is usually applied to the patient in one or another prior to health-related situation [51].

49.5.2.1 Contact and Airborne Infection

Rooms, equipment, ventilation and other patients and personnel can be contaminated and infected with MRSA before test results are available [12, 18, 52–56]. Contamination and spread of MRSA may lead to carrier states: the nose, and sometimes the throat, in the perineum, around the wrists, hands, hair, ears and other parts of the body [18, 23, 24].

MRSA-infected patients are often contaminated on hands and therefore constitute major infectious sources for direct contact and the environment [18, 23, 57]. A study of 82 patients colonized with MRSA demonstrated that 82% had MRSA on hands and that hand disinfection was ineffective in 40% of the cases [57].

Carriers of MRSA on multiple anatomical sites on the body are more prone to infection than those with MRSA only on one place [58]. Large amounts of MRSA in the patient is more easily transmitted to the environment [46]. Contamination of environment and air in the room of MRSA patients happens very quickly—within 10 h [18, 52–55]. Therefore, personnel should use infection control equipment when entering the room, and patients should be isolated for suspected MRSA from admittance to hospital.

49.5.2.2 Contact Isolation (Contact Precaution = CP)

Contact isolation, defined by CDC (use of gloves, gown and the patient in isolate/private room), is used in high-endemic areas where 5–10% of hospitalized patients are infected [12]. Effect of CP is discussed [59–67]. Many studies are poor in terms of documentation and compliance [59]. Some studies are worth noting.

- Huang et al. found that CP led to significant reduction in bacteraemia in ICU (ICU): 75%, in non-ICU, 40%, and throughout the hospital, 67% reduction of MRSA cases [60].
- Robiscek et al. conducted PCR MRSA screening on admission and CP and eradication (sanitation) of MRSA positive patients, with significant reduction of MRSA disease during stay and 30 days after discharge [61]. MRSA was detected in 8.3% of 3300 patients admitted to the ICU and in 6.3% of the total of 62,000 patients tested, as is endemic conditions [61].
- Harris et al. showed significant reduction of MRSA under endemic conditions (10% MRSA infection among hospitalized patients), among 26, 200 patient admissions to 20 ICUs' [62]. Overall CP treatment of patients resulted in 40% reduction of MRSA, and a targeted isolation of only proven MRSA cases led to 15% reduction [62]. The more use of the CP, the less prevalence of MRSA in the units [62].
- A two-phase study from Australia was conducted at a medical ICU where prevalence of MRSA was 6.9%, and 60% became infected with MRSA during their stay [63]. In phase 1, MRSA patients were treated as other patients (no use of CP or isolation), although they were MRSA positive. In phase 2, CP was utilized for all MRSA positive patients, with use of a single room or cohort with other MRSA-infected patients [63]. All patients in the Phase 1 and 2 were MRSA screened on arrival (PCR), and in phase 2, all MRSA findings were reported

telephonic. There were about 2200 ICU patients in each phase. CP and isolation resulted in 60% reduction of MRSA infections acquired in the ICU [63]. *This is the only known "pure study" where the contact isolation are compared with no isolation.*

- Mangini et al. showed significant reduction of nosocomial MRSA when using CP and further reduction when using masks in addition to CP, for healthcare personnel working within 3 feet of the MRSA patient [64].
- A couple of large studies from the healthcare chain, Veterans Affairs, hospitals and long-term institutions in the United States, showed that with universal MRSA nose testing (96%) at admission, contact isolation of MRSA cases, hand hygiene and cultural changes in the institutions led to a sharp reduction of MRSA [65, 66].
  – In long-term institutions of Veterans Affairs (12,000 places), the reduction of MRSA cases was 36% [65].
  – In hospitals of Veterans Affairs (approximately two million admissions), 93–96% were nose tested at admission, and 13.6% were MRSA positive, an endemic situation [66]. During the period 2007–2010, a 62% reduction in MRSA infections in ICU's and 45% reduction in non-ICU's were found [66].
  – The large and robust studies showed significant effect of CP combined with hand hygiene and identification of MRSA positive patients.
- Good networking concerning infection control among hospitals may lead to less spread of infection [67].
- MRSA screening, isolation and eradication are important to reduce the spread of MRSA, even in hyperendemic areas [60–70].
- At the University Hospital of Basel, Switzerland, Widmer et al. (2015) described that the same procedures for strict isolation of MRSA cases had been used for 20 years [71]. There was targeted testing of patients and personnel and routine decontamination of infected persons. During a period of 20 years, approximately 540,700 blood cultures were studied. *S. aureus* was detected in blood cultures of 1200 patients, of which 34 were MRSA cases (2.7%). During the whole period, there had been a stable, low MRSA rate, without significant changes of the presence of MRSA in blood cultures [71].
- Similar experiences, with strict disease control measures and low rate of MRSA bacteraemia, have been recorded in Norway and other Scandinavian countries [18].

49.5.3 MRSA Testing and Screening

One single test is not good enough. Today, MRSA screening, only from a single anatomic site, the nose, is rather "bad medicine". At least 50% of nasal samples may be negative, even if the patient is an infection disperser to the environment [18, 23, 52, 72–75]. The greater the number of MRSA colonizing the nose, the greater the chance of finding MRSA elsewhere on the body [74]. In case of MRSA patients with skin and soft tissue infections, which occur most often outside healthcare (CA-MRSA), samples from the nose are often negative for MRSA [52, 72]. Among the 290 MRSA patients with skin and soft tissue infections, only 41% of nasal samples were positive [72].

Hands/wrist-testing MRSA patients often have contamination on hands and transmit the infection via contact to the environment [18, 23, 53, 57]. Among 82 patients colonized with MRSA, 82% had MRSA on hands, and hand disinfection was ineffective in 40% [57]. Therefore, hands/wrists should be included by MRSA testing of patients and personnel, as a routine used at United States during the past 20 years [13–24].

Universal test, targeted test, rapid test, universal decontamination without testing, etc. are different methods used to prevent the spread of MRSA. This is especially discussed in areas with endemic occurrence of MRSA [76–80]. The problem is that unstructured and half-hearted infection control measures over time have prepared the ground for serious endemic MRSA [59]. Under such conditions, it may pay to do universal testing, isolation and decontamination of MRSA cases, as shown by Jain et al. in the United States [66, 67]. Ireland, having one of the highest rates of MRSA both in Europe and compared to the United States, reports that MRSA screening—universal or targeted—is better than no screening because it results in fewer MRSA infections [79]. All measures that reduce MRSA lead to savings, not just MRSA but also with regard to other resistant microbes [79]. Targeted screening and isolation is probably most effective in countries with more stress on infection control over the MRSA situation.

Rapid tests are successful. A prerequisite for successful screening and savings is that rapid tests are used as real quick tests on a daily basis, combined with the culture and PCR response within a few hours [18, 23, 51, 61, 63]. Patient rooms may be contaminated within a few hours to a day and thus fellow patients are at risk for infection [45, 51]. MRSA are detected in the air in most hospital rooms where MRSA patients are staying [55]. Colonized persons are greater infection spreaders than patients with clinical infections [55]. Therefore it is important to isolate patients from the start and use rapid tests to quickly clarify infectious condition.

49.5.4 Sanitation and Eradication of MRSA in Patients and Personnel

Without sanitation measures, MRSA may disappear spontaneously in approximately 10% of the cases within 1 month. In a study of 365 patients with prolonged admission and infected or colonized with MRSA and/or VRE, MRSA disappeared spontaneously in 11% after a median of 23 days and VRE in 18% after a median of 26.5 days [81]. Many persons are carriers of MRSA for years if sanitation is not performed, documented by several studies [18].

Daily baths of patients in chlorhexidine, regardless of MRSA status, are becoming popular in the United States but miss good documentation [82–88]. The main study included 74,000 patients at 74 ICUs for adults and showed that daily chlorhexidine bath reduced sepsis in patients infected with MRSA by 23% [82, 83]. If all were sanitized with chlorhexidine bath, regardless of MRSA status, the MRSA sepsis was reduced by 37% and all sepsis cases with 44% [82, 83]. There are a number of important objections to this survey with regard to quality and documentation [84, 85]. A good global used disinfectant which is also used as surgical handwashing may not be used indiscriminately as a substitute for good infection control. There is a documented risk of developing resistance to chlorhexidine.

Sanitation (disinfection of person and environment) and eradication of cases infected/colonized with MRSA may be difficult and need often to be repeated several times before effect. Among 351 MRSA carriers who got institutional clearance of MRSA, most 70% were negative after 2 years, while about 30% relapsed [89]. However, the carrier state was only controlled by nasal samples [89]. It is especially important to eradicate MRSA in healthcare personnel and in patients that is going to be treated in the healthcare [23]. Among 510 healthcare personnel with MRSA, 88% successful eradication was reported by Albrich and Harbarth [90].

Chlorhexidine sanitation for clearance of carrier state of MRSA may eradicate the risk of infectious attack and transmission and prevent the skin and soft tissue infections. Among 3090 military with MRSA skin infections, the reduction of infections was 64% after implementation of chlorhexidine gluconate wash/shower on arrival at training camp and with six consecutive repetitions with chlorhexidine during their stay, in addition to advice on personal hygiene [88]. During high-endemic conditions, eradication of MRSA in infected patients may be very effective [91, 92]. Screening and sanitation of healthcare workers are best utilized and targeted, especially when it comes to superspreaders [18, 71, 92].

It is often recommended to have 5 days of sanitation, but experience suggests 10–14 days to get rid of the microbe [13–18]. Patients and personnel are then monitored so that the "isolation time" can be minimized.

49.5.5 Contamination of Environment, Equipment and Textile Uniforms

49.5.5.1 Environmental Infection

It is often a very fast contamination of rooms via contact and air from patients with MRSA [45, 51, 55]. More than 80% of environmental samples from patient rooms of MRSA patients may be positive [45]. MRSA carriers are transmitting MRSA as much to the environment as patients with infections do [93]. MRSA-type USA300 has great ability to contaminate and survive in the hospital environment and in homes [94]. Therefore environmental sanitation is important. Gas disinfection is recommended in difficult local conditions with a lot of equipment and with medical devices that cannot be cleaned internally [18, 95–97].

49.5.5.2 Personnel Attire Is Contaminated

During all care, examination and treatment, personnel most often have a close contact with the patients, which may lead to the transmission of the patient's flora to the uniform—especially on the front and sleeves of staff's outfits. The use of private clothes in healthcare entails increased carrying state of microbes [98–101]. Resistant bacteria are commonly detected in clothes and other textiles, particularly at high patient occupancy and high rates of bacterial resistance in the department [99, 100]. Universal gowning and gloving and good hand hygiene when caring for patients have shown a reduced transmission of the patient's microbes to the staff clothing by 70% [99].

MRSA is easily transmitted in intensive care with a respirator, a catheter and contact with the head/neck area of the patient [101]. Gloves used "everywhere" without change pose a serious source of infection [102]. The healthcare workers use and change of uniforms is considered as "the emerging frontier" in epidemiologically important environmental surfaces [103].

49.5.5.3 Healthcare Worker

Outbreaks in hospitals are often linked to overcrowding, understaffing and increased workloads for staff [18, 21]. Healthcare personnel is considered as "source, vector or victim" with regard to MRSA infections [90]. Up to 5% of personnel in Northern Europe may be infected with MRSA [90]. In Paris, MRSA was detected in 10% of healthcare providers, associated with a high incidence among patients. Nurses who were most in contact with the patients had the greatest risk of becoming infected [104]. Carrier state on hands is common in MRSA-colonized persons, and hand disinfectant may fail, which makes testing of the hands and wrists necessary also by healthcare professionals [18, 53, 57, 105, 106].

49.5.5.4 Hand Hygiene and Use of Gloves

Hand hygiene is a problem in busy departments with understaffing, overcrowding and many patients on the corridor without access to washing or other hygiene, as observed by Norwegian hospitals that generally have occupancy rate of more than 100%. Infection barrier is the first thing that falls in busy departments. This is expensive for the healthcare system. More and more new and dangerous nosocomial microbes are spread in the hospital, including MRSA. Hand disinfection with alcohol 70% v/v was ineffective against MRSA in 40% of the cases, also earlier documented [26, 105, 106]. Therefore, good disposable gloves should always be used for any suspected infection, hand hygiene before and after using gloves.

References

1. Norwegian Board of Health. Advice for the application of the infection act § 3-3 advance examination of patients- infectious diseases. IK-28/96. Oslo: Norwegian Board of Health; 1996.
2. Norwegian Board of Health. Regulations concerning advance examination of workers in health care – antibiotic resistant bacteria. Issued by the Health and Social Affairs July 5, 1996 pursuant to the Act of 5 August 1994 No. 15 concerning protection against infectious diseases § 3.2. FOR 1996-07-05 No. 700. Norway.
3. Norwegian Board of Health. Hospitals Act §18A-hospital infections that may significant damage the patient. Oslo: Norwegian Board of Health, 2000.
4. Norwegian Board of Health. Law on protection against infectious diseases by 5 Aug 1994. no 55.

5. Regulations on infection control in health care. Adopted by Royal. Res. 17 June 2005 pursuant to the Act of 5 August 1994. 55 on protection against infectious diseases §§ 4-7, 7-11, Law 19 November 1982 no. 66 Municipal Health §1-3 fifth paragraph, law 2 July 1999 no. 61 relating to the specialist health care with more § 2-1a fifth paragraph and law on 18 May 2001 no. 24 on health registers and processing of health information § 6, third paragraph. Promoted by the Ministry of Health and Social Affairs.
6. Norwegian Board of Health. Use of isolation to prevent spread of infection in hospitals. Oslo: Directorate of Health; 1988. p. 2–88.
7. Norwegian Board of Health. Isolation guideline. Health and Social Affairs, 2003.
8. Measures to discourage antibiotic resistance (2000–2004). Oslo: Health and Social Affairs; 2000.
9. MRSA Guide. National guidelines for preventing the spread of methicillin-resistant *Staphylococcus aureus*(MRSA) in health institutions. Norwegian Board of Health and National Public Health, in 2002, 2004 and 2009.
10. Directorate for Labor Inspection. Regulations for protection against exposure to biological agents (bacteria, viruses, fungi, etc.) in the workplace, 19 Dec 1997.
11. European Parliament – and Council Directive 2000/54/EC of 18 September 2000 on the protection of workers from the risks related to exposure to biological agents at work.
12. Calfee DP, Salgado CD, Milstone AM, et al. Strategies two preventer methicillin-resistant *Staphylococcus aureus* transmission and infection in acute care hospitals: 2014 update (from 2008). Infect Control Hosp Epidemiol. 2014;35:772–96.
13. Andersen BM. Methicillin-resistant *Staphylococcus aureus* (MRSA). In: Handbook of hygiene and infection control. Ullevål sykehus. 1996. p. 156–8.
14. Andersen BM. Methicillin-resistant *Staphylococcus aureus* (MRSA). In: Handbook of hygiene and infection control. Ullevål sykehus. 1999. p. 214–20.
15. Andersen BM. Methicillin-resistant *Staphylococcus aureus*. In: Bacteria and disease. Epidemiology, infection and infection control. Gyldendal Academic. 2005. p. 110–57.
16. Andersen BM. Methicillin-resistant *Staphylococcus aureus*(MRSA). In: Håndbok in hygiene and infection control. Ullevål University Hospital. 2003. p. 259–69.
17. Andersen BM, Rasch M Hochlin K, Tollefsen T, Seljordslia B. Prevention of MRSA infection. In: Handbook of hygiene and infection control for hospitals. Ullevål University Hospital.2008. p. 422–50.
18. Andersen BM. Methicillin-resistant *Staphylococcus aureus*. MRSA. Handbook of hygiene and infection control in hospitals. Part 1: Microbiology and infection protection. Fagbokforlaget. 2014. p. 39–57.
19. Andersen BM, Bergh K, Steinbakk M, Syversen G, Magnes B, Dalen H, Bruun JN. A Norwegian nosocomial outbreak of methicillin-resistant *Staphylococcus aureus* resistant to fusidic acid and susceptible to other antistaphylococcalagents. J Hosp Infect. 1999;41:123–32.
20. Andersen BM, Syversen G. Methicillin-resistant *Staphylococcus aureus* in Oslo in 2000. Tidsskr Nor Legeforen. 2001;121:1844–7.
21. Andersen BM, Lindemann R, Bergh K, Nesheim BI, Syversen G, Solheim N, Laugerud F. Spread of methicillin-resistant *Staphylococcus aureus* in a neonatal intensive unit associated with underpinning, overcrowding and mixing of patients. J Hosp Infect. 2002;1:1–7.
22. Andersen BM, Rasch M, Syversen G. Is an increase of MRSA in Oslo, Norway, associated with changed infection control policy? J Infect. 2007;55:531–8.
23. Andersen BM, Tollefsen T, Seljordslia B, Hochlin K, Syversen G, Jonassen Ø, Rasch M. Rapid MRSA test in exposed persons: costs and savings in hospitals. J Infect. 2010;60:293–9.
24. Andersen BM. MRSA infection control in a low-endemic area. www.webbertraining.com. 24 Oct 2013.
25. Kvittingen J, Tryme A. Hospital-endemia with methicillin-resistant staphylococci. Tidsskr Nor Legeforen. 1977;97:813–6.
26. Promed-mail, 18 July 2015. *Staphylococcus aureus* (MRSA) – UK: Meat products, human, ST398.

27. David MZ, Daum RS. Community-associated methicillin-resistant *Staphylococcus aureus*: epidemiology and clinical consequences of an emerging epidemic. Clin Microbiol Rev. 2010;23:616–87.
28. Shallcross LJ, Fragaszy E, Johnson AM, Hayward A. The role of the Panton-Valentine leucocidin toxin in staphylococcal disease: a systematic review and meta-analysis. Lancet Infect Dis. 2013;13:43–54.
29. Otter JA, French GL. Molecular epidemiology of community-associated methicillin-resistant *Staphylococcus aureus* in Europe. Lancet Infect Dis. 2010;10:227–39.
30. Peterson AE, Davis MF, Julian KG, et al. Molecular and phenotypic characteristics of healthcare- and community-associated methicillin-resistant *Staphylococcus aureus* at a rural hospital. PLoS One. 2012;7:e38354.
31. Dikema DJ, Richter SS, Heilmann KP, et al. Continued emergence of USA300 methicillin-resistant *Staphylococcus aureus* in the United States: results from a nationwide surveillance study. Infect Control Hosp Epidemiol. 2014;35:285–92.
32. Zarpellon MN, Gales AC, Sakasaki A, et al. Survival of vancomycin-intermediate *Staphylococcus aureus* on hospital surfaces. J Hosp Infect. 2015;90:347–50.
33. Tosh PK, Agolory S, Strong BL, et al. Prevalence and risk factors associated with vancomycin-resistant *Staphylococcus aureus* precursor organism colonization among patients with chronic lower-extremity wounds in Southeastern Michigan. Infect Control Hosp Epidemiol. 2013;34:954–60.
34. Sievert DM, Boulton ML, Stoltman G, Johnson D, et al. *Staphylococcus aureus* resistant to vancomycin – United States, 2002. MMWR. 2002;51:565–7.
35. Prince JR, Golubchik T. Cole Ket al. Whole-genome sequencing shows that patient to patient transmission rarely accounts for acquisition of *Staphylococcus aureus* in an intensive care unit. Clin Infect Dis. 2014;58:609–18.
36. Azarian T, Cook RL, Johnson JA, et al. Whole-genome sequencing for outbreak investigation of methicillin resistant *Staphylococcus aureus* in the neonatal intensive care unit: time for routine practice? Infect Control Hosp Epidemiol. 2015;36:777–85.
37. Sciortino CV, Kemper M Parthasathy L, Lay J. Surveillance of methicillin-resistant *Staphylococcus aureus* mupirocin resistance in a Veterans Affairs Hospital. Infect Control Hosp Epidemiol. 2015;36:235–6.
38. ECDC. WSummary of the latest data on antibiotic resistance in the European Union. EARS-Net surveillance data. Nov 2017.
39. Lewis SS, Walker VJ, Lee MS, et al. Epidemiology of methicillin-resistant *Staphylococcus aureus* pneumonia in community hospitals. Infect Control Hosp Epidemiol. 2014;35:1452–7.
40. Creech CB, Litzner B, Talbot TR, Schaffner W. Frequency of detection of methicillin-resistant *Staphylococcus aureus* from rectovaginal swabs in pregnant women. Am J Infect Control. 2010;38:72–4.
41. Chaffrey AR, LaPlante KL. Changing epidemiology of methicillin-resistant *Staphylococcus aureus* in the Veterans Affairs Healthcare System, 2002–2009. Infection. 2012;40:291–7.
42. Lee BY, Wiringa AE, Bailey RR, et al. The economic effect of screening orthopedic surgical patients preoperatively for methicillin-resistant *Staphylococcus aureus*. Infect Control Hosp Epidemiol. 2010;31:1130–8.
43. Lee BY, Song Y, McGlone SM, et al. The economic value of screening haemodialysis patients for methicillin-resistant *Staphylococcus aureus* in the United States. Clin Microbiol Infect. 2011;17:1717–26.
44. Wassenberg M, Kluytmans J, Erdkamp S, et al. Costs and benefits of rapid screening of methicillin-resistant *Staphylococcus aureus* carriage in intensive care units: a prospective multicenter study. Crit Care. 2012;16:R22.
45. Brooks HL, Hodson J, Richardson SJ, et al. Improving the timeliness of methicillin-resistant *Staphylococcus aureus* antimicrobial decolonization therapy administration: a descriptive account. J Hosp Infect. 2014;86:209–15.

46. French GL, Otter JAS, Shannon KP, Adams NMT, Parks MJ, Watling D. Tackling contamination of the hospital environment by methicillin resistant *Staphylococcus aureus* (MRSA): a comparison between conventional terminal cleaning and hydrogen peroxide vapour decontamination. J Hosp Infect. 2004;57:31–7.
47. Livorsi DJ, Arif S, Garry P, et al. Methicillin-resistant *Staphylococcus aureus*(MRSA) nasal real-time PCR: a predictive tool for contamination of hospital environment. Infect Control Hosp Epidemiol. 2015;36:34–9.
48. Tacconelli E, Pop-Vica AE, D'Agata EMC. Increased mortality among elderly patients with methicillin-resistant *Staphylococcus aureus* bacteraemia. J Hosp Infect. 2006;64:251–6.
49. Kaasch AJ, Barlow G. Edgeworth et al. *Staphylococcus aureus* bloodstream infection: a pooled analysis of five prospective, observational studies. J Infect. 2014;68:242–51.
50. Yaw LK, Robinson JO, Ho KM. A comparison of long-term outcomes after methicillin-resistant and methicillin-sensitive *Staphylococcus aureus* bacteraemia: an observational cohort study. Lancet Infect Dis. 2014;14:967–75.
51. McKinnell JA, Miller LG, eell SJ, Cui E, Huang SS. A systematic literature review and meta-analysis of factors associated with methicillin-resistant *Staphylococcus aureus* colonization at time of hospital or intensive care unit admission. Infect Control Hosp Epidemiol. 2013;34:1077–86.
52. Chang S, Sethi AK, Stiefel U, Cadnum JL, Donskey CJ. Occurrence of skin and environmental contamination with methicillin-resistant *Staphylococcus aureus* before results of polymerase chain reaction that hospital admission become available. Infect Control Hosp Epidemiol. 2010;31:607–12.
53. Yang ES, Tan J, Eells S, Rieg G, Tagudar G, Miller LG. Body site colonization in patients with community-associated methicillin-resistant *Staphylococcus aureus* and other types of *S aureus*skin infections. Clin Microbiol Infect. 2010;16:425–31.
54. Bhalla A, Pultz NJ, Gries DM, et al. Acquisition of nosocomial pathogens on hands after contact with environmental surfaces near hospitalized patients. Infect Control Hosp Epidemiol. 2004;25:164–7.
55. Gehanno JF, Louvel A, Nouvellon M, Caillard JF, Pestel-Caron M. Aerial dispersal of methicillin-resistant *Staphylococcus aureus* in hospital rooms by infected or colonised patients. J Hosp Infect. 2009;71:256–62.
56. Masclaux FG, Sakwinska O, Charriere N, Semaani E, Oppliger A. Concentration of airborne *Staphylococcus aureus* (MRSA and MSSA), total bacteria, and endotoxins in pig farms. Ann Occup Hyg. 2013;57:550–7.
57. Sunkensula V, Kundrapu S, Macinga DR Donskey CJ. Efficacy of alcohol gel for removal of methicillin-resistant *Staphylococcus aureus* from hands of colonized patients. Infect Control Hosp Epidemiol. 2015;36:229–31.
58. Sim BLH, McBryde E Street AC, Marshall C. Multiple site surveillance cultures as a predictor of methicillin-resistant *Staphylococcus aureus* infections. Infect Control Hosp Epidemiol. 2013;34:818–24.
59. Morgan DJ, Murthy R, Munoz-Price LS, et al. Reconsidering contact precautions for endemic methicillin-resistant *Staphylococcus aureus* and vancomycin-resistant *Enterococcus*. Infect Control Hosp Epidemiol. 2015;36(10):1163–72.
60. Huang SS, Yokoe DS, Hinrichsen VL, et al. Impact of routine intensive care unit surveillance cultures and resultant barrier precautions on hospital-wide methicillin-resistant *Staphylococcus aureus* bacteremia. Clin Infect Dis. 2006;43:971–8.
61. Robicsek A, Beaumont JL, Paule SM, et al. Universal surveillance for methicillin-resistant *Staphylococcus aureus* in 3 affiliated hospitals. Ann Intern Med. 2008;148:409–18.
62. Harris AD, Pinel L, Belton B, et al. Universal glove use and acquisition of antibiotic-resistant bacterial in the ICU. A randomized trial. JAMA. 2013;310:1571–80.
63. Marshall C, Richards M, McBryde E. Do active surveillance and contact precautions reduceMRSA acquisition? A prospective interrupted time series. PLoS One. 2013;8:e58112.
64. Mangini E, Segal-Maurer S, Burns J, et al. Impact of contact and droplet precautions on the incidence of hospital-acquired methicillin-resistant *Staphylococcus aureus* infection. Infect Control Hosp Epidemiol. 2007;28:1261–6.

65. Evans ME, Kralovice SM, Simbartl L, et al. Nationwide reduction of healthcare-associated methicillin-resistant *Staphylococcus aureus* infections in veterans affairs long-term care facilities. Am J Infect Control. 2014;42:60–2.
66. Jain R, Kralovice SM, Evans ME, et al. Veterans affairs initiative to prevent methicillin-resistant *Staphylococcus aureus* infections. N Engl J Med. 2011;364:1419–30.
67. Lee BY, Barsch SM, Wong KF, et al. Simulation shows hospitals that cooperate on infection control obtain better results than hospitals acting alone. Health Aff (Millwood). 2012;31:225–2303.
68. Luk S, Ho AY, Ng TK, et al. Prevalence, prediction, and clonality of methicillin-resistant *Staphylococcus aureus* carriage at admission to medical units in Hong Kong, China. Infect Control Hosp Epidemiol. 2014;35:42–8.
69. Fisher D, Tambyah PA, Lin RTP, et al. Sustained methicillin-resistant *Staphylococcus aureus* control in a hyper-endemic tertiary acute care hospital with infrastructural challenge in Singapore. J Hosp Infect. 2013;85:141–8.
70. Deeny SR, Cooper CS, Cookson B, Hopkins S, Robotham JV. Targeted versus universal screening and decolonization to reduce healthcare-associated methicillin-resistant *Staphylococcus aureus* infection. J Hosp Infect. 2013;85:33–44.
71. Widmer F, Lakatos B, Frei R. Strict infection control leads to low incidence of methicillin-resistant *Staphylococcus aureus* bloodstream infection over 20 years. Infect Control Hosp Epidemiol. 2015;36:702–9.
72. Ellis MW, Schlett CD, Millar EV, et al. Prevalence of nasal colonization and strain concordance in patients with community-associated *Staphylococcus aureus* skin and soft-tissue infectons. Infect Control Hosp Epidemiol. 2014;35:1251–6.
73. Muerman O, Routamaa M, Peltonen R. Screening for methicillin-resistant *Staphylococcus aureus*: which anatomical sites two culture? J Hosp Infect. 2005;61:351–3.
74. Mermel LA, Cartony JM, Covington P, Maxey G, Morse D. Methicillin-resistant *Staphylococcus aureus* colonization at different body sites: a prospective, quantitative analysis. J Clin Microbiol. 2011;49:1119–21.
75. Gibson KE, McNamara SE, Cassone M, et al. Methicillin-resistant *Staphylococcus aureus*: site of acquisition and strain variation in high-risk nursing home residents with indwelling devices. Infect Control Hosp Epidemiol. 2014;35:1458–65.
76. McKinnell JA, Huang SS, Eeells SJ, Cui E, Miller LG. Quantifying the impact of extra nasal testing of body sites for methicillin-resistant *Staphylococcus aureus* colonization at the time of hospital or intensive care unit admission. Infect Control Hosp Epidemiol. 2013;34:161–70.
77. Otter JA, Herdman MT, Williams B, Tosas O, Edgeworth JD, French GL. Low prevalence of methicillin-resistant *Staphylococcus aureus* carriage at hospital admission: implication for risk-factor-based vs universal screening. J Hosp Infect. 2013;83:114–21.
78. McKinnell JA, Bartsch SM, Lee BY, Huang SS, Miller LG. Cost - benefit analysis form the hospital perspective of universal active screening followed by contact precautions for methicillin-resistant *Staphylococcus aureus* carriers. Infect Control Hosp Epidemiol. 2015;36:2–13.
79. O'Riordan MT, Harrington P, Mac Lellen K, Ruan M, Humphreys H. Response to McKinnell et al.'s original article cost – benefit analysis form the hospital perspective of universal active screening followed by contact precautions for methicillin-resistant *Staphylococcus aureus* carriers. Infect Control Hosp Epidemiol. 2015;36:856–8.
80. Kang J, Smith KJ, Bryce CL, Muto CA. Economic analysis of universal active surveillance screening for methicillin-resistant *Staphylococcus aureus*: perspective matters. Infect Control Hosp Epidemiol. 2015;36:14–6.
81. Gosh A, Jiao L, Al-Mutawa F, et al. Value of active surveillance policy to document clearance of methicillin-resistant *Staphyloccoccus aureus* and vancomycin-resistant enterococci amongst inpatients with prolonged admissions. J Hosp Infect. 2014;88:230–3.
82. Huang SS, Septimus E, Kleinman K, et al. Targeted versus universal decolonization to prevent ICU infection. N Engl J Med. 2013;368:2255–65.

83. Huang SS, Septimus E, Avery TL, et al. Cost savings of universal decolonization to prevent intensive care unit infection: implications of the REDUCE MRSA trial. Infect Control Hosp Epidemiol. 2014;35:23–31.
84. Kirby A. Universal decolonization to prevent intensive care unit methicillin-resistant *Staphyloccoccus aureus* infection. J Hosp Infect. 2014;88:179–80.
85. Derde LPG, Dautzenberg MJD, Bonten MJM. Chlorhexidine body washing to control antimicrobial-resistant bacteria in the intensive care unit: a systematic review. Intensive Care Med. 2012;38:931–9.
86. Viray M, Morley JC, Coopersmith CM, et al. Daily bathing with chlorhexidine-based soap and the prevention of *Staphylococcus aureus* transmission and infection. Infect Control Hosp Epidemiol. 2014;35:243–50.
87. Quach C, Milstone AM, Perpete C, et al. Chlorhexidine bathing in a tertiary care neonatal intensive care unit: impact on central-line-associated bloodstream infections. Infect Control Hosp Epidemiol. 2014;35:158–63.
88. Morrison SM, Blaesing CR, Millar EV, et al. Evaluation of methicillin-resistant *Staphylococcus aureus* skin and soft-tissue infection preventing strategies at a military training center. Infect Control Hosp Epidemiol. 2013;34:841–3.
89. Valencia Rey PA, Strymish J, Robillard E, et al. Survival time of methicillin-resistant *Staphylococcus aureus*- free status after institutional clearance. Infect Control Hosp Epidemiol. 2014;35:1271–6.
90. Albrich WC, Harbarth S. Health-care workers: source, vector, or victim of MRSA? Lancet Infect Dis. 2008;8:289–301.
91. Fraser TG, Fatica CF, Scarpelliu M, et al. Decrease in *Staphylococcus aureus* colonization and hospital-acquired infection in a medical intensive care unit after institution of an active surveillance and decolonization program. Infect Control Hosp Epidemiol. 2010;31:779–83.
92. Gurieva TV, Bootsma MCJ, Bonten MJM. Decolonization of patients and healthcare workers to control nosocomial spread of methicillin-resistant *Staphylococcus aureus*. BMC Infect Dis. 2012;12:302.
93. Knelson LP, Williams DA, Gergen MF, et al. A comparison of environmental contamination by patients infected or colonized with methicillin-resistant *Staphylococcus aureus* or vancomycin-resistant enterococci: a multicenter study. Infect Control Hosp Epidemiol. 2014;35:872–5.
94. Eeells SJ, David MZ, Taylor A, et al. Persistent environmental contamination with USA300 methicillin-resistant *Staphylococcus aureus* and other pathogenic strain types in households with *S aureus*skin infections. Infect Control Hosp Epidemiol. 2014;35:1373–82.
95. Andersen BM, Rasch M, Hochlin K, Jensen FH, Wismar P, Fredriksen JE. Decontamination of rooms, medical equipment and ambulances, using a dry mist of hydrogen peroxide disinfectant. J Hosp Infect. 2006;62:149–55.
96. Andersen BM, Hochlin K, Daling JP. Cleaning and decontamination of reusable medical equipments, includingthe use of hydrogen peroxide dry-mist gas decontamination. J Microbiol Biochem Technol. 2012;4:57–62.
97. Deshpande A, Mana TSC, Cadnum JL, et al. Evaluation of sporicidal peracetic acid/hydrogen peroxide-based daily disinfectant cleaner. Infect Control Hosp Epidemiol. 2014;35:1414–6.
98. Koh KC, Husni S, Tan CW an ASL. High prevalence of methicillin-resistant *Staphylococcus aureus* (MRSA) on doctors' neckties. Med J Malaysia. 2009;64:185–6.
99. Williams C, McGraw P, Schneck EE, et al. Impact of universal gowning and gloving on healthcare worker clothing contamination. Infect Control Hosp'Epidemiol. 2014;35:1–7.
100. Boutin MA, Thom KA, Zhan M, Johnson JK. A randomized crossover trial to decrease bacterial contamination of hospital scrubs. Infect Control Hosp Epidemiol. 2014;35:1411–3.
101. Snyder GM, Thokm KA, Furuno JP, et al. Detection of methicillin-resistant *Staphylococcus aureus* and vancomycin-resistant enterococci by healthcare workers on infection control gown and gloves. Infect Control Hosp Epidemiol. 2008;29:583–9.
102. Loveday HP, Lynam S, Singleton J, Wilson J. Clinical glove use, healthcare workers' actions and perceptions. J Hosp Infect. 2014;86:110–6.

103. Mitchell A, Spencer M, Edminston JRC. Role of healthcare apparel and other healthcare textiles in the transmission of pathogens: a review of the literature. J Hosp Infect. 2015;90:285–92.
104. Legrand J Temime L, Lawrence C, et al. Occupational determination of methicillin-resistant *Staphylococcus aureus* colonization among healthcare workers. A longitudinal study in a rehabilitation center. Infect Control Hosp Epidemiol. 2015;36:767–76.
105. Kjølen H, Andersen BM. Handwashing and disinfection of heavily contaminated hands-effective or ineffective? J Hosp Infect. 1992;21:61–71.
106. Andersen BM, Rasch M. When normal hand washing is not sufficient. Tidsskr Nursing. 2001;11:52–7.

Vancomycin-Resistant Enterococci Prevention

50

Abstract

Multidrug-resistant enterococci are selected by antibiotics, combined with lack of hygiene and infectious barriers and promoted by infected patients and carriers. The most common and serious types today are vancomycin-resistant enterococci, VRE, most commonly associated with *Enterococcus faecium*. From a few imported cases each year, VRE has become a large global problem in healthcare institutions. VRE is more than conventionally resistant against antibiotics and disinfectants and can withstand high temperatures encapsulated in biological material. Some types may be harder to control than the other, can cause more problems and have a very long environmental survival—up to 4 years. The infection is transmitted via direct and indirect contact, via faecal oral infection, via equipment, environment and textiles and occasionally via air. Everyone should be protected against infection with VRE since it is a highly preventable infectious disease. The following chapter is focused on practical measures to detect and prevent transmission of VRE in healthcare institutions.

Keywords

VRE · Vancomycin-resistant enterococci · *Enterococcus faecium* · Imported from abroad · Admission control · Pre-examination · Information · Screening · Isolation PPE · Decontamination of environment · Eradication · Nosocomial infections Infection control · Hygiene · Prevention

50.1 Purpose

To prevent transmission of VRE between patients, staff, visitors, equipment, textiles and the environment [1–9]. In accordance with international and national laws and guidelines, neither patients nor personnel shall be subjected to unnecessary risk of infection with resistant and potentially dangerous bacteria such as VRE [1, 6, 7, 10–24].

B. M. Andersen, *Prevention and Control of Infections in Hospitals*, https://doi.org/10.1007/978-3-319-99921-0_50

50.2 Comprise

All close contacts of patients (patients in the same room, personnel, visitors, etc.) and all patient-related equipment, textiles, waste, etc.

50.3 Responsibility

The hospital's management is ensuring appropriate testing, isolation, control and treatment of patients with suspected/detected VRE infection.

The department's management has overall responsibility for the follow-up of routines and to report to the Director if preventive routines are not followed up, such as lack of isolation, contaminated equipment, lack of expertise and personnel and the like [1, 8, 9].

Employees are responsible for following the department's routines in suspected VRE infection.

Information. Medical doctor or other healthcare provider/home care/hospital department/other healthcare institution is obliged to report known or suspected/exposed VRE (current or previously proven) to the recipient and to others who are going to treat/investigate the patient.

50.4 Practical Measures

Note: The treatment facilities (investigation, care) should not be weakened if infected with VRE.

Preliminary examination. Ask the patient, relatives or referring physician *before* admission/check, etc. if the patient has been infected or exposed to VRE [1, 6, 8].

If detected infection/exposed to infection, there are at least two possibilities: (a) wait for admission/treatment until the infection status is cleared; (b) isolate and treat the patient as infectious until infection status has been clarified.

50.4.1 The VRE-Infected Patient Is Isolated as for MRSA-Positive Patients

- Isolate as contact infection in a single room—immediately.
- Wear protective clothing, gloves and surgical mask/cap. Room-bound shoes or shoe covers are recommended. Learn to take on and off personal protective equipment (PPE).

50.4.2 Screening for VRE

- All import patients, patients who have been hospitalized/treated in the health service abroad for the last 12 months [1, 6, 8, 9, 12].
- All patients who have been admitted/treated at healthcare institution with ongoing VRE outbreaks for the last 12 months.
- All patients who have been exposed to VRE infection, i.e. been in the same room and/or used the same equipment as a VRE-infected person.
- Faeces test or perineal swab test.
- Rapid test for VRE is recommended.
- Inform the laboratory and ask for a telephone answer.
- For more quicker answer, do not send the sample by mail!

50.4.3 Proven VRE-Infected Patient

The VRE patient is isolated and treated as MRSA-positive patients [1, 6, 8, 9].

- If several cases of VRE in the ward, evaluate intake of new patients (like MRSA), and test all patients.
- Inform all healthcare institutions and departments that have been in contact with the patient.
- Avoid transport/transfer of VRE-positive patients between wards/departments/ institutions.
- *Flagging and control.* VRE-positive patients should be isolated and checked for VRE when readmitted to health institutions.
- *The journal is labelled* VRE under critical information.
- *Cohort in a separate unit* with own services; store rooms for textiles and equipment, which are only used by the unit. A separate competent personnel should be attached to the unit and not participate in care/treatment elsewhere. Do *not* mix VRE-positive patients with MRSA-positive patients!
- Ready-treated patients (for basic disease) can be transferred to the home if patient/relatives, home care and primary healthcare services are well-informed about infection prevention and enhanced environmental hygiene.

50.4.4 VRE-Exposed Patients

- Patients exposed to infection are tested and isolated separately (as for MRSA).
- Isolated in single room with own toilet/shower until infection has been clarified.
- Declared as not infected if four consecutive rectal samples/faeces (+ clinical samples) taken on separate days are negative in a patient who has not been on

antibiotics for the past 14 days and has previously not been VRE-positive. If these samples are negative, there is little risk of infection.
- In uncertain and persistent exposure to infection in the ward, implement control specimens for exposed patients every 14 days to once per month for 6 months.

50.4.5 Other Patients at the Ward with Outbreak of VRE

- Other patients at the department may be exposed to infection if they are taken care of by the same VRE-exposed personnel, common service room, living room, kitchen, serving, etc. When submitting clinical samples to the laboratory, mark them with "VRE". Evaluate testing of all in-patient patients and contact infection control personnel.
- Non-infected patients in the department must be protected from infection by VRE-exposed employees by being treated with "protective isolation"; use surgical mask/cap, gloves and gown during the period of the outbreak (see MRSA).

50.4.6 Large Outbreaks

- Close the ward for new admissions until tracing is finished and the measures are organized.
- Divide the ward into three units:
  - Isolation unit for all VRE-positive patients.
  - Isolation unit for all VRE-exposed patients.
  - Unit for patients who are not/have not been exposed to VRE infection.

Staff are informed about infection, but not tested:

- Employees are informed of infection protection, PPE and good hand hygiene and must comply strictly with the prescribed isolation measures.
- Personnel working on a VRE-infected unit with direct patient care do not participate in serving of food, cleaning or other common service work.
- Personnel shall not work in other units while working in a VRE device. If necessary, inform the department manager/infection control personnel.
- Employees are not tested for VRE infection and may therefore be spreaders in the environment.
- In case of repeated outbreaks associated with some of the staff, testing may be applicable. This must be discussed with the infection control doctor/the hospital's medical officer since there are no good routines for sanitation/disinfection of VRE, as the bacterium is part of normal intestinal flora [1, 13, 18–20].

50.4.7 Environmental Sanitation and Eradication Is Important!

- VRE is resistant to several disinfectants and to heat. Dishwashers and decontaminators must have a temperature above 85 °C!
- *Extra daily disinfection and cleaning* of floors and surfaces in the patient's room is carried out. In addition, all contact points are treated with alcoholic wipes three times/day. As a disinfectant use 5% chloramine or peracetic acid or other chemical that has proven effect on VRE. Virkon may have an uncertain effect. All cleaning equipment must be treated as contaminated and treated in a decontaminator. VRE can survive in the environment for 3–4 years if not removed well enough [1, 2, 25].
- *Final disinfection* after termination of stay is carried out with thorough decontamination of the rooms the patient has used. Optionally, hydrogen peroxide gas can be used in rooms with a lot of equipment, followed by good disinfection of all surfaces.
- Disinfect all rooms where the patient has stayed before infection was detected!
- Cleaners must follow routines for using PPE equipment: surgical mask/cap, gloves, gown, room-bound shoes/shoe covers—learn taking on and off PPE! See routines for MRSA!
- Final disinfection is also assessed at other parts of the department since employees are not tested.

50.4.8 Control

- Antibiotics and type of antibiotics should be checked on units where VRE occurs. Reduce the use of third-generation cephalosporins, carbapenems and other broad spectrums, as well as metronidazole. Do not use vancomycin and similar preparations, if unnecessary. Contact infection medicine physician/infection control doctor for advice.
- Workload and patient care ratio are known risk factors and must be checked where VRE occurs [1].
- Update personnel with regard to hand hygiene and infection protection, isolation measures and treatment of infectious waste/equipment/clothing, etc.

50.4.9 Transport and Transfers

- For examinations, treatment etc. elsewhere, message about VRE is sent in advance to the recipient. The patient arrives in a clean bed with clean clothes and a surgical mask is used if there is cough. The recipient treats the patient as contact precaution (see above) and with decontamination of the room afterwards.

- When transferring between healthcare levels, healthcare personnel must be informed in advance of infection status. This includes ambulance transport.
- The patient and possibly relatives are informed of the duty to provide information in the health service.
- Visitors/relatives follow the infection protection regime of the institution and do not use the hospital's common rooms.

50.4.10 Follow-Up of VRE-Infected Patient

Prolonged condition and carrier state are usually not disinfected! Negative faeces in between positive findings is natural, also after attempting disinfection [26–28]. A carrier period of at least 45–50 days is common (median 42 days), and it may last for almost 2 years with relapses [1, 26–28]. Reinfection in a contaminated home environment or patient room, etc. cannot be excluded since the bacterium survives for many years in the environment [25]. Therefore, environmental sanitation and eradication is very important. In the case of new antibiotic cures, such strains are most often selected in the faeces. Chronic carrier state may be relevant.

- In the case of proven VRE, four consecutive test sets taken at 1-week intervals shall be negative before the person is defined as *low VRE risk.* Prerequisite is that the sampling starts at least 14 days after the end of the use of antibacterial agents (and at least 10 days after completion of disinfection if this is completed).
- *After four consecutive negative VRE samples,* follow-up of the patient is started for 1 year to ensure that the infection disappears. Initially, samples are often taken to prevent spread of infection to patients, personnel and the environment. If at least 20 consecutive tests are negative during 1 year and no positive tests in between, the patient is considered to be a noncarrier of VRE.

50.4.11 Important Information

If there has been a significant spread of infection in the environment of a department, repeated patient checks may occur, in addition to common routines.

In long-term institutions such as nursing homes, VRE can spread a large extent if no special measures are taken over time. See special measures for infection monitoring of VRE-positive patients at long-term institutions [8].

50.5 Background Information

Antibiotics, combined with lack of hygiene and infectious barriers and infected patients, promote selection of multidrug-resistant enterococci [1, 2]. The most common and serious type today is vancomycin-resistant enterococci (VRE), especially *Enterococcus faecium* [1, 2]. From a few imported cases each year, VRE has become a problem at health institutions all over the world, including Scandinavia [1–9].

- In accordance with international and national laws and guidelines, neither patients nor personnel shall be subjected to unnecessary risk of infection with resistant and potentially dangerous bacteria such as VRE [1, 6, 7, 10–24].
- *The infection is* transmitted via direct and indirect contact, faecal-oral infection, via equipment, environment and textiles and occasionally via air [1, 7].
- Enterococci are normal skin and intestinal bacteria in humans and rarely cause infections in healthy subjects [1]. They are very robust, long-term survivors, up to 4 years in the environment—on bedside tables, bedside borders and other contact points—and they are naturally resistant to a variety of common antibiotics, chemicals and heat treatment [1, 2, 25].
- Enterococci in the intestine have been able to absorb and give rise to different resistance genes/signals to other bacteria. High consumption of antimicrobial agents leads to the selection and development of special antibiotic-resistant enterococci like VRE [1]. VRE can at the same time be resistant to ampicillin and gentamicin, which reduces treatment options [29].
- Clinical VRE infection is particularly related to urinary tract infections, sepsis, endocarditis and postoperative wound infection—especially in the abdominal region—in elderly long-term patients with kidney disease, haematological disease or cancerous diseases [1, 2, 30, 31].
- As in most other countries in Europe, VRE is an increasing problem in Norwegian health institutions and in home nursing care [1, 8]. Therefore, the measures to prevent spread of infection are extra strict here [8]. There is no search for VRE outside the healthcare service. VRE poses no risk to healthy persons and usually low risk to patients with normal infection defences.

50.5.1 Occurrence, Costs and Mortality

VRE was first detected in Europe in the 1980s in connection with the use of a vancomycin-like growth enhancer, avoparcin, in chicken feed, which was then banned around 1995 in Norway and in 1997 in Europe [1, 30–34]. Some years later, VRE-positive patients were detected in hospitals in the United States, linked to a high consumption of vancomycin in patients with *Clostridium difficile* infections and to lack of isolation measures around such patients [1, 30, 31].

For the last 10–15 years, VRE has caused increasing problems for a large number of patients in the United States, Europe and the rest of the world, especially related to hospital outbreaks and outbreaks in long-term institutions [1, 4, 7, 24, 29–31, 34–41].

In Sweden and Denmark, VRE has had a dramatic increase in patients, with a high environmental pollution of VRE in animal production (chicken, pigs) and in sewage, in the last 5–10 years [24, 29, 35–39]. The same increase is observed in Germany, England, Ireland and a number of other countries (see Fig. 50.1, source: ECDC) [35, 42]. In Sweden, the outbreak started in 2007, and in Denmark there was an increase among hospital patients registered in 2010 [29].

In Norway, VRE was until 2010 largely an imported infection with 0–8 cases annually [3]. In 2010, a VRE (vanB) hospital outbreak started at Haukeland

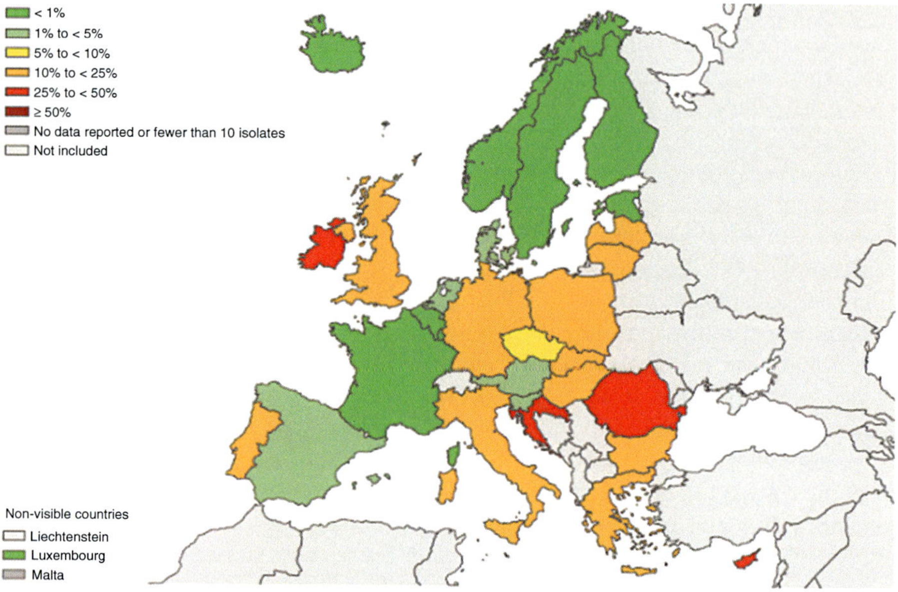

Fig. 50.1 Percentage (%) of invasive *Enterococcus faecium* isolates resistant to vancomycin, by country, EU/EEA countries, 2015. *Source: ECDC, January 2017* [35]

University Hospital, Bergen, with more than 150 cases [4, 5]. The same type had been registered a few years earlier. From 2011 on, there have been several minor outbreaks of VRE (vanA) at hospitals and nursing homes in Eastern Norway and in Central Norway [7, 9, 34].

Food industry has the control. A significant problem today is that food manufacturers and government authorities do not stop the development of severe antibacterial resistance in food and animal production. From 1994 on, the regular control of all food and drink done by Norwegian Food Safety Authority was shut down. Instead the food industry itself took over the control, which led to a reckless profit in the food industry, strongly linked to the unjustifiable consumption of growth-stimulated substances with antimicrobial effects [43, 44].

Mortality. The combination of VRE- and ESBL-producing *Enterobacteriaceae* in the intestine in patients with haematological and other cancer diseases is associated with sepsis and increased mortality with these agents, and therefore faeces screening is recommended for such patients [45]. Multidrug-resistant enterococci is also a serious risk of surgery [46]. A study of end-stage renal failure did not show increased mortality associated with VRE, but extended admission time [47]. Compared to vancomycin-sensitive enterococci, VRE has about twice as high mortality [1, 30].

Costs generated by VRE infection (prolonged stay in hospital, isolation, medication, etc.) are high, and most measures that reduce spread of infection are cost-effective [1, 30, 31, 48, 49].

50.5.2 Infection Risk

Transmission of VRE occurs mainly through direct and indirect contact, faecal-oral infections (foods, hands, etc.), via equipment, textiles, uniform and occasionally via air; by re-aerosols from treatment, examination and care and by cleaning. The environment contamination is widespread and lasting and is a risk to fellow patients if not removed [1, 25, 27, 28, 50–54].

VRE is a threat to nursing homes and long-term institutions due to lack of isolation and lack of competent healthcare personnel, combined with unusually robust and resistant bacteria with long survival in the environment. Long-term problems in some countries are an increase in patients that are at the same time infected with a mixture of multidrug-resistant bacteria, such as VRE, MRSA, *C. difficile*, ESBL and/or multidrug-resistant gram-negative rod bacteria and which eventually develop combined "worst-case microbes" like vancomycin-resistant MRSA during major antibiotic pressure [26, 35, 45, 55–58].

Patient groups who often have infections and use a lot of antibiotics that affect the intestinal flora for long periods are prone to infections/carrier state with more resistant bacteria, such as VRE [1]. Single room with own toilet and bath and good environmental hygiene around patients who use a lot of antibiotics will generally reduce the spread of resistant microbes.

Patients from abroad are more likely to be infected/colonized with VRE and other resistant bacteria.

Clostridium difficile infections treated with vancomycin are associated with the risk of developing VRE [1, 21, 22, 26, 30, 31].

In endemic areas for VRE, risk is particularly related to haemodialysis patients, elderly patients and MRSA-infected patients during the last year, admitted to long-term institutions and admittance to the hospital during the past year [30].

50.5.3 Control Over VRE: Isolation and Testing

VRE is a preventable infectious disease if recommendations are followed [1, 6, 8, 15, 21–24]. CDC recommended in its isolation guide of VRE (1994) contact isolation, training in infection protection, enhanced hand hygiene, screening for VRE and careful use of certain types of antibiotics [21–23]. Now it also generally recommended isolation and screening on *suspicion* of VRE (pre-emptive contact isolation), i.e. high-risk cases such as patients from the health service abroad last 12 months, previous VRE-positive patients or patients exposed to VRE infection [1, 6, 8, 21–23, 30, 31, 41, 48]. Nevertheless, there has been a global spread of VRE over many years, and the guidelines are often not followed [59].

50.5.3.1 Contact Isolation (Contact Precaution, CP): Not Effective Enough

In highly endemic areas where 3–10% of hospitalized patients are infected/carriers with VRE, the use of CP (gloves, gown and isolate/single room) is discussed—if it has any protective effect against the spread of VRE in hospitals [30, 31, 60–63]. Many studies are inadequate with regard to documentation and isolation conditions or have low compliance with the use of hand hygiene and personal protection equipment, etc. [31, 60]. Examples of some studies are shown below.

- About 26,200 patients at 20 ICUs in the United States were tested for MRSA and VRE during arrival and discharge during a period of 10 months [61]. The control group of patients was contact- isolated using CP (gloves and gown) if detected infection (MRSA or VRE), according to recommendations from CDC [23]. All patients in the intervention group were universally contact-isolated with CP, regardless of infection status. Both in the control and intervention group, a non-significant reduction of MRSA or VRE infections while the patients were in the department were recorded [61]. For MRSA alone, there was a significant but low effect, while for VRE infection separately, there was no difference in effect between the two groups. However, the general CP routine (intervention) for all patients led to fewer visits to the patient's room, increased compliance with hand hygiene when leaving the room and no significant adverse effects on the patients [61].
- Another American study demonstrated high transmission of VRE infection among patients admitted to a medical intensive care unit, and no effect of CP isolation [62]. Patient samples were taken upon admission, while in-patient and at the discharge. During a 3-month phase, VRE-positive patients became CP-isolated (CDC) [23, 62]. During the next 3-month phase, all patients were treated with only general glove use and no isolation. During the stay in ICU, 18% (35/192) were VRE infected in phase one using CP, against 0.5% (1/192) when admitted. In phase two, with glove use on all patients, 14% (35/257) were infected, against 0/257 when admitted! [62]. It was concluded that the use of only gloves for all patients in the ICU gave the same result as CP isolation of patients with proven infection [62]. Isolation procedures were not effective enough.
- Two ICU groups of a total of approximately 9000 patients were compared [63]. The intervention group were using CP isolation in all patients with proven VRE/MRSA and universal glove use for contact with all other patients, as well as rapid information on test results upon admission [63]. The control group used CP isolation for known infections of MRSA and VRE; they were also tested at admittance, but no response was given on the result to the ward. There was no difference between the two groups—both with CP in their "arm". However, there was a low compliance with the use of CP. The proportion infected was approximately the same upon entry as at discharge, in contrary to the former study [62, 63].

50.5.3.2 Rapid Control in Case of Minor Outbreaks and Intensive Measures

- Lucet et al. describe a VRE outbreak in Paris in 2007, with a total of 39 VRE cases before the outbreak stopped after 4 weeks [64]. The index patient had urinary tract infections with VRE and infected fellow patient in the same room. Screening was carried out, and two new cases were found, and after a new screening round of the department, three new cases were discovered. The index patient had moved to another ward before VRE findings were known, and there he infected three new patients. All patients were isolated, the staff were informed and trained in infection control and tracing and a screening program was followed up over time for high-risk units, defined as intensive medicine, renal medicine, haemodialysis, rehabilitation and infection units [64]. A separate cohort unit for patients with VRE was established, with own personnel and equipment and with environmental disinfection twice a day. VRE patients were followed up when readmitted. It was recommended to avoid the use of third-generation cephalosporins, glycopeptides and amoxicillin—clavulanic acid, imipenem, piperacillin-tazobactam and metronidazole [64]. Readmitted VRE carriers (flagged out) were CP-isolated until three rectal samples at 1 week interval were negative [64].

- An outbreak at Ullevål University Hospital, spring 2011, included 13 VRE cases in an open haemodialysis department that had 70 patients for dialysis treatment on 22 treatment sites [9]. The index patient had been admitted to all four hospitals in Oslo (OUS), had received a lot of antibiotics over time and was known as VRE-positive. Because of some misunderstanding, the person was not isolated during dialysis treatments and divided dialysis site with a number of other patients who eventually became infected. The ward was run down and heavily overcrowded [9]. The outbreak stopped within 1 month after the infection was detected, using strict isolation of infected carriers (PPE: gloves, gown, surgical mask/cap), as well as general use of gown, gloves and surgical mask/cap on contact with all other patients. There was no intake of new patients, but all 70 previous patients were still treated by the unit under strict hygiene measures. No more cases were registered than the 13, and 1 year later, all were negative [9].

50.5.3.3 Contact- and Airborne Isolation as by MRSA Is Recommended

Contact isolation for VRE has not led to effective infection control in endemic VRE infection, although most studies are inadequate [33, 31, 60–63].Therefore, these patients should be isolated as MRSA by contact- and airborne isolation and with strict enhanced environmental hygiene [1, 2, 8, 9, 64, 65].

50.5.3.4 Testing for VRE

Routine testing for VRE has been discussed and is recommended today for risk patients while personnel should usually not be tested [7–9, 48, 64, 66, 67].

50.5.4 Spread of VRE Via Personnel/Visitors/Attendees, Equipment, Textiles and Environment

VRE is more than conventional resistant against antibiotics, disinfectants (chloramine 5% and peracetic acid have good effects) and against heat (usually killed after a certain treatment time above 85 °C but can withstand higher temperatures encapsulated in biological material) [1]. Some VRE types may be harder to control than others. Vancomycin-*resistant Enterococcus faecium* can cause more problems than *E. faecalis*, associated with a very long environmental survival of *E. faecium* for 4 years [25, 40].

VRE is like other bacteria in the intestine, does usually not give disease in a healthy person but survives in the intestine for a long time and easily reaches the skin and hands. Infection is transmitted primarily by contact. This means that the infection is transmitted through unclean hands or that an infected patient has "left" the bacterium on items like washing, toilet, door handles or the like. Equipment such as BT apparatus, stethoscope and the like are prone to infection unless routine infection is performed between patients.

Carriers of the bacterium usually have no symptoms and should not be treated with antibiotics. Some sanitation attempts have been done, including the use of Bacitracin 30,000 IU three times for 15 days or whole body wash with chlorhexidine [68, 69]. Studies of 82 VRE carriers showed a carrier period of median 42 days, maximum measured was 708 days [28]. Antibiotics are only given to patients with clinical VRE infection, which occurs relatively rarely. There are a number of good antimicrobial medicaments that can be used if there should be a clinical infection.

Hygiene and environmental control provide good protection against infection [70]. Good cleaning and disinfection of rooms, surfaces and equipment can stop the spread of infections [70]. There is, however, a high risk of transmission to fellow patients, even after apparently good disinfection and cleaning before the next patient [30]. The more colonized by VRE, the more environmental contamination and infection pressure; especially in faecal incontinence and when using certain types of antibiotics [30, 70–72]. Good environmental sanitation and routine disinfection of equipment such as stethoscopes, blood pressure devices, etc., lead to a significant decrease in VRE in endemic areas [30, 53, 54, 70]. Therefore, environmental sanitation is a core area for measures against VRE infection [30, 53, 54, 70, 73–75].

Transport, patient relocation, overcrowding, many patients on same room, etc. are known factors that increase the risk of cross contamination and spread of infections [9]. Information is important when moving patient with VRE.

Workload and too high patient-nurse ratio are very well-known risk factors. Excessive activity often leads to a breach of hygiene barriers; patients get infections, then they receive antibiotics for infections, then they spread to others because of infectious barriers are breached, then workload increases on employees, then more patients are infected and must be isolated, etc., and the activity is stopped up.

Healthcare personnel are prone to be contaminated via hands and uniforms, other textiles and equipment [30]. VRE is found on both gloves and gown in larger or smaller numbers after treatment of VRE-infected patients [76–84]. Although hand hygiene is not always 100% effective [83, 84], employee should constantly be encouraged to and given time to this important procedure in all work with patients.

References

1. Andersen BM. Enterokokker. Håndbok i hygiene og smittevern for sykehus. Del 1: Mikrobiologi og smittevern. Fagbokforlaget. 2014. p. 59–64.
2. Andersen BM. Enterococcus. I: Bakterier og sykdom. Epidemiologi, infeksjoner og smittevern. Gyldendal Akademisk. 2005. p. 157–171.
3. Simonsen GS, Andersen BM, Digranes A, et al. Low fecal carrier rate of vancomycin resistant enterococci in Norwegian hospital patients. Scand J Infect Dis. 1998;30:465–8.

4. Oma D, Stenhaug Kilhus K. Pågående utbrudd av vankomycinresistente enterokokker ved Haukeland Universitetssjukehus. 2010, fhi.no. Oppdatert 14.2.2012.
5. Nasjonalt Folkehelseinstitutt. Haukeland Universitetssjukehus; Pågående utbrudd av vankomycinresistente enterokokker (VRE); en oppdatering og råd om screening av pasienter. FHI. no. 09.06.2011.
6. Nasjonalt Folkehelseinstitutt. Nasjonal anbefaling: Håndtering av vankomycinresistente enterokokker (VRE) ved norske sykehus og sykehjem. 25.8.2011. fhi.no.
7. Nasjonalt Folkehelseinstitutt. Oppdatering om forekomst av vankomycinresistente enterokokker (VRE) i Norge. Fhi.no. 12.06.2012.
8. Andersen B. Enterokokker resistente mot vankomycin – VRE. Håndbok i hygiene og smittevern. Sykehjem og langtidsinstitusjoner. Oslo: Akademika forlag; 2013. p. 281–98.
9. Andersen BM, Seljordslia B, Hochlin K, Rasch M, Syversen G. A predicted outbreak in an overcrowded, administratively neglected and run-down haemodialysis unit as an offer of «New Public Management» in Norwegian hospitals. J Hosp Admin. 2013;2:15–24.
10. Lov om vern mot smittsomme sykdommer av 5. august 1994 nr. 55.
11. Forskrift om smittevern i helsetjenesten. Fastsatt ved kgl. Res. 17. juni 2005 med hjemmel i lov 5. august 1994 nr. 55 om vern mot smittsomme sykdommer §§ 4–7, 7–11, lov 19. november 1982 nr.66 om helsetjenesten i kommunene §1–3 femte ledd, lov 2.juli 1999 nr. 61 om spesialisthelsetjenesten med mer § 2-1a femte ledd og lov 18.mai 2001 nr. 24 om helseregistre og behandling av helseopplysninger § 6 tredje ledd. Fremmet av Helse- og omsorgsdepartementet.
12. Statens helsetilsyn. Råd for anvendelse av smittevernloven § 3–3 forhåndsundersøkelse av pasienter – smittsomme sykdommer. IK-28/96. *Statens helsetilsyn*, Oslo: 1996.
13. Forskrift om forhåndsundersøkelse av arbeidstakere innen helsevesenet antibiotikaresistente bakterier. Fastsatt av Sosial- og helsedepartementet 5 juli 1996 med hjemmel i lov av 5. august 1994 nr 15 om vern mot smittsomme sykdommer § 3–2. FOR 1996-07-05 nr 700.
14. Sykehusloven §18A-sykehusinfeksjoner som betydelig skade på pasient. Oslo: *Statens helsetilsyn,* mars 2000.
15. Helsedirektoratets veiledningsserie: Bruk av isolering til å forebygge smittespredning i sykehus. *Helsedirektoratet,* Oslo: 2–88, 1988.
16. Isolasjonsveilederen. *Sosial- og helsedepartementet* 2003.
17. Tiltak for å motvirke antibiotika resistens (2000–2004). Sosial- og helsedepartementet. 2000.
18. Helsepersonelloven. Sosial og helsedepartementet. Lov 1999-07-02 nr 64: Lov om helsepersonell. 2001.
19. Arbeidstilsynet. Forskrift om vern mot eksponering for biologiske faktorer (bakterier, virus, sopp med mer) på arbeidsplassen, av 19 desember 1997.
20. Europaparlamentets- og Rådsdirektivet 2000/54/EF av 18 september 2000 om vern av arbeidstakerne mot fare ved å være utsatt for biologiske agenser på arbeidsplassen.
21. CDC Management of multidrug-resistant organisms in healthcare settings, 2006. CDC. 2006. p. 1–72.
22. CDC. Prevention of transmission of multidrug resistant organisms 2009. CDC 2009.
23. Siegel JD, Rhinehart E, Jacksom M, et al. 2007 Guideline for isolation precautions: preventing transmission of infectious agents in healthcare settings. CDC. 2007.
24. Smittskyddsinstitutet. Vården kan minimera spridningen av VRE. SMI, Sweden. 2011.
25. Wagenvoort JHT, De Brauwer EIGB, Penders RJR, Willems RJ, Top J, Bonten MJ. Environmental survival of vancomycin-resistant *Enterococcus faecium*. J Hosp Infect. 2011;77:274–83.
26. Garbutt JM, Littenberg B, Evanoff BA, Sahm D, Mundy LM. Enteric carriage of vancomycin-resistant *Enterococcus faecium* in patients tested for *Clostridium difficile*. Infect Control Hosp Epidemiol. 1999;20:664–70.
27. Lee WG, Park IJ, Jin HY, Park MH. Relapse and reacquisition of rectal colonization by vancomycin-resistasnt *Enterococcus faecium* after decolonization. Epidemiol Infect. 2010;138:1449–53.
28. Henard S, Lozniewski A, Aissa N, Jouzeau N, Rabaud C. Evaluation of the duration of *van*A vancomycin-resistant *Enterococcus faecium* carriage and clearance during a large-scale outbreak in a region of eastern France. Am J Infect Control. 2011;39:169–71.

29. Viden om vancomycin-resistente enterokokker. *Statens Seruminstitut*, Danmark, 17 mars 2015.
30. Tacconelli E, Cataldo MA. Vancomycin-resistant enterococci (VRE): transmission and control. Int J Antimicrob Agents. 2008;31:99–106.
31. De Angelis G, Cataldo MA, De Waure C, et al. Infection control and prevention measures to reduce the spread of vancomycin-resistant enterococci in hospitalized patients: a systematic review and meta-analysis. J Antimicrob Chemother. 2014;69:1185–92.
32. Borgen K, Simonsen GS, Sundsfjord A, Wasteson Y, Olsvik Ø, Kruse H. Continuing high prevalence of vanA-type vancomycin-resistant enterococci on Norwegian poultry farms three years after avoparcin was banned. J Appl Microbiol. 2000;89:478–85.
33. Kruse H, Johansen BK, Rørvik LM, Schaller G. The use of avoparcin as a growth promotor and the occurrence of vancomycin-resistant *Enterococcus* species in Norwegian poultry and swine production. Microb Drug Resist. 1999;5:135–9.
34. Anonymous. Human clinical isolates. Is the epidemiology of vancomycin resistant enterococci in Norway changing? NORM/NORM-VET 2013. p. 79.
35. ECDC. Surveillance report 2017. Antimicrobial resistance surveillance in Europe. 2015.
36. Schouten MA, Hoogkamp-Korstanje JAA, Meis JFG, Voss A, et al. Prevalence of vancomycin resistant enterococci in Europe. Eur J Clin Microbiol Infect Dis. 2000;19:816–22.
37. Sahlstrøm L, Rehbinder V, Albhin A, Aspan A, Bengtsson B. Vancomycin resistant enterococci (VRE) in Swedish sewage sludge. Acta Vet Scand. 2009;51:24.
38. Søderblom T, Aspevall O, Erntell M, et al. Alarming spread of vancomycin resistant enterococci in Sweden since 2007. Euro Surveill. 2010;15 pii: 19620
39. Nilsson O. Vancomycin resistant enterococi in farm animals – occurrence and importance. Infect Ecol Epidemiol. 2012;2:16959.
40. Pereira GH, Muller PR, Zanella RC, et al. Outbreak of vancomycin-resistant enterococci in a tertiary hospital: the lack of effect of measures directed mainly by surveillance cultures and differences in response between *Enterococcus faecium* and *Enterococcus faecalis*. Am J Infect Control. 2010;38:406–9.
41. Pearman JW. 2004 Lowbury lecture: the Western Australian experience with vancomycin-resistant enterococci- from disaster to ongoing control. J Hosp Infect. 2006;63:14–26.
42. Gastmeier P, Schrøder C, Behnke M, Meyer E, Geffers C. Dramatic increase in vancomycin-resistant enterococci in Germany. J Antimicrob Chemother. 2014;69:1660–4.
43. Andersen BM. Matsmitte er et forsømt problem. Næringsmiddelkontrollen i Norge er så dårlig at det kan gå ut over helsen vår. *Aftenposten Viten* 28 oktober 2014. og ap.no/viten.
44. Midtvedt T. Bekymringsmelding om antibiotika i kyllingfor. Tidsskr Nor Legeforen. 2015;135:742.
45. Liss BJ, Vereschild JJ, Cornely OA, et al. Intestinal colonisation and blood stream infections due to vancomycin-resistant enterococci (VRE) and extended-spectrum beta-lactamase-producing *Enterobacteriaceae* (ESBLE) in patients with haematological and oncological malignancies. Infection. 2012;40:613–9.
46. Low DE, Willey BM, McGeer AJ. Multidrug-resistant enterococci: a threat to the surgical patient. Am J Surg. 1995;169:8–12.
47. Garner SE, Polkinghorne KR, Kotsanas D, Kerr PG, Korman TM, Stuart RL. Vancomycin-resistant enterococi colonization does not increase mortality in end-stage kidney failure: a case-control study. J Hosp Infect. 2013;85:289–96.
48. Mayhall CG. Control of vancomycin-resistant enterococci: it is important, it is possible, and it is cost-effective. Infect Control Hosp Epidemiol. 2002;23:420–3.
49. Song X, Srinivasan A, Plaut D, Perl TM. Effect of nosocomial vancomycin-resistant enterococcal bacteremia on mortality, length of stay, and costs. Infect Control Hosp Epidemiol. 2003;24:251–6.
50. Hamel M, Zoutman D, O'Callaghan C. Exposure to hospital roommates as a risk factor for health care-associated infection. Am J Infect Control. 2010;38:173–81.
51. Bonilla HF, Zervos MJ, Kauffman CA. Long-term survival of vancomycin-resistant *Enterococcus faecium* on a contaminated surface. Infect Control Hosp Epidemiol. 1996;17:770–1.
52. Noskin GA, Stosor V, Cooper I, Peterson LR. Recovery of vancomycin-resistant enterococci on fingertips and environmental surfaces. Infect Control Hosp Epidemiol. 1995;16:577–81.

53. Knelson LP, Williams DA, Gergen MF, et al. A comparison of environmental contamination by patients infected or colonized with methicillin-resistant *Staphylococcus aureus* or vancomycin-resistant enterococci: a multicenter study. Infect Control Hosp Epidemiol. 2014;35:872–5.
54. Perugini MRE, Nomi SM, Lopes GK, et al. Impact of the reduction of environmental and equipment contamination on vancomycin-resistant enterococcus rates. Infection. 2011;39:587–93.
55. Johnston BL, Bryce E. Hospital infecton control strategies for vancomycin-resistant *Enterococcus,* methicillin-resistant *Staphylococcus aureus* and *Clostridium difficile*. Can Med Assoc J. 2009;180:627–31.
56. Hayakawa K, Marchaim D, Vidaillac C, Lephart P, et al. Growing prevalence of vancomycin-resistant *Enterococcus faecalis* in the region with the highest prevalence of vancomycin-resistant *Staphylococcus aureus*. Infect Control Hosp Epidemiol. 2011;32:922–4.
57. Rossi F, Diaz L, Wollam A, et al. Transferable vancomycin resistance in a community-associated MRSA lineage. N Engl J Med. 2014;370:1524–31.
58. McKinnell JA, Kunz DF, Chamot E, et al. Association between vancomycin-resistant enterococci bacteremia and ceftriaxone usage. Infect Control Hosp Epidemiol. 2012;33:718–24.
59. Willems RJL, Top J, van Santen M, et al. Global spread of vancomycin-resistant *Enterococcus faecium* from distinct nosocomial genetic complex. Emerg Infect Dis. 2005;11:821–8.
60. Morgan DJ, Murthy R, Munoz-Price LS, et al. Reconsidering contact precautions for endemic methicillin-resistant *Staphylococcus aureus* and vancomycin-resistant *Enterococcus*. Infecty Control Hosp Epidemiol. 2015;36:1163–72.
61. Harris AD, Pineles L, Belton B, et al. Universal glove use and acquisition of antibiotic-resistant bacterial in the ICU. A randomized trial. JAMA. 2013;310:1571–80.
62. Bearman GML, Marra AR, Sessler CN, et al. A controlled trial of universal gloving versus contact precautions for preventing the transmission of multidrug-resistant organisms. Am J Infect Control. 2007;35:650–5.
63. Huskins WC, Huckabee CM, O'Grady NP, et al. Intervention to reduce transmission of resistant bacteria in intensive care. N Engl J Med. 2011;364:1407–18.
64. Lucet J-C, Armand-Lefevre L, Laurichesse JJ, et al. Rapid control of an outbreak of vancomycin-resistant enterococci in a French university hospital. J Hosp Infect. 2007;67:42–8.
65. Andersen BM. Luftsmitteisolasjon. Håndbok i hygiene og smittevern for sykehus. 2008. p. 234–9.
66. Humphreys H. Controlling the spread of vancomycin-resistant enterococci. Is active screening worthwhile? J Hosp Infect. 2014;88:191–8.
67. Gosh A, Jiao L, Al-Mutawa F, et al. Value of active surveillance policy to document clearance of methicillin-resistant *Staphyloccoccus aureus* and vancomycin-resistant enterococci amongst inpatients with prolonged admissions. J Hosp Infect. 2014;88:230–3.
68. Brossier F, Lefrancois S, Paute J, et al. Decolonisation for early control of an outbreak of vancomycin-resistant *Enterococcus faecium* in a geriatric rehabilitation care facility. J Hosp Infect. 2010;76:354–72.
69. Derde LPG, Dautzenberg MJD, Bonten MJM. Chlorhexidine body washing to control antimicrobial-resistant bacteria in intensive care units: a systematic review. Intensive Care Med. 2012;38:931–9.
70. Grayson ML, Mahony AA, Grabsch EA, et al. Marked reductions in rates of vancomycin-resistant enterococci (VRE) colonization and disease associated with introduction of a routine hospital-wide bleach cleaning program. *BMC Proc*. 2011;5:24.
71. Grabsch EA, Mahony AA, Cameron DRM, et al. Significant reduction in vancomycin-resistant enterococcus colonization and bacteraemia after introduction of a bleach-based cleaning-disinfection programme. J Hosp Infect. 2012;82:234–42.
72. Bonten MJ, Slaughter S, Ambergen AW, et al. The role of «colonization pressure» in the spread of vancomycin-resistant enterococci: an important infection control variable. Arch Intern Med. 1998;158:1127–32.
73. Donskey CJ, Chowdhry TK, Hecker MT, et al. Effect of antibiotic therapy on the density of vancomycin-resistant enterococci in the stool of colonized patients. N Engl J Med. 2000;343:1925–32.

74. Andersen BM, Rasch K, Hochlin F-H, Jensen P, Wismar J-E, Fredriksen. Decontamination of rooms, medical equipment and ambulances, using a dry mist of hydrogen peroxide disinfectant. J Hosp Infect. 2006;62:149–55.
75. Andersen BM, Hochlin K, Daling J-P. Cleaning and decontamination of reusable medical equipments, including the use of hydrogen peroxide dry-mist gas decontamination. J Microbiol Biochem Technol. 2012;4:57–62.
76. Deshpande A, Mana TSC, Cadnum JL, et al. Evaluation of sporicidal peracetic acid/hydrogen peroxide-based daily disinfectant cleaner. Infect Control Hosp Epidemiol. 2014;35:1414–6.
77. Snyder GM, Thokm KA, Furuno JP, et al. Detection of methicillin-resistant *Staphylococcus aureus* and vancomycin-resistant enterococci by healthcare workers on infection control gown and gloves. Infect Control Hosp Epidemiol. 2008;29:583–9.
78. Williams C, McGraw P, Schneck EE, et al. Impact of universal gowning and gloving on health care worker clothing contamination. Infect Control Hosp Epidemiol. 2014;35:1–7.
79. Boutin MA, Thom KA, Zhan M, Johnson JK. A randomized crossover trial to decrease bacterial contamination of hospital scrubs. Infect Control Hosp Epidemiol. 2014;35:1411–3.
80. Mitchell A, Spencer M, Edminston JRC. Role of healthcare apparel and other healthcare textiles in the transmission of pathogens: a review of the literature. J Hosp Infect. 2015;90:285–92.
81. Morgan DJ, Rogawski E, Thom KA, et al. Transfer of multidrug-resistant bacteria to healthcare workers' gloves and gowns after patient contact increases with environmental contamination. Crit Care Med. 2012;40:1045–51.
82. Hayden MK, Blom DW, Lyle EA, Moore C, Weinstein RA. Risk of hand or glove contamination after contact with patients colonized with vancomycin-resistant Enterococcus of the colonized patients' environment. Infect Control Hosp Epidemiol. 2008;29:149–54.
83. Kjølen H, Andersen BM. Handwashing and disinfection of heavily contaminated hands – effective or ineffective? J Hosp Infect. 1992;21:61–71.
84. Andersen BM, Rasch M. Når vanlig håndvask ikke er tilstrekkelig. Tidsskr sykepleien. 2001;11:52–7.

51 Multidrug-Resistant Gram-Negative Rods

Abstract

Overuse of antibiotics, lack of infection control and increased mobility in the population result in the spread of multidrug-resistant (MDR or MDRO resistant to many types of antibiotics) gram-negative bacteria. *Escherichia coli* are present in intestines and faeces and present in the environment (toilet, bathrooms, etc.). Others, like *Klebsiella* sp., *Enterobacter* sp., *Serratia*, *Proteus*, *Citrobacter*, *Pseudomonas* sp., *Acinetobacter* sp., *Burkholderia cepacia*, *Stenotrophomonas maltophilia*, etc. may be contaminants in the environment and sometimes colonize or infect the patient. MDR bacteria may be resistant to all penicillins and cephalosporins (ESBL), all carbapenems (CRE) or quinolones or aminoglycosides. They are robust survivors who migrate between humans, animals and the environment and may tolerate dry conditions, antibiotics and disinfectants. The most vulnerable to infections are persons with reduced infection defence, elderly and new-borns, and the main arena is usually in the healthcare system. Good infection control with removal of microbes from the environment and equipment is among the best preventive measures against the spread of these bacteria. The following chapter is focused on practical measures to detect and prevent transmission of multidrug-resistant gram-negative rods in healthcare institutions.

Keywords

Gram-negative bacteria · Multidrug resistance · MDR · Multidrug-resistant organisms · MDRO · Gram-negative rod · *Enterobacteriaceae* · *Escherichia coli* *Klebsiella* sp. · *Serratia* · *Enterobacter* sp. · *Pseudomonas* · *Acinetobacter* *Burkholderia cepacia* · ESBL · Extended beta-lactamases · CRE · Carbapenemase production · Super resistance · NDM-1 · Aminoglycosides · Fluoroquinolone Cephalosporins · Imported from abroad · Admission control · Pre-examination Information · Screening · Isolation · PPE · Decontamination of environment Eradication · Nosocomial infections · Infection control · Hygiene · Prevention

B. M. Andersen, *Prevention and Control of Infections in Hospitals*,
https://doi.org/10.1007/978-3-319-99921-0_51

51.1 Purpose

Prevent transmission of resistant gram-negative rod bacteria to patients, staff and the environment. Prevent imported infection of super resistant bacteria through patients, personnel and/or visitors.

51.2 Comprise

- All close contacts (patients in the same room, nursing staff, relatives, others).
- Patient room and equipment, toilet, ward office, living room, disinfection room, storage rooms, kitchen, etc.

51.3 Responsibility

The hospital's management is responsible, according to law and regulations [1–9], to ensure proper isolation and control of patients with suspected/proven infection with resistant microbes and that written procedures are available.

The department management has the overall responsibility for the follow-up of routines and to report to the director if preventive infection control routines are not followed up for suspected/detected cases with multidrug-resistant bacteria, such as lack of isolation, disinfection routines, lack of expertise and use of PPE and the like [10] (see isolation routines).

Employees are responsible for following the department's routines.

Information is a duty. Medical doctor or other healthcare provider/home care/hospital department/healthcare institution is obliged to report known or suspected/exposed multidrug-resistant bacteria (current or previously proven) to the recipient and to others who are going to treat/examine the patient.

51.4 Practical Measures

Overuse of antibiotics, lack of infection control and increased mobility in the population results in the spread of multidrug-resistant (MDR) microbes (resistant to many antibacterial agents) as gram-negative rods [10–12]. Gram-negative rods are robust survivors in the environment, migrating between humans, animals and the environment and tolerating drying, antibiotics and disinfectants [10–46].

- Infection control measures are same for all MDR gram-negative bacteria.
- Patients should be examined and treated properly and isolation should be facilitated in the best possible way.
- The general hygiene standard should be high with a prudent use of antibiotics.

51.4.1 Check upon Admission

Patient receipt form should contain current questions regarding infection. See admittance to hospital.

51.4.2 Notification

Notification of proven multidrug-resistant gram-negative bacteria should be sent immediately to relevant health contacts at all levels that have received, examined or treated patients exposed to infection. The ambulance unit that serves the relevant institution in which it is infected must also be notified.

Outbreaks are reported to the infection control personnel, the hospital director, the county doctor and the National Public Health Institute.

51.4.3 Screening at Admittance/Readmittance

- Patients contact with healthcare abroad during the last 12 months.
- Patients have been in a health institution with ongoing outbreak of resistant, gram-negative bacteria or previously infected.
- Screened as for MRSA, + any clinical samples.
- Personnel only screened if they are patients (or in special situations).
- *Remember:* Request the laboratory for examination of resistant bacteria—written on the referral!

51.4.4 Admittance/Treatment/Examination

The patient is immediately isolated. Exposed rooms are disinfected and cleaned (only where the patient has been). Microbial sampling is done.

51.4.4.1 Good General Hand Hygiene

The patient's and staff's hand hygiene prevents spread of infection. Also include visitors.

51.4.4.2 Good Information About Infection Prevention

To all employees, including extra workers and informed, and to the patient and visit to the patient.

51.4.4.3 Isolation and Use of Personal Protective Equipment (PPE)

- *Infected patient or carrier* with multidrug-resistant bacteria is isolated in a single room with its own toilet/shower. The infection or carrier state is often prolonged and alternates between positive and negative test findings. A well-equipped negative air pressure isolate with good space and direct entrance is a good long-term solution.

- *Exposed patients* are also isolated in single room with own toilet/shower until the infection state has been clarified. Declared non-infected if *three* consecutive rectum pencils/faecal samples and clinical samples from drain, urine catheter, wound, etc. taken on separate days are negative, in a patient who has not been on antibiotic past 14 days and not previously infected with multidrug-resistant bacteria.
- *Cohort isolation.* Patients who are infected with the same multiresistant bacterium can be isolated in the same room, if they not have any other infection at the same time (MRSA, VRE, etc.).
- *Infection control equipment.* Personnel who treat/clean/visit infected or exposed patients use surgical mask, cap, gown with long sleeves and cuff and gloves. Room-bound shoes and shoe covers may be used. A chlorine mat outside the door can be used.
- Take off used PPE in anteroom or sluice or, if not, at the door in the patient's room. Learn taking off PPE! Never take off used PPE outside—on a common corridor—and never deposit used, contaminated equipment on the corridor!
- *Protect the uniform and hair/head* to avoid contamination. Use disposable equipment.
- *Visitors* follow the department's routines. See Chaps. 14–16 on isolation routines.

51.4.4.4 Personnel in Work with Multidrug-Resistant Cases

- *Staff* who care and treat these patients do not participate in work with serving foodstuffs, cleaning or other common service work.
- *Staff* should not work at other wards at the same time.
- *Testing of personnel* is not recommended. Exceptions may be suspected of repeated spread. Should be discussed with infection control personnel.
- *In case of personnel infected.* If the person is healthy and has a proper personal hygiene, there should be no work restriction, except for repeated outbreaks associated with the same person.
- *Transmission of infection to healthcare professionals and family/visitors* is likely to occur unless the use of PPE and other measures is carried out in a proper manner.

51.4.4.5 Disinfection and Cleaning

- *Multidrug-resistant bacteria have varyingly resistance* to disinfectants (can even grow in disinfectants) and to heat. Dishwashers and decontaminators must have temperatures above 85 °C! Textiles should be washed at temperatures above 85 °C (10 min × 2).
- *Extra daily cleaning* of floors and surfaces in the patient's room is carried out. In addition, all contact points are wiped over with alcohol three times a day. As a disinfectant use 5% chloramine, chlorine, household bleach, or per-acetic acid. "Virkon" may have an uncertain effect. All cleaning equipment must be treated

as infectious. Multiresistant bacteria can survive in the environment for several months to years if not removed well enough.

- *Final disinfection* after completion of stay is carried out with thorough decontamination, possibly by hydrogen peroxide gas with spore control, followed by main cleaning in the rooms the patient has used [47–50]. *See Isolation regimes.*

51.4.4.6 Transport and Transfer

- For examinations, treatment, etc. elsewhere, message about multidrug-resistant bacteria is sent in advance to the recipient. The patient arrives in a clean bed with clean clothes and a surgical mask is used if coughing. The recipient treats the patient as contact precaution (see above) and with decontamination of the room afterwards.
- When transferring between healthcare levels, healthcare personnel must be informed in advance of infection status. This includes ambulance transport.
- The patient and possibly relatives are informed of the duty to provide information in the health service.
- Visitors/relatives follow the infection protection regime of the institution and do not use the hospital's common rooms.

51.4.4.7 Check and Control

- Antibiotics consumption and type of antibiotics should be checked. Reduce the use of broad-spectrum agents (cephalosporins, carbapenems, ciprofloxacin). Contact infection medicine physician/infection control doctor for advice.
- Carrier status should not usually be treated with antibiotics.
- Workload and patient/care ratio are known risk factors and must be checked.
- Update personnel with regard to hand hygiene and infection protection, isolation measures and treatment of infectious waste/equipment/clothing, etc.
- Overcrowding and corridor-beds pose a risk of spreading! [26]
- Training/review of infection protection, isolation measures and treatment of infectious waste/equipment/clothes, etc. are important.

51.4.5 Unexpected Finding of Multidrug-Resistant Bacteria in the Ward

- Consider intake stop while infection tracing is in progress.
- The patient and exposed patients are isolated separately.
- At least three rectal samples (+ any clinical material from the wound, drain, urine, catheters) on separate days from each exposed patient.
- Eventually, samples from all patients in the same department. Clinical samples are examined for these bacteria, inform about the problem in the referral to the laboratory.
- Notify the units that have treated/examined the patient for the last 12 months. Contact infection control personnel for advice.

- If several cases are infected, extend the infection tracing to the units that have treated/examined the patient for the last 12 months.
- It is not recommended to take samples from the staff.
- While infection tracing is in progress, the ward is treated as with MRSA outbreaks with use of PPE in the care of all patients. The patients are staying in their own rooms and have no common activities with other patients on the ward.
- Buffet service ceases, including coffee and other vending machines in the actual ward.

51.4.6 Major Outbreaks of Multidrug-Resistant Bacteria

- Admission stop until infection tracing is complete and the department/hospital is organized.
- Divide the patients eventually into three units:
  - Cohort isolation unit for all patients with proven infection
  - Cohort isolation unit for all patients exposed to infection—until status is clarified
  - Unit for nonexposed/exposed patients

51.4.7 Microbial Sampling

Rectal pencil, faeces sample and any clinical trial material (urine, drain, wound) are sent for growth on selective media for 24–48 h. The laboratory calls out findings of multiresistant bacteria. Rapid sampling and test response are required to stop major outbreaks.

Exposed patients: minimum three rectal samples (+ clinical trials) in 3 separate days. If the samples are negative, there is little likelihood of infection.

51.4.8 Follow-Up of Patients Still Exposed to Multiresistant Bacteria

In case of uncertainty and persistent exposure to infection in the ward, control tests are carried out over a period of approximately 6 months, depending on the infection and in collaboration with the infection control doctor. Clinical samples from the department are labelled. Note multiresistant bacteria.

51.4.9 Follow-Up of Patients with Multidrug-Resistant, Gram-Negative Bacteria

- *Prolonged condition: the patient is usually not decontaminated.* Negative faeces samples in between positive are natural. In any case, it may be considered as a long-term infectious disease for some months—depending on the type of gram-negative bacteria and use of antibiotics.

- Reinfection in the home environment/patient room, etc. cannot be excluded. In the case of antibiotic treatment, such strains are selected in the environment.
- *Patients are isolated like MRSA routines* and checked for multiresistant bacteria upon admission to another health institution.
- *Cohort in a separate infection control unit* can be used in case of outbreak where several persons are infected/carrier with the same bacterial type. The unit must have its own service rooms, stockpiles, sterile storage rooms, waste rooms, kitchens, etc., which are only used by the unit. Own competent personnel should be affiliated with the unit and shall not participate in care/treatment elsewhere. Do *not* mix patients with multidrug-resistant gram-negative bacteria with MRSA- or VRE-positive patients!
- *Patient journal is flagged out*—critical information.
- *Negative control* tests are *followed* up for 1 year with samples taken after 3, 6, 9, and 12 months. If at least 15 consecutive tests are negative during 1 year, the patient is considered to be free of the actual microbe.

51.4.10 When to Terminate Isolation?

Infected patients with risk factors, repeated carrier state or infection, wounds, drainage, eczema, etc., should be isolated until several controls have been completed. There is a release of, from the skin and hair, bedclothes, own clothes and equipment, relatively large amounts of bacteria, some of which may be multiresistant. A very good daily cleaning with daily disinfection of floors, surfaces and central points and good patient hygiene are important. In hospitals, the patient should be isolated during the admission period.

Infected patients with reduced risk. First-time infected with multidrug-resistant bacteria and *without* wounds/drainage/skin disorders. After *three consecutive negative* test sets are taken properly (sampling starts at least 14 days after discontinuation of antibacterial agents), the likelihood of infection risk is reduced. A carrier state of several months is common as is relapse after shorter or longer time. A careful transition from isolation to fewer infection prevention measures is necessary in order not to infect other patients and personnel.

Special measures for *follow-up are* conducted at home care, nursing homes and long-term institutions [11].

51.5 Background Information

Multidrug-resistant (MDR) gram-negative bacteria are challenges in European hospitals with absence of guidelines, isolation capacity and lack of competent healthcare professionals (Figs. 51.1 and 51.2). In many countries, there is, in addition, an increase in patients that are infected at the same time with a mixture of

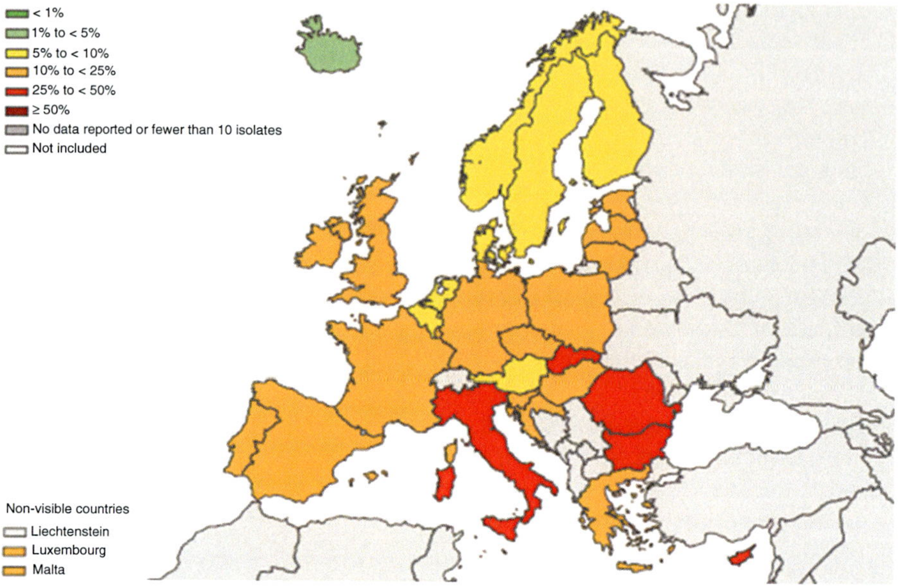

Fig. 51.1 ESBL resistance in invasive *E. coli* isolates in EU/EEA countries, 2015. Source: ECDC, 2017 [43]

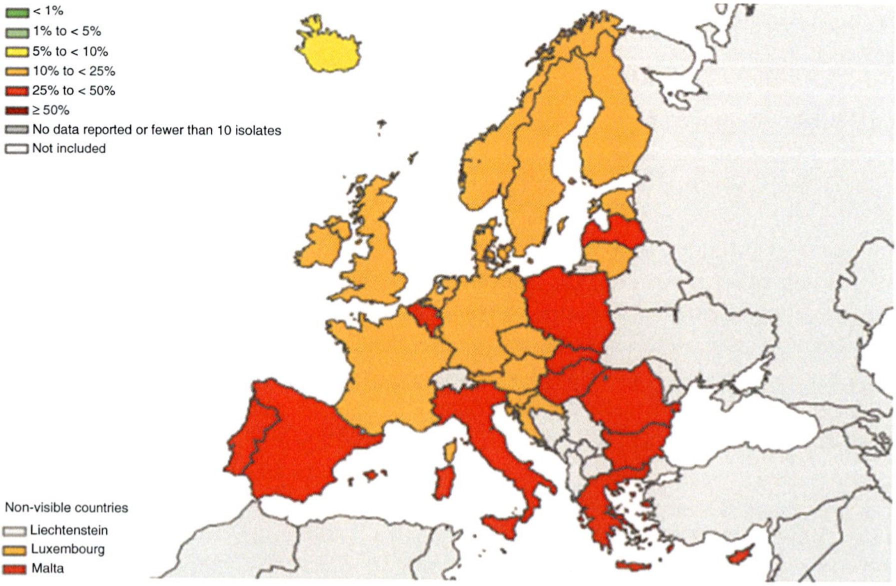

Fig. 51.2 Invasive *E. coli* isolates with resistance against fluoroquinolones in EU/EEA countries, 2015. Source: ECDC, 2017 [43]

multidrug-resistant organisms (MDRO) such as VRE, MRSA, *C. difficile* and/or multidrug-resistant gram-negative rod bacteria. Such problems are present also in countries with more prudent use of antibiotics [10, 20, 21].

The most vulnerable to this type of infection are persons with reduced defence against infections, elderly and new-borns, and the main arena is usually in the healthcare system. Good infection control with removal of microbes from environment and equipment is among the best preventive measures against the spread of these bacteria [10–12].

51.5.1 ESBL (Extended-Spectrum Beta-Lactamase) Bacteria

E. coli, *Klebsiella*, *Enterobacter*, *Citrobacter*, *Serratia* and other *Enterobacteriaceae* may develop resistance to all beta-lactam antibiotics: all penicillins, cephalosporins and carbapenems (when used) [10]. The ESBL enzyme breaks down and destroys all beta-lactam antibiotics [10–13]. Treatment failures for a variety of infections may occur [14–21]. Transmission (contact and air borne) of resistant strains may follow infected or colonized patients between levels of healthcare, causing urinary tract infections, sepsis and lower respiratory tract infections [10–12, 14–19, 21–30]. ESBL-producing bacteria can be detected in drinking water sold locally in a variety of countries [10, 29].

Relatives, in the same household as patients with ESBL, are easily infected and become carriers of ESBL: 24–50%. Most carriers are asymptomatic, but in some cases severe infectious disease is reported in relatives and other contacts [10].

Healthcare workers. ESBL transmission is described from a sick healthcare worker (gall bladder infection) to relatives who developed pyuria and renal failure with the same MDR-resistant *E. coli* strain [10].

In Norway, ESBL is an increasing problem with significant increase in prevalence of ESBL in *E. coli* blood culture isolates, "from 3.5% in 2011 to 5.8% in 2014–2015 and 5.1% in 2016", and in *Klebsiella pneumoniae* isolates, "from 2.0% in 2011 to 6.3% in 2014 and 4.4% in 2016" (NORM) [21]. The increasing ESBL problem at Norwegian hospitals is transmitted to patients in primary care.

51.5.2 Carbapenemases and Super Resistance that Break Down All Antibiotics

Carbapenemases are enzymes breaking down all types of beta-lactam antibiotics, including imipenem, meropenem and other carbapenems (CRE bacteria). *Klebsiella pneumoniae* and other carbapenemase (KPC)-producing bacteria within the family *Enterobacteriaceae* are spread widely in most countries in Europe and America, today, and is also a problem in Norway [10, 11, 21, 32–37, 43]. Several resistance mechanisms are forming these bacteria. Different resistance genes are spread between bacteria types like a very contagious epidemic. This happens in the intestines, but also in an environment burdened by a bad hygienic standard. Little by little, this will occur as local nosocomial outbreaks in primary healthcare and spread between different healthcare levels with frequent patients exchanges.

Super-resistant, gram-negative bacteria are often completely resistant to common antimicrobial agents due to special resistance genes that are easily transmitted between bacteria [10–12]. New Delhi metallo-beta-lactamase 1 (NDM-1) gene has led to almost complete antibiotic-resistant environmental bacteria, first discovered in Asia (New Delhi) in 2007, and is now spread all over the world [31–42]. Up to 40% of cases dies [10, 35, 38–42]. Medical tourism is spreading microbes worldwide and nosocomial between health institutions in Europe [43]. Patients from areas with NDM-1 bacteria are recommended to be isolated, screened and handled as with MRSA [10, 11, 20, 35, 44–46].

E. coli may be infected by the NDM gene that is easily spread between bacteria types. Since *E. coli* is one of the common causes of serious infections inside and outside hospitals, like urinary tract infection, sepsis, lower respiratory tract infections, postoperative wound infections, osteomyelitis, etc., its development is very serious for the global health. The NDM gene is detected in drinking water in New Delhi. Especially exposed to infection are people living in India, Pakistan and Bangladesh. It is assumed that up to 20% of the population in some areas of Pakistan are carriers of NMD-1-producing bacteria [10]. Cholera bacteria (*Vibrio cholerae*) with NDM-1 gene have been detected in India. This can cause major problems since cholera is an additional serious infection disease spread through contaminated drinking water in large areas [10]. Polymyxin (colistin) resistance is developing and is causing even greater therapeutic problems. One case of NMD-1 was detected in Norway in 2010.

51.5.3 Other Important Resistance Types Among Gram-Negative Rods

Aminoglycosides. Resistance to aminoglycosides is a major problem in countries around the Mediterranean, especially Greece [10, 12, 43]. It is the result of overuse of aminoglycosides and lack of infection control, i.e. to "treat bad hygiene with antibiotics", mostly imported problems from the defined areas.

Always resistant bacteria at risk. Some gram-negative rods—mainly environmental bacteria—are always resistant (or are becoming) against many commonly used antimicrobials. Most problems are done by *Pseudomonas aeruginosa*, *Acinetobacter*, *Stenotrophomonas*, *Burkholderia*, *Serratia* sp., *Citrobacter*, *Enterobacter* sp., etc.,—all present in the environment of most health institutions all over the world [10–12, 14–19, 21, 32].

51.5.4 Disease of Multidrug-Resistant Gram-Negative Rod Bacteria [10]

Resistant bacteria spread between healthcare levels cause many types of infections [10–12, 14–19, 21–30]:

- Urinary tract infection—especially associated with catheter use
- Postoperative wound infection or pressure ulcer infection
- Pneumonia or other infections in the middle or lower respiratory tract like COPD/cystic fibrosis—chronic lung disease
- Bacteraemia and septicaemia—especially in the case of reduced infection defence
- Osteomyelitis or joint infection
- Diarrhoea or other intestine disorders
- Infections in patients with severe immune deficiency

51.5.5 Ways of Transmission

- *Contact* via hands and equipment.
- *Contact* transmission can often become *air* transmission (bed linen and other activities)!
- From own bowel and skin flora.
- Pus that infects equipment, hands and wounds. Lack of cleaning of technical equipment.
- Infected bandages, drainage and intravascular equipment.
- Urinary catheterization, catheter and open drainage.
- Contaminated diapers.
- Patients with gram-negative pneumonia and cough/expectorate may especially cause airborne transmission.
- Highly contaminated environment—floors, surfaces and focal points.

51.5.6 Isolation [10, 11]

Contact- and airborne isolation in particularly resistant bacteria:

- Always isolation when resistant bacteria: *Pseudomonas*, *Serratia*, *Stenotrophomonas*, *Acinetobacter* or other gram-negative bacteria that are proven to be resistant to one of the groups below:
- Three-generation cephalosporins

- Aminoglycosides
- Carbapenem (meropenem, imipenem)
- *Airborne isolation* when super-resistant gram-negative bacteria such as NDM-1 bacteria and highly resistant *Acinetobacter* sp. and *Burkholderia cepacia*—at uncontrolled amounts of pus and pneumonia [10, 11, 30]. Internationally, patients with NDM-1 bacteria are recommended to be isolated as with MRSA.
- *Airborne, infectious* multiresistant bacteria (MDRO) has been detected in 67% of patients' rooms of patients colonized with MDRO [30].

51.6 Remember!

- Gram-negative rod bacteria can have a very long life in the environment for up to several years. Therefore, decontamination and other disinfection are particularly important! [47–51].
- Note that some resistant bacteria may be more resistant also to chemical disinfectants [10].
- Textiles, gloves, coat and equipment around the patient are usually contaminated [52–55].
- Studies show that after wearing gloves and before hand hygiene, hands can be contaminated with resistant bacteria [56].
- Medical equipment is an increasing problem due to defects/deficiencies in decontamination [48, 51].
- Transport, patient relocation, overcrowding, patients on corridors, etc. are known factors that increase the risk of cross contamination and spread of infections. Information is important when moving patient with infections.
- Resistant bacteria usually occur in hospitals but are at the highest risk of spread in nursing homes and home nursing that receive these patients for further treatment.
- Persistent carrier status is not uncommon and three negative test sets can later be followed by positive in 10–25% of patients [57].
- Workload and patient/nurse ratio are very well-known risk factors. Excessive activity often leads to breach of hygiene barriers; patients get infections and receive resistance-driving antibiotics for their infections that are further spread to others because of broken infection barriers [10].

References

1. Norwegian Board of Health. Law on protection against infectious diseases by 5 August 1994. no 55.
2. Regulations on infection control in health care. Adopted by Royal. Res. 17 June 2005 pursuant to the Act of 5 August 1994. no.55 on protection against infectious diseases §§ 4-7, 7-11, law 19 November 1982 no. 66 Municipal Health care §1-3 fifth paragraph, law 2 July 1999 no. 61

relating to the specialist health care with more § 2-1a fifth paragraph and law on 18 May 2001 no. 24 on health registers and processing of health information § 6, third paragraph. Promoted by the Ministry of Health and Social Affairs.

3. Norwegian Board of Health. Advice for the application of the Infection Act § 3-3 advance examination of patients—infectious diseases. IK-28/96. Oslo: Norwegian Board of Health; 1996.
4. Norwegian Board of Health. Regulations concerning advance examination of workers in health care—antibiotic resistant bacteria. Issued by the Health and Social Affairs July 5, 1996 pursuant to the Act of 5 August 1994 No. 15 concerning protection against infectious diseases § 3.2. FOR 1996-07-05 No. 700. Norway.
5. Norwegian Board of Health. Hospitals Act §18A-hospital infections that may significant damage the patient. Oslo: Norwegian Board of Health; 2000.
6. Measures to discourage antibiotic resistance (2000–2004). Oslo: Ministry of Health and Social Affairs; 2000.
7. Healthcare personnel law. Law 1999-07-02 no 64: Law about healthcare personnel. Oslo: Ministry of Health and Social Affairs; 2001.
8. Directorate for Labor Inspection. Regulations for protection against exposure to biological agents (bacteria, viruses, fungi, etc.) in the workplace, Oslo; 1997.
9. European Parliament—and Council Directive 2000/54/EC of 18 September 2000 on the protection of workers from the risks related to exposure to biological agents at work.
10. Andersen BM. Gram-negative rod bacteria in intestine and environment. In: Handbook in hygiene and infection control for hospitals. Part 1. Microbiology and infection control. Norway: Fagbokforlaget; 2014. p. 85–95.
11. Andersen BM. Multidrug-resistant, gram-negative rod bacteria. In: Handbook in hygiene and infection control for nursing homes and long-term institutions. Akademika forlag; 2013. p. 299–317.
12. Andersen BM. Multidrug-resistant, gram-negative rod bacteria. In: Bacteria and infections. Epidemiology, infections and infection control. Oslo: Gyldendal Akademisk; 2005. p. 437–48.
13. Andersen BM. Bacterial resistance mechanisms against beta-lactam antibiotics. Tidsskr Nor Laegeforen. 1990;110:2333–9.
14. Olafsen K, Hotvedt R, Andersen BM, Almdahl SM, Søprlie D. Nosocomial infection with resistant *Enterobacter cloacae*. Tidsskr Nor Laegeforen. 1989;109:332–6.
15. Andersen BM, Sørlie D, Hotvedt D, Almdahl SM, Olafsen K, George RC, Gilfillian A. Multiply beta-lactam resistant *Enterbacter cloacae* infections linked to the environmental flora in a unit of cardiothoracic and vascular surgery. Scand J Infect Dis. 1989;21:181–91.
16. Andersen BM, Almdahl SM, Sørlie D, Hotvedt R, Backer-Christensen J, Nicolaysen RB, Solem OI. *Enterobacter cloacae* infections at Regionsykehuset in Tromsø. Tidsskr Nor Lægeforen. 1990;110:342–7.
17. Onarheim H, Høivik T, Harthug S, Digranes A, Mylvaganam H, Vindenes HA. Outbreak of infections with multiresistant *Acinetobacter baumannii*. Tidsskr Nor Laegeforen. 2000;120:1028–33.
18. Andersen BM. Concern about resistant gram-negative rods. Dagens medisin; 16 august 2001.
19. Bukholm G, Tannæs T, Kjelsberg ABB, et al. An outbreak of multidrug-resistant *Pseudomonas aeruginosa* associated with increased risk of patient death in an intensive care unit. Infect Control Hosp Epidemiol. 2002;23:441–6.
20. National Public Health. Prevention and control of spread of multiresistant gram-negative rod bacteria and ESBL-bacteria in healthcare institutions. Oslo: Norwegian Institute of Public Health; 2013.
21. NORM-VET. Usage of antimicrobial agents and occurrence of antimicrobial resistance in Norway. 2012–2016.
22. D'Agata EMC, Venkataraman L, DeGirolami P, Samore M. Molecular epidemiology of ceftazidime-resistant gram-negative bacilli on inanimate surfaces and their role in cross-transmission during non-outbreak periods. J Clin Microbiol. 1999;37:3065–7.

23. Catalano M, Quelle LS, Jeric PE, Di Martino A, Maimone SM. Survival of *Acinetobacter baumannii* on bed rails during an outbreak and during sporadic cases. J Hosp Infect. 1999;42:27–35.
24. Engelhart S, Krizek L, Glasmacher A, Fischnaller E, Marklein G, Exner M. *Pseudomonas aeruginosa* outbreak in a hematology-oncology unit associated with contaminated surface cleaning equipment. J Hosp Infect. 2002;52:93–8.
25. Denton M, Wilcox MH, Parnell P, Green D, Keer V, Hawkey PM, et al. Role of environmental cleaning in controlling an outbreak of *Acinetobacter baumannii* on a neurosurgical intensive care unit. J Hosp Infect. 2004;56:106–10.
26. Hamel M, Zoutman D, O'Callaghan C. Exposure to hospital roommates as a risk factor for health care-associated infection. Am J Infect Control. 2010;38:173–81.
27. Cotter M, Boyle F, Khan A, Boo TW, O'Connell B. Dissemination of extended-spectrum beta-lactamase-producing *Escherichia coli* at home: a potential occupational hazard for healthcare workers? J Hosp Infect. 2012;80:100–1.
28. Lo WU, Ho PL, Chow KH, et al. Fecal carriage of CTXM type extended-spectrum beta-lactamase—producing organisms by children and their household contacts. J Infect. 2010;60:286–92.
29. De Boeck HD, Miwaqnda B, Lunguya-Metlia O, et al. ESBL-positive *Enterobacteria* isolates in drinking water. Emerg Infect Dis. 2012;18:1019–20.
30. Bernard MC, Lanotte P, Lawrence C, Goudeau A, Bernard L. Air contamination around patients colonized with multidrug-resistant organisms. Infect Control Hosp Epidemiol. 2012;33:949–51.
31. Naparstek L, Carmeli Y, Chemelnitsky I, Banin E, Navon-Venezia S. Reduced susceptibility to chlorhexidine among extremely-drug-resistant strains of *Klebsiella pneumoniae*. J Hosp Infect. 2012;81:15–9.
32. Samuelsen O, Naseer U, Tofteland S, et al. Emergence of clonally related *Klebsiella pneumoniae* isolates of sequence type 258 producing plasmid-mediated KPC carbapenemase in Norway and Sweden. J Antimicrob Chemother. 2009;63:654–8.
33. Nordmann P, Naas T, Poirel L. Global spread of carbapenemase-producing *Enterobacteriaceae*. Emerg Infect Dis. 2011;17:1791–8.
34. Patel G, Huprikar S, Factor SH, Jenkins SG, Clafee DP. Outcomes of carbapenem-resistant *Klebsiella pneumoniae* infection and the impact of antimicrobial and adjunctive therapies. Infect Control Hosp Epidemiol. 2008;29:1099–106.
35. CDC. Guidance for control of cabapenem-resistant *Enterobacteriaceae* (CRE); 2012.
36. Promed-mail 17 februar 2012. Gram negative bacilli, multidrug resistant – Brazil, KPC, nosocomial.
37. Promed-mail 18 mars 2012. Gram negative bacilli, MDR-Chile: ex Italy, KPC, nosocomial.
38. Promed-mail 18 februar 2012. NDM-1 carrying Enterobacteriaceae – Irland: 1st rep, ex India.
39. Promed-mail 20 februar 2012. NDM-1 carrying Acinetobacter – Czech Rep, ex Egypt.
40. Promed-mail 21 juni 2012. NDM-1 carrying Enterobacteriaceae – USA: ex Viet Nam.
41. Promed-mail 18 mai 2012. NDM-1 carrying bacilli. Canada: nosocomial, fatal. ex India.
42. Promed-mail 28 juli 2012: NMD-1 carrying Vibrio cholerae-India.
43. ECDC. Surveillance report. Antimicrobial resistance surveillance in Europe, 2015. 2017.
44. CDC. Management of multidrug-resistant organisms in healthcare settings, 2006. CDC; 2006. p. 1–72.
45. CDC. Prevention of transmission of multidrug resistant organisms 2009. CDC; 2009.
46. Siegel JD, Rhinehart E, Jacksom M et al. 2007 Guideline for isolation precautions: preventing transmission of infectious agents in healthcare settings. CDC; 2007.
47. Andersen BM, Rasch M, Hochlin K, Jensen F-H, Wismar P, Fredriksen J-E. Decontamination of rooms, medical equipment and ambulances, using a dry mist of hydrogen peroxide disinfectant. J Hosp Infect. 2006;62:149–55.
48. Andersen BM, Hochlin K, Daling J-P. Cleaning and decontamination of reusable medical equipments, including the use of hydrogen peroxide dry-mist gas decontamination. J Microbiol Biochem Technol. 2012;4:57–62.

49. Deshpande A, Mana TSC, Cadnum JL, et al. Evaluation of sporicidal peracetic acid/hydrogen peroxide-based daily disinfectant cleaner. Infect Control Hosp Epidemiol. 2014;35:1414–6.
50. Rutala WA, Weber DJ. Environmental interventions to control nosocomial infections. Infect Control Hosp Epidemiol. 1995;16:442–3.
51. Promed-mail 18 august 2015. Antibiotic-resistant Enterobacteriaceae – USA. Endoscopic retrograde cholangiopancreatography endoscopes, FDA, Update.
52. Williams C, McGraw P, Schneck EE, et al. Impact of universal gowning and gloving on health care worker clothing contamination. Infect Control Hosp Epidemiol. 2014;35:1–7.
53. Boutin MA, Thom KA, Zhan M, Johnson JK. A randomized crossover trial to decrease bacterial contamination of hospital scrubs. Infect Control Hosp Epidemiol. 2014;35:1411–3.
54. Mitchell A, Spencer M, Edminston C Jr. Role of healthcare apparel and other healthcare textiles in the transmission of pathogens: a review of the literature. J Hosp Infect. 2015;90:285–92.
55. Morgan DJ, Rogawski E, Thom KA, et al. Transfer of multidrug-resistant bacteria to healthcare workers' gloves and gowns after patient contact increases with environmental contamination. Crit Care Med. 2012;40:1045–51.
56. Morgan DJ, Liang SY, Smith CL, et al. Frequent multidrug-resistant *Acinetobacter baumannii* contamination of gloves, gowns, and hands of healthcare workers. Infect Control Hosp Epidemiol. 2010;31:716–21.
57. Lewis JD, Enfield KB, Mathers AJ, Gianetta ET, Sifri CD. The limits of serial surveillance cultures in predicting clearance of colonization with carbapenemase-producing *Enterobacteriaceae*. Infect Control Hosp Epidemiol. 2015;36:835–7.

Gastrointestinal Infections

52

Abstract

Gastroenteritis with vomiting and/or diarrhoea frequently occurs in healthcare institutions, caused by bacteria, viruses or parasites, either brought into hospitals or spread within hospitals. Symptoms may include vomiting, abdominal pain, diarrhoea, or frequent bowel movements, and often fever. Late autumn, winter and early spring may be periods of epidemics of norovirus, and other viruses occur both inside and outside health institutions, while *Clostridium difficile* (CD) diarrhoea is associated with antibiotic treatment. *Listeria* may be a serious risk in special vulnerable patient groups, associated to unpasteurized food or beverages. Travelling to other countries with lower state of hygiene or consuming contaminated food and drinks may cause outbreaks of entero-pathogenic bacteria like *Salmonella*, *Shigella*, *Yersinia*, entero-pathogenic *Escherichia coli*, *Campylobacter* and others. Outbreaks of cholera have been associated with catastrophes like earthquake, tsunami, war, starvation and breakdown of sanitary functions. However, in hospitals in developed countries, gastrointestinal outbreaks are most often caused by CD or norovirus. The following chapter is focused on practical measures to detect and prevent transmission of infections associated with gastroenteritis, vomiting and diarrhoea in healthcare institutions.

Keywords

Gastroenteritis · Vomiting · Diarrhoea · Abdominal pain · Frequent bowel movements · Entero-pathogenic bacteria · *Salmonella* · *Shigella* · *Yersinia* Entero-pathogenic *Escherichia coli* · EHEC · *Campylobacter* · *Cholera* *Clostridium perfringens* · *Bacillus cereus* · *Staphylococcus aureus* · *Listeria* Bacterial toxins · Entero-pathogenic viruses · Entero-pathogenic protozoa Food and beverage control · Imported · Admission control · Pre-examination Information · Screening · Isolation · PPE · Decontamination · Environment Eradication · Nosocomial infections · Infection control · Hygiene · Prevention

B. M. Andersen, *Prevention and Control of Infections in Hospitals*,
https://doi.org/10.1007/978-3-319-99921-0_52

52.1 Purpose

Prevent transmission of gastroenteritis-inducing microorganisms to other patients, personnel and the environment [1–9].

52.2 Comprise

All close contacts of patients (patients in the same room, personnel, visitors, etc.) and equipment, textiles, fixtures, rooms, etc. that the patient has been in direct or indirect contact with. Also includes the hospital's kitchen, ward office and the serving of food and drink, in case of suspected food-borne infection.

52.3 Responsibility

Hospital management ensures procedures for isolation and control of patients with suspected gastrointestinal infections.

The department management implements routines and reports to the director in the absence of resources (isolate, expertise, personnel) that may expose patients, personnel or visitors to unnecessary infection.

Employees follow routines and guidelines.

52.4 Practical Measures [2, 3]

Gastroenteritis with vomiting and/or diarrhoea frequently occurs in healthcare institutions, caused by bacteria, viruses or parasites, either brought into hospitals or spread within hospitals [1–7]. Symptoms may include vomiting, abdominal pain, diarrhoea, or frequent bowel movements, and often fever.

- See also Clostridium difficile, Chap. 53 and norovirus, Chap. 54.

1. Check before and upon admission:
   - Patient receipt form should contain current questions regarding infection. See admittance to hospital.
   - *If detected infection/exposed to infection*, there are at least two possibilities: (a) wait for admission/treatment until the infection status is cleared; (b) isolate and treat the patient as infectious until infection status has been clarified.
2. Clinical tips on type of infection and cause:
   Initially, it is often unclear what type of infection the patient has. Fast and drastic measures from the start prevent larger spread. Once the infectious agent is known, special measures may be implemented.

- Acute vomiting and/or diarrhoea, short incubation time, one after another becomes acutely ill, and there is an epidemic going on in the society as a whole—think of norovirus or other intestinal pathogenic viruses (see separate chapter).
- Single cases of diarrhoea in connection with antibiotics (cephalosporins, clindamycin, ciprofloxacin), long-term healthcare, elderly patients—think of *Clostridium difficile* (see separate chapter).
- After staying abroad, think about intestinal bacteria: *Salmonella*, *Shigella*, entero-pathogenic *E. coli*, *Campylobacter*.
- *Campylobacter* is often a summer disease in most countries, associated with grilling, unprocessed meat and contaminated water. Often convulsive pain attacks and bloody diarrhoea in the lower part of abdomen.
- Acute gastric problems with vomiting and diarrhoea and stomach ache, many ill at the same time; think about common food or drinking sources and food poisoning with bacterial toxins (toxins from *Staphylococcus aureus*, *Salmonella*, *Clostridium perfringens*, *Bacillus cereus*, etc.).
- Diarrhoea and sepsis-like symptoms, meningitis and endocarditis in immunosuppressed, pregnant, new-borns and people with intestinal diseases; unpasteurized food and drink—check *Listeria*.
- Waterborne, large outbreaks—think of entero-pathogenic protozoa, *Campylobacter*, *Shigella*, *Vibrio cholerae (cholera)* (in special areas) and entero-pathogenic virus (norovirus/sapovirus).

3. The patient is isolated:
    - Directly in contact isolation or single room with priority and separate toilet/bathroom attached to the room. The door of the room must be marked. See separate Chap. 16 on isolation.
    - Infection gown (gown to protect), gloves and eventual surgical mask/cap/face shield by vomiting or splashing and preferably room-bound shoes or shoe covers. Learn to take on and off PPE.
    - The hands are washed with soap and water—also after removing of gloves, mask/cap/gown and shoes.
    - More patients with the same symptoms should preferably not share rooms due to reinfection! In difficult circumstances may patients be isolated in cohort [2, 5, 6]
    - Inform all (patient, personnel, visitors) that hand washing with soap and water is important after toilet visits, before and after meals, etc.
    - Visitors of the infectious patient should be informed, follow routines for PPE, and not stay in rooms with other patients.
4. Sampling—investigation phase:
    - Sampling usually *only from patients with symptoms*. In case of large sample numbers, contact the microbiological laboratory in advance.
    - Common faeces test for bacteriological examination and faeces test (or vomitus) in dry vials for viral examination.
    - Take the sample as early as possible during the course of disease and rapid transport to the microbiological laboratory (same day).

- Greater infection tracing is carried out in cooperation with infection control personnel. Microbiological laboratory is informed due to the number of samples and organization.
- Sampling from food, drinks and environment may be actual in some cases.

5. General infection control measures:
   - Avoid shared dining; no serving of food and drinks on corridors.
   - Note: ice machines, water tanks, coffee machines, fruit and the like for shared use may be risks!
   - Limit the visitor number.
   - Check drinking water—if necessary, contact the water system administration for information of quality, and apply bottled water, in case of suspected waterborne infection.
   - Check foods; unpasteurized cheeses/butter/other dairy products should not be served in hospitals; food buffets are not compatible with good food hygiene; cut meat must be replaced in good time before the date of expiry.
6. Patients exposed to infection:

   Isolated in the same way as patients with known infection until incubation time for infection is over (e.g. 2 days for norovirus) or samples show that the patient is not infected.
7. Other patients without exposure to infection:
   - Treat with a patient-bound gown (changed daily) for each patient and increased focus on the patient's personal hygiene.
   - Patients are informed about hand washing after toilet visits, before and after meals, before and after medication, etc.
8. Personnel with symptoms:
   - Sick leave and follow-up until free of infection, according to the infection type.
   - In the case of viral gastroenteritis: norovirus—recommended to stay at home 2 days after free of symptoms.
   - If personnel is infected or have carrier state of *Salmonella*, *Shigella*, *Yersinia*, epidemic *E. coli* or *Campylobacter*, tracing among others in the ward may be done. Faeces samples should be negative before returning to work.
9. Information [2, 3]:
   - The staff, patients and relatives must get accurate information about the risk of infection and specific measures.
   - Other departments, hospitals and institutions that have been in contact with the patient are informed according to the current agent.
   - Personnel should not work elsewhere as long as infection tracing/other measures take place. Extra workers and other personnel (supervision, etc.) must be informed of outbreak at the ward. Contact hygiene nurse for advice.
   - The ward should be closed for walking through or for new admissions while the outbreak is going on.
   - Cleaning staff are informed about infection protection and to avoid work elsewhere during outbreaks of norovirus.

10. Cleaning/disinfection [2, 3]:
    The responsible leader provides a rapid implementation of disinfection and cleaning of relevant rooms and objects according to guidelines for contact infection and in cooperation with the hygiene nurse. Sharpen the general and personal hygiene of the ward. Disinfection is directed against the specific agent detected/suspected. See chapters on isolation regimens and on decontamination of rooms Chaps. 14–16 and 66.
    - Environment that is easily contaminated like beds, bedside tables, water faucets, on and off buttons and door handles must be disinfected daily.
    - Toilets, washbasins and door handles to the toilets are disinfected one to four times a day. Cloths or wipes soaked with alcohol (75–85%) can be used.
11. Textiles, waste, reusable equipment, service, and cutlery (see isolation routines Chaps. 14–16)
12. Notification procedures:
    - Report to infection control unit in case of suspected outbreak of gastrointestinal infection.
    - Report suspected infections via *food or water*—to the local authority the same day. The food safety department (national) is also notified.
    - Several cases of illness from the same source of infection should be notified to the National Institute of Public Health.
    - Nominal reporting may be obligated for diseases in different risk groups (A and B), according to legislation.
13. Consider admission stop at the ward:
    - If two or more patients or one employee and one patient are suspected to be infected with the same microbial agent or have the same symptoms.
14. Follow-up on infection:
    Carrier or source of infection
    Hospital staff with positive findings of *Salmonella/Shigella/Yersinia/Campylobacter*/intestinal pathogens of *E. coli* are reported and followed up by the occupational health services/general practitioner in cooperation with the infection control unit.
    Patients are isolated during repeated admissions at the hospital.
    Isolation is lifted
    - After cessation of symptoms and after negative samples from faeces.
    - In case of major outbreaks, the need of further isolation is considered according to infection type and control.

    Exception for isolation in hospital—special cases
    In special cases, the patient may leave the single room if he/she:
    - Understand and follow precautions not to spread infectious agents
    - Does not have diarrhoea, vomiting and uncontrolled incontinence
    - Does not have norovirus infection—up to 2 days after freedom of symptoms
    - Does not stay in a common room with other patients or use a common toilet/bath
    - Does not use “corridor service” or other shared serving (coffee machines, etc.)

- Performs good hand hygiene, and this is done in agreement with the hospital's infection control unit.

15. Control samples after entero-pathogenic bacteria:
    A minimum of three negative faeces samples should be taken with 2–3 days intervals, starting 14 days after any discontinuation of antibacterial treatment. Five negative faeces samples are recommended for *Salmonella typhi and Salmonella paratyphi* A and B, as well as one duodenal aspirate.
    - Control of faeces: *Salmonella*, *Shigella*, *Yersinia*, entero-pathogenic *E. coli*, *Campylobacter*, etc. First check is taken 2–3 days after symptom freedom.
    - If treated with antibiotics, control samples should be taken at least 14 days after discontinuation.
    - In case of negative findings, further check tests may be taken at least 2 days apart.
    - After three negative tests, the patient can be declared non-contagious.
    - In case of positive findings, the next check should be taken after 1 week.
    - Employees who work with food or patients should be on sick leave as long as they are culture positive. At least three negative samples are required before they can return to work after infection with intestinal bacteria: *Salmonella*, *Shigella*, *Yersinia*, entero-pathogenic *E. coli* or *Campylobacter*.

    Registration and information

    Patient/staff with proven *Salmonella*/*Shigella*/*Campylobacter*/*Yersinia*/ entero-pathogenic *E. coli* or other entero-pathogenic bacteria can be carriers and contagious for 1–3 months after undergoing infection (rarely for a longer time). The patient is informed about this, about the importance of good personal hygiene and about special conditions for kitchen hygiene, healthcare and care/contact with children and people with impaired general condition.
    - Healthy carriers (no symptoms) of entero-pathogenic bacteria are seen frequently after *Salmonella*, *Shigella* or *Campylobacter* infections. Some may have the bacteria in the faeces for several years after the infection, which represent a risk to their environment.
    - Those who still secret *Shigella*, *Campylobacter or Salmonella* after 3–6 months should as a rule be investigated and, if appropriate, treated with antibacterial agents and referred to specialist in infectious diseases.

52.5 Background Information

The most common entero-pathogenic bacterial groups are *Salmonella*, *Shigella*, *Campylobacter*, *Yersinia* and various types of entero-pathogenic *Escherichia coli* (including entero-haemorrhagic *E. coli* (EHEC)) and *Listeria* [1–5, 8, 9]. The highest mortality is recorded after food poisoning with *Salmonella* and *Clostridium perfringens*. Norovirus is usually causing the largest outbreaks [6].

- *Gastroenteritis* is most commonly caused by viruses (norovirus, sapovirus, rotavirus, bocavirus etc.), entero-pathogenic bacteria or toxins [1, 6].

- *Food-borne gastroenteritis* from the hospital's kitchen may occur (*Bacillus cereus, Salmonella, Clostridium perfringens, S aureus*, etc.). In 2004, 75 people were infected with *Salmonella infantum* from the hospital's kitchen at a hospital in the South of Norway [4]. Food-borne infections are often linked to poor food control, low hygiene and people that have been abroad [4].
- *Food poisoning* causes gastroenteritis with varying incubation time (2–18 h), caused by the ingestion of bacteria and bacterial toxins (the same as above) from infected foods or beverages [1–4].
- *Entero-pathogenic bacteria* are not normal flora in the intestines of people living in northern parts of Europe. Spread in hospitals occurs rarely because of contact isolation [4]. Increased food contamination and travel activity may increase the risk in hospitals [1, 4]. The situation in Norway, for example, is the following for ca 5.5 million inhabitants in 2014:
  - *Salmonella*: 1100 cases, mainly *S. typhimurium* and *S. enteritidis*; 70% were imported; 10% were multidrug resistant (MDR to five antibiotic groups), and there were a few dangerous types such as *S. typhi* (7 isolates) and *S. paratyphi* (8 isolates) [9]. A total of 65 isolates were detected in blood cultures (0.5%) [9].
  - *Shigella*: 96 cases, mainly *S. sonnei* and *S. flexneri*; 85% were imported; 50–90% were MDR [9].
  - *Yersinia enterocolitica*: 65 cases; 50% were mainly serogroup 3 from Norway, with exception of ampicillin—mostly antibiotic sensitive [9].
  - *Campylobacter*: 3386 cases; 46% were imported; MDR varied, highest among imported cases [9].
  - *E. coli* enteritis and EHEC: 334 cases of *E. coli* enteritis and 148 of EHEC [10]. The increase is worrying (see Fig. 52.1).

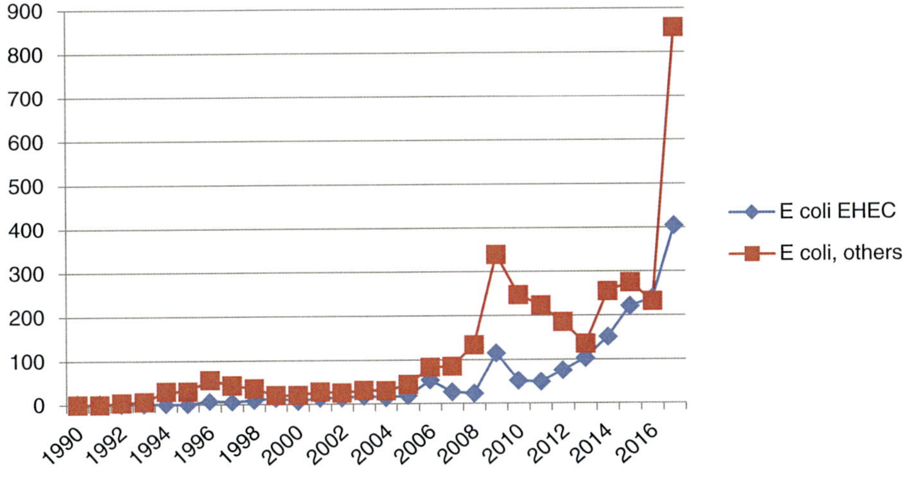

Fig. 52.1 Entero-pathogenic *E. coli*—development in Norway, 1990–2017 (Source: MSIS, National Public Health Institute)

- *Helicobacter pylori* is associated with dyspepsia, gastric ulcer and rarely development of cancer [5]. Infections in hospitals are unknown, transmission may occur by poor hygiene [5].
- *Listeria monocytogenes* is a normal intestinal flora in animals and can be found on all types of uncooked foods, vegetables, cold cuts and fruit (in melons) and in water (internally in waterborne amoebas) and grow well in the refrigerator temperature [8, 11]. Gastroenteritis and sepsis may be a risk for patients with immune deficiency, pregnant women, new-borns and cancer patients, especially colon cancer [8]. In 2007, 17 patients were infected with *Listeria*, of which 3 died, at a hospital for cancer patients in Oslo (Radiumhospitalet). The source of infection was camembert cheese made from pasteurized milk, but probably re-infected in the late production phase [8].
- Norovirus and other entero-pathogenic viruses show a high tendency to spread like a conflagration in and outside hospitals [2, 3, 6].
- *Giardia lamblia and Cryptosporidium* are the most common intestinal protozoa (*Entamoeba histolytica* in tropical areas) spread through infected water, food, bad hygiene and in person-to-person contact, especially in institutions with close contact [2, 7].

52.5.1 Risk Factors in Hospitals

- Poor hygiene and lack of isolation.
- Lack of hygienic control with food and beverages
- Uncritical use of broad spectrum antimicrobial agents
- Impaired general condition, chronic bowel disease, diabetes, kidney failure, immune deficiency and in ventricular operated patients
- Travel to endemic areas without preventive hygiene measures

52.5.2 Message

In case of outbreaks and in connection with primary findings, contact department management and infection control personnel. In case of negative microbiological findings, but more patients/staff (three to four) with similar symptomatology in a short period of time (approximately 1 week), contact the same instances.

In case of *major outbreaks*, the number of new patients is registered each day and sent via the department management to infection control personnel (telephone or mail). The department also contacts microbiological laboratory if there are unusually large sample numbers. Remember nominative notification regarding *Salmonella, Shigella, Yersinia, Campylobacter*, entero-pathogenic *E. coli* and cholera.

Food-borne infections—National aggregated registration and surveillance are essential [9, 11].

52.5.3 Sampling: Extended

Sampling of faeces is recommended on suspicion of:

- Infectious spread in the hospital (nosocomial spread—norovirus in particular).
- Food poisoning.
- *Clostridium difficile.*
- Serious infections and import infection.
- Control of previous findings, chronic carrier status and environmental studies.
- In case of outbreak, samples of up to three first patients are taken (usually).

Samples are taken as early as possible and examined for viruses and bacteria:

- Faeces containing mucus or blood when this occurs—or by vomiting.
- Sent the same day or stored in a refrigerator until the next day.
- In suspected virus- or parasite-related gastroenteritis, the stool sample is sent on sterile container without addition.
- In suspected bactericidal gastroenteritis, the faeces sample is sent in Cary-Blair transport medium or delivered in sterile container directly to the microbiological department immediately after sampling.
- In suspected infection with *Clostridium difficile*, the faeces sample is sent in sterile container without addition directly to the laboratory.

Avoid the use of antibiotics that may prolong and worsen the condition.

- Antibacterial agents; contact specialist in infection medicine.

Note! special conditions like intestinal infections in patients with immunodeficiency, prostheses or grafts or with known aneurysm. Contact specialist in infection medicine for advice on treatment.

References

1. Andersen BM. Bacteria and disease. Epidemiology, infections and infection protection. Gyldendal Academic; 2005. p. 56–78, 222–70, 342–48.
2. Andersen BM. Prevention of bacterial gastroenteritis. In: Handbook for hygiene and infection control for hospitals. Ullevål University Hospital; 2008. p. 451–4.
3. Andersen BM. Prevention of gastrointestinal infections. In: Handbook in hygiene and infection control for nursing homes, long-term institutions. Akademika; 2013. p. 229–40.
4. Andersen BM. Gastrointestinal and intestinal bacteria. In: Handbook for hygiene and infection control for hospitals. Part 1: microbiology and infection protection. Fagbokforlaget; 2014. p. 95–107.
5. Andersen BM. Other potentially gastric and intestinal pathogenic bacteria. In: Handbook for hygiene and infection control for hospitals. Part 1: microbiology and infection protection. Fagbokforlaget; 2014. p. 108–15.

6. Andersen BM. Gastrointestinal virus infections. In: Handbook for hygiene and infection control for hospitals. Part 1: microbiology and infection protection. Fagbokforlaget; 2014. p. 248–54.
7. Andersen BM. Entero-pathogenic protozoa. In: Handbook for hygiene and infection control for hospitals. Part 1: microbiology and infection protection. Fagbokforlaget; 2014. p. 356–63.
8. Andersen BM. Listeriose—*Listeria monocytogenes*. In: Handbook for hygiene and infection control for hospitals. Part 1: microbiology and infection protection. Fagbokforlaget; 2014. p. 150–3.
9. Nordstrøm M, Slettemeås JS, Urdahl AM, Wester AL. Zoonotic and non-zoonotic entero-pathogenic bacteria. NORM/NORM-VET; 2014. p. 43–57.
10. MSIS. Norwegian National Public Health Institute. 2015.
11. Henao OL, Jones TF, Vugia DJ, Griffin PM, et al. Foodborne disease active surveillance network—2 decades of achievements, 1996–2015. Emerg Infect Dis. 2015;21:1529–36.

Clostridium difficile 53

Abstract

Clostridium difficile infections (CDIs) are among the most serious and widespread hospital infections in Europe and the United States and are related to the use of antibiotics combined with lack of hygiene and infection protection. CD is gram-positive, anaerobic, spore-forming rod bacteria, adhesive to mucosa, and may have enzymes and toxins. Only *toxin-producing* CD can cause antibiotic-associated diarrhoea and pseudomembranous colitis. The bacteria die in air. The CD spores survive outside the body for years. Spores are inactivated by autoclaving or treated with certain disinfectants. Virulent CD types may be associated with serious disease, even in young people without contact with the healthcare system. CD is normally found in the intestines and perineum, is transient flora of the hands and skin and is asymptomatic present in many new-borns and in 3–4% of healthy persons. In case of antibiotic treatment, 40–50% may have CD in the intestine due to selection. Environmental contamination is large both with and without symptoms. CDI is associated with prolonged, antibacterial treatment. "Drivers" are third-generation cephalosporins, clindamycin and quinolones. The following chapter is focused on practical measures to detect and prevent transmission of CDI in healthcare institutions.

Keywords

Clostridium difficile · CD · CDI · CD infection · Toxin-producing · Colitis Diarrhoea · Abdominal pain · Frequent bowel movements · Bacterial toxins Antibiotics · Admission control · Pre-examination · Information · Screening Isolation · PPE · Decontamination · Environment · Eradication · Nosocomial infections · Infection control · Hygiene · Prevention

B. M. Andersen, *Prevention and Control of Infections in Hospitals*,
https://doi.org/10.1007/978-3-319-99921-0_53

53.1 Purpose

Prevent transmission of toxin-producing *Clostridium difficile* to other patients, personnel and the environment [1–10].

53.2 Comprise

All close contacts of patients (patients in the same room, personnel, visitors, etc.). All equipment, textiles, fixtures, rooms and surfaces the patient has been in direct or indirect contact with, as well as food and beverages contaminated with toxin producing CD bacterial spores.

53.3 Responsibility

The hospital's management provides written procedures for detecting and isolating patients with CD and for monitoring of antibiotic use at the hospital.

The department management ensures that personnel, patients and visitors are informed of infection prevention measures by CD infection and report to the director if resource shortages (capacity, isolation, etc.) cause patient, personnel and visitors to be exposed to CD infection.

Employees follow routines and guidelines for infection protection.

53.4 Practical Measures

53.4.1 Routines for All Admission/Outpatient Clinics/ Day Surgery [5–8]

Preliminary examination: ask patient, relatives and physician *before* admission; check if the patient or people in the local area have symptoms of enteritis.

If suspected or confirmed CD, there are at least two possibilities: (a) wait for admission until the patient's recovery/infection status has been resolved; (b) isolate the patient until infection status has been clarified.

53.4.2 Isolation and Other Preventive Measures [5–8]

- The index patient is contact isolated immediately with private toilet and decontaminator. Do not share toilet/bath or patient room with others.
- Patients in the same room as the index patient are isolated in separate rooms and treated as possible infected.
- Personal protective equipment (PPE) is taken on and off properly to prevent spread of infection to others and environment.

  - Donning (dressing) of PPE takes place in a defined clean area in the sluice or anteroom of the insolation unit or on the corridor outside the patient room. *Only clean, unused equipment must be on the corridor outside the isolation unit!*
    - Wash or disinfect your hands before donning.
    - Gown—disposable—with long sleeves and cuffs. Single use.
    - Gloves pulled over the coat's cuff.
    - Room-bound shoes (or disposable cover). Room-bound shoes should be machine washed at 85 °C or autoclaved (due to CD spores).
    - Cap and surgical mask, especially important when bedding and cleaning the room, when the patient is assisted in the toilet and at other major activities that can swirl CD spores up in the air.
  - Doffing (undressing) of PPE after use is carried out in a defined area of the isolation unit's sluice or in the patient's room at the exit door (should be avoided). *Never undress PPE on the corridor!*
    - Shoes, room-bound, or disposable shoe covers must be removed first. Gloves are used when gently removing the shoe covers and placed in contaminated waste.
    - Remove the gloves. Learn to undress gloves!
    - Hand hygiene.
    - The gown is taken off by opening behind the back—avoid touching the front and arms—learn to undress gown!
    - Hand hygiene.
    - Remove surgical mask by loosening back in the neck—learn undressing mask.
    - Remove the cap by taking off from back, not in front—learn undressing cap.
    - Hands are finally washed with soap and water.
    - Use eventually a "cloth" with chloramine 5% in anteroom/sluice for wiping off shoes. Replaced each shift.
- *The CD spores* firmly adhere to the skin. There is no complete effect of either hand wash or hand disinfection on CD spores. Hand wash with soap and water can have a slightly better effect than hand disinfection and is therefore used for CD. The use of gloves and a good hand hygiene before and after wearing gloves are therefore central.
- *Visitors* follow the same routine as personnel and leave the department directly—not in the living room/corridor and the like.
- *Self-service drinks, food,* etc. *on the corridor are removed.* Ice and coffee machines, etc. on the corridor are emptied, decontaminated and washed. Should not be used during outbreaks.

53.4.3 Disinfection of Rooms and Surfaces

There is a heavy contamination of CD spores in the environment and equipment around the CD patient, which often can be detected even after disinfection [11, 12]. The spores are killed by autoclaving (equipment, etc.) or by disinfection with 5%

chloramine for a minimum of 5 min [4, 8]. Also household bleach 10% or peracetic acid kills spores. Afterwards, clean with soap and water.

- *Disinfection daily* with 5% chloramine disinfection or peracetic acid; wipe over fixtures, door handles, on and off knots etc., wipe over the floor, and cleaning with soap and water immediately afterwards. Disinfection of the entire room, including the floor when termination the isolation, see isolation regimens Chaps. 14–16.
- *Hydrogen peroxide gas/aerosol* can effectively kill CD spores if used properly; use spore control for terminal disinfection [8, 13–15].

53.4.4 Isolation Time, Readmissions and Transfers

- *The patient is isolated throughout the hospital stay* even after the diarrhoea is stopped [5–8, 16].
- *In case of readmission* during the first 3–4 following months, the patient is isolated as a CD patient. This is especially important if the patient is going to be treated with antibiotics and/or cancer medicines.
- *When transferring to another health institution*, inform about CD infection, including for CD-exposed patients. After CD infection, use of antibiotics (clindamycin, cephalosporins, ciprofloxacin) or cytostatics can easily trigger a new outbreak of diarrhoea—at least the first half of the year after CD.

53.4.5 Infection Transmission

- *Contact transmission*: via hands, faecal-oral, equipment, environment, dust, etc.
- *Airborne transmission:* an air transmission in the toilet room has been detected when it is pulled down and the toilet lid is open. [9] CD spores are detected in the air 25 cm above the toilet opening and around the toilet room. [9] Close the toilet bowl before it is pulled down! Helpers use cap and surgery mask in addition to gloves, gown and room-bound shoes.
- Patients should generally be advised not to walk barefoot on the floor of the nursing room in order not to pull bacteria and spores into the bed.

53.4.6 Risk of Infection

- Overcrowding and understaffing [8].
- Airborne spread of spores [8–10].
- Lack of isolation.
- Overuse of selective antibacterial agents (clindamycin, cephalosporins, fluoroquinolones).

- Cytostatics.
- Reservoir development in nursing homes, other health institutions and home nursing, with spread to hospitals [8].
- Large workload and lack of glove use when caring for CD patients may cause one in four healthcare professionals to get CD spores on their hands [17].

53.4.7 Disease Manifestation: Varying

Incubation period is 2–3 days or longer. Varying from asymptomatic CD to diarrhoea that is partly bloody, mucous and painful; pseudomembranous colitis; toxic mega-colon; and perforation of the intestine [4, 8].

53.4.8 Diagnosis

- Diarrhoea:
  - Six aqueous in 36 h
  - Three unformed/24 h for 2 days
  - Eight unformed for 2 days
- Pseudomembranous (continuous mucous membranes)
- Toxin detection (only at diarrhoea)
- Growth of *C. difficile* (anaerobic cultivation—CFA—medium) just by diarrhoea
- No other cause of diarrhoea

53.4.9 Sampling

Preferably, take only aqueous, loose faeces, if not epidemiological examination. Pencil samples are not good enough because of a too small volume for toxicity studies (can be used in epidemiological studies). Lumen content v/operative treatment is applicable. Always ask for the cultivation and identification of CD due to increasing incidence of more virulent CD types.

53.4.10 Personnel Are Not Tested

Personnel caring for patients with CD are usually not becoming ill (except for colonization, use of antibiotics, colon disease, etc.), but may be important spreader if infection prevention measures are not implemented. Hypervirulent strains can attack healthy people, including healthcare professionals [8].

53.5 Background Information

Clostridium difficile (CD) is gram-positive, anaerobic, spore-forming rod bacteria, adhesive to mucosa, and may have enzymes and toxins [4, 5, 8]. Only toxin-producing CD can cause antibiotic-associated diarrhoea and pseudomembranous colitis. The CD bacteria dies when coming out in air (oxygen). The CD spores survive outside the body for a long time—for years—but are inactivated by autoclaving or treatment with 5% chloramine for a minimum of 5 min, household bleach 10% or peracetic acid. CD bacteria are usually sensitive (may be killed) to medicaments like vancomycin and metronidazole. Virulent CD types are associated with serious disease, even in young people, without contact with the healthcare system (ribotype variants NAPI/O27/III, 106, 001, etc.) [4, 8].

Exotoxin produced by CD bacteria is a protein with a toxic A part and a cytotoxic B part, produced in the growth phase of the bacteria. Toxin A is an enterotoxin that increases fluid secretion in the intestine; toxin B, cytotoxin, has a strong cellular affection on the mucous membrane in the colon. Another factor reduces intestinal motility. Toxin-producing CD was associated with the use of antibiotics, especially clindamycin in 1980, and was first called "clindamycin diarrhoea" [4, 5, 8]. The CD infection (CDI) in the colon occurs in 90% of the cases in the sigmoideum and destroys intestinal epithelium and lamina propria with infiltration of leukocytes, erythema and oedema and formation of white to green plaques.

Normal intestine flora contaminates the environment. CD is normal flora in the intestines and perineum and transient flora of the hands and skin. It is asymptomatic present in many new-borns, in 3–4% of healthy persons over 2 years and at 15–25% of hospital patients. In case of antibiotic treatment, 40–50% may have CD in the intestine due to selection. Environmental contamination is large when CD, both with and without symptoms [8–12].

CD infection (CDI) is most often antibiotic-induced diarrhoea. CDI is associated with prolonged, antibacterial treatment. Clindamycin selects for CD, and that does also cephalosporins (third-generation), ciprofloxacin, ampicillin, etc. Compared with penicillin V, causes penicillinase -stable penicillins more frequent CD diarrhoea (×8), cephalosporins even more frequent (×40), and clindamycin most frequently (×70) [8]. Use of antibiotics may increase the risk of CD infection 7–10 times for up to 1 month after discontinuation of antibiotics. Then there is a threefold increase in risk for the next 2 months [2, 4]. "Drivers" for CDI are third-generation cephalosporins, clindamycin and ciprofloxacin (quinolones) [3, 4, 8, 18, 19].

53.5.1 Risk

Risk score for CDI in endemic hospitals constitutes contamination pressure, elderly patients, previous institutional admittance, previous CD infection, intensive treatment and a variety of clinical parameters [2, 20]. Patients with leukaemia in hospitals have a greater (2×) risk of CD infection than non-leukaemia patients, and the CDI results in increased mortality, longer hospital stays and higher hospital expenses. [21] At Ullevål University Hospital, Oslo, there was a CD outbreak in 2003 among many children with leukaemia and other forms of cancer. [8] The outbreak came quickly under control; none of the children died. Isolation and "home hospital treatment" were established, the antibiotic therapy was changed and parents and employees understood and followed the hygiene measures [8].

Good terminal disinfection of rooms and equipment reduces CD in hospitals by approximately 20% [2].

53.5.2 Occurrence, Costs and Mortality

Monitoring of CDI is important as it is done in several places in the United States and Europe [22]. In 2013, 20 states in the United States reported to the health authorities [22]. In endemic areas, CD is defined by where the infection has occurred, "hospital onset" or "community onset", which results in an economic and therapeutic responsibility [23]. Monitoring of CDI started in Norway in 2013, with approximately 1400 cases in 2014 and a doubling to 3000 cases in 2017 (Fig. 53.1. *MSIS, National Public Health*).

Spread with transport and interaction. CD is a typical institution-bacterium, spread between hospitals, other healthcare institutions and primary healthcare in general, by extensive patient transport between the different treatment levels as shown in the United States [24]. This may expose other patients to infection [25].

Global outbreak of virulent strains. In recent years there have been global outbreaks of ciprofloxacin-resistant CD 027 with high mortality rates, 20–25% within 60 days, and with relapse in approximately 15% or more of the cases within 40 days [4, 8, 26].

Large relapse hazard and prolonged stay in hospital. There is a high chance of relapse within 30 days after discharge, ca. 20–30% [4, 8, 27, 28]. Extended length

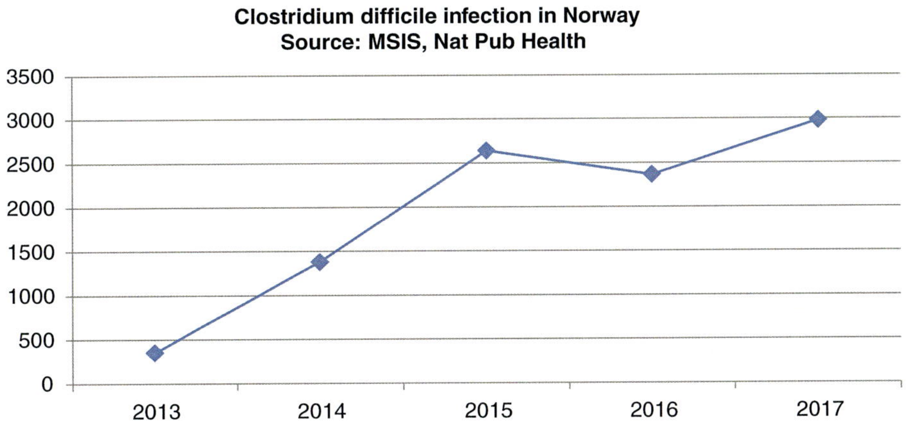

Fig. 53.1 *Clostridium difficile* infections are increasing in Norway (ca. 5.5 million inhabitants). Source: MSIS, Nat Pub Health

of time in hospital depends on the severity of the disease. A study of 43, 500 CD cases in the United States showed an average of 14 additional days in hospital due to the disease, while a multistate model came to less extra days. [29]

Endemic conditions and death. In the United States, CDI is endemic with 1 of 100 (1.3%) hospitalized patients in 2008. In 2011, half a million patients in the United States had CDI, and approximately 29,000 died [30]. In 2012, the incidence, mortality and cost of CDI reached "historical heights" in the United States, with more than 14,000 deaths/year (4.7/100,000 inhabitants) [2, 3].

Hospital-associated CDI costs 5000–7200 USD per patient, with a national expense of 0.9–1.3 billion USD/year [2, 3]. Proper measures over a 5-year period will prevent more than 500,000 CD cases, 82,000 deaths and a national savings of 2.5 billion USD [31]. Such measures are profitable; cost benefit to the society.

In Europe, mortality rate 30 days after start of the CDI varies from 2% in France to 42% in the UK [32].

Restriction of antibiotics The United Kingdom has registered about 60% reduction of CDI from 2008 to 2012, with a simultaneous reduction of use of cephalosporins and quinolones [33]. A multifaceted model was used with the restriction of certain types of antibiotics, patient isolation, hand hygiene and environmental management, as well as control [1].

At an orthopaedic department in Mexico, a 92% restriction of clindamycin—without increase of other antimicrobials—led to approximately 90% reduction of CD infection [19]. Studies show that fidaxomicin treatment can reduce environmental contamination around CD patients, compared with the use of metronidazole and/or vancomycin [34].

References

1. Anonymous. *Clostridium difficile* infection: how to deal with the problem. London: DH Department of Health, Health Protection Agency; 2008. p. 1–131.
2. McDonald LC, Lessa F, Sievert D, et al. CDC. Vital signs: preventing *Clostridial difficile* infections. MMWR Morb Mortal Wkly Rep. 2012;61:157–62.
3. Dubberke ER, Carling P, Carrico R, et al. Strategies to prevent *Clostridial difficile* infections in acute care hospitals: 2014 update. Infect Control Hosp Epidemiol. 2014;35:628–45.
4. Gerding DN, Young VB. Clostridial infection. In: Mandell, Douglas, and Bennett's principles and practice of infectious diseases, vol. 2. 8th ed. Philadelphia: Saunders/Elsevier Churchill Livingstone; 2015. p. 2744–56.
5. Andersen BM. *Clostridium difficile.* In: Bacteria and disease. Epidemiology, infections and infection protection. Oslo: Gyldendal Akademisk, Gyldendal Norsk Forlag; 2005. p. 56–78.
6. Andersen BM. Prevention of *Clostridium difficile*. In: Handbook for hygiene and infection control for hospitals. Oslo: Ullevål University Hospital; 2008. p. 455–8.
7. Andersen BM. Prevention of *Clostridium difficile* (CD). In: Handbook for hygiene and infectious care for nursing homes, long-term institutions. Oslo: Akademika Forlag; 2013. p. 229–40.
8. Andersen BM. *Clostridium difficile*. In: Handbook for hygiene and infection control for hospitals. Part 1: microbiology and infection protection. Bergen: Fagbokforlaget; 2014. p. 108–11.
9. Best EL, Sandoe JAT, Wilcox MH. Potential for aerosolization of *Clostridium difficile* after flushing toilets: the role of toilet lids in reducing environmental contamination risk. J Hosp Infect. 2012;80:1–5.

10. Macve JC, Weinbren MJ. Dirty utility room design and aerosolization of organisms. J Hosp Infect. 2012;81:66–7.
11. Ali S, Moore G, Wilson GR. Spread and persistence of *Clostridium difficile* spores during and after cleaning with sporicidal disinfectants. J Hosp Infect. 2011;79:97–8.
12. Speight S, Moy A, Macken S, et al. Evaluation of the sporicidal activity of different chemical disinfectants used in hospitals against *Clostridium difficile*. J Hosp Infect. 2011;79:18–22.
13. Andersen BM, Rasch M, Hochlin K, Jensen FH, Wismar P, Fredriksen JE. Decontamination of rooms, medical equipment and ambulances, using a dry fog or hydrogen peroxide disinfectant. J Hosp Infect. 2006;62:149–55.
14. Barbut F, Yezli S, Otter JA. Activity in vitro or hydrogen peroxide vapour against *Clostridium difficile* spores. J Hosp Infect. 2012;80:85–7.
15. Andersen BM, Hochlin K, Daling JP. Cleaning and decontamination of reusable medical devices, including the use of hydrogen peroxide gas decontamination. J Microb Biochem Technol. 2012;4:57–62.
16. Jinno S, Kundrapu S, Guerrero DM, et al. Potential for transmission of *Clostridium difficile* by asymptomatic acute care patients and long-term care facility residents with prior *C difficile* infection. Infect Control Hosp Epidemiol. 2012;33:638–9.
17. Landelle C, Verachten M, Legrand P, et al. Contamination of healthcare workers' hands with *Clostridium difficile* spores after caring for patients with *C difficile* infection. Infect Control Hosp Epidemiol. 2014;35:10–5.
18. Yip C, Loeb M, Salama S, Moss L, Olde J. Quinolone use as a risk factor for nosocomial *Clostridial difficile* -associated diarrhea. Infect Control Hosp Epidemiol. 2002;22:572–5.
19. Cruz-Rodriguez N, Hernandez-Garcia R, Salinas-Caballero AG, et al. The effect of pharmacy restriction of clindamycin on *Clostridium difficile* infection rates in an orthopaedics ward. Am J Infect Control. 2014;42:e71–3.
20. Tabac YP, Johannes RS, Sun X, Nunez CM, McDonald LC. Predicting the risk of hospital-onset *Clostridial difficile* infection (HO-CDI) at the time of inpatient admission: HO-CDI risk score. Infect Control Hosp Epidemiol. 2015;36:695–701.
21. Luo R, Greenberg A, Stone CD. Outcomes of *Clostridium difficile* infection in hospitalized leukemia patients: a nationwide analysis. Infect Control Hosp Epidemiol. 2015;36:794–801.
22. Reagan J, Herzig CTA, Pogorzelska-Maziarz M, et al. State law mandates for reporting healthcare-related *Clostridium difficile* infections in hospitals. Infect Control Hosp Epidemiol. 2015;36:350–2.
23. Pakyz AL, Patterson JA, Motzkus-Feagans C, et al. Performance of the present—on-admission indicator for *Clostridial difficile* infection. Infect Control Hosp Epidemiol. 2015;36:838–40.
24. Simmering JE, Polgreen LA, Campell DR, Cavanaugh JE, Polgreen PM. Hospital transfer network structure as a risk factor for *Clostridium difficile* infection. Infect Control Hosp Epidemiol. 2015;36:1031–7.
25. Hamel M, Zoutman D, O'Callaghan C. Exposure to hospital roommates as a risk factor for healthcare-related infection. Am J Infect Control. 2010;38:173–81.
26. Scardina T, Labuszewski L, Pacheco SM, et al. *Clostridium difficile* infection (CDI) severity and outcome among patients infected with the NAP1/BI/027 strain in a non-epidemic setting. Infect Control Hosp Epidemiol. 2015;36:280–6.
27. Zilberberg MD, Shorr AF, Micek ST, Kollef MH. *Clostridium difficile* recurrence is a strong predictor of 30-day rehospitalization among patients in intensive care. Infect Control Hosp Epidemiol. 2015;36:273–9.
28. Deshpande A, Pasupuleti V, Thota P, et al. Risk factors for recurrent *Clostridial difficile* infection: a systematic review and meta-analysis. Infect Control Hosp Epidemiol. 2015;36:452–60.
29. Stevens VW, Khader K, Nelson RE, et al. Excess length of stay attributable to *Clostridial difficile* infection (CDI) in the acute care setting: a multistate model. Infect Control Hosp Epidemiol. 2015;36:1024–30.

30. Lessa FC, Bamberg WM, Beldavs ZG, et al. Burden of *Clostridial difficile* infection in the United States. N Engl J Med. 2015;372:825–34.
31. Slayton RB, Scott IIRD, Baggs J, Lessa FC, McDonald LC, Jernigan JA. The cost-benefit of Federal investment in preventing *Clostridium difficile* infections through the use of a multifaceted infection control and antimicrobial stewardship program. Infect Control Hosp Epidemiol. 2015;36:681–7.
32. Wiegand PN, Nathwani D, Wilcox MH, Stephens J, Shelbaya A, Haider S. Clinical and economic burden of *Clostridial difficile* infection in Europe: a systematic review of healthcare-facility-acquired infection. J Hosp Infect. 2012;81:1–14.
33. Marufu O, Desai N, Aldred D, Brown T, Eltringham I. Analysis of interventions to reduce the incidence of *Clostridial difficile* infection at a London teaching hospital trust, 2003-2011. J Hosp Infect. 2015;89(1):38–45.
34. Biswas JS, Patel A, Otter JA, et al. Reduction on *Clostridium difficile* environmental contamination by hospitalized patients treated with fidaxomicin. J Hosp Infect. 2015;90:267–70.

Norovirus and Other Viral Gastroenteritis

54

Abstract

New and old entero-pathogenic viruses are increasing in the society and in the healthcare, like the *Calicivirus* family (*Norovirus*, *Sapovirus*, *Astrovirus*), *Reovirus* family (*Rotavirus*) (especially infant, toddler and elderly) and rarely other viral types such as adenovirus (especially serotype 40, 41), bocavirus, parechovirus, enterovirus and a variety of other types. In all types of gastroenteritis, infection prevention measures are performed as with norovirus, described below. The following chapter is focused on practical measures to detect and prevent transmission of entero-pathogenic viruses in healthcare institutions.

Keywords

Entero-pathogenic viruses · Norovirus · Sapovirus · Rotavirus · Viral gastroenteritis, enteritis, vomiting, diarrhoea · Abdominal pain, frequent bowel movements Admission control · Pre-examination · Information · Screening · Isolation · PPE Decontamination · Environment · Eradication · Nosocomial infections Infection control · Hygiene · Prevention

54.1 Purpose

- To prevent transmission of viral gastroenteritis to patients, staff and the environment.
  - The infections are transmitted via contact, faecal-oral and/or air (droplets, aerosol).
  - Actual virus types are norovirus, sapovirus, astrovirus, rotavirus and rarely other viral types such as adenovirus (especially serotype 40, 41), bocavirus, parechovirus, enterovirus and a variety of other types [1–4].
  - For all types of viral gastroenteritis, infection prevention measures are performed as with norovirus, described below [4–7].

B. M. Andersen, *Prevention and Control of Infections in Hospitals*,
https://doi.org/10.1007/978-3-319-99921-0_54

54.2 Comprise

All close contacts of patients (patients in the same room, personnel, visitors, etc.)

All equipment, textiles, rooms and surfaces the patient has been in contact with.

54.3 Responsibility

The hospital's management provides written procedures for detecting, isolating and controlling infectious patients with norovirus and other infectious gastrointestinal viruses.

Department management implements guidelines and ensures that personnel, patients and visitors are informed of infection prevention measures in connection with outbreaks of norovirus and other viral gastroenteritis and reports to the Director about resource problems (personnel, expertise, isolates) that may expose other patients, personnel and visitors to infection.

Employees follow routines and guidelines for infection protection.

54.4 Practical Measures

54.4.1 Routine at All Admissions/Outpatient Clinics/Day Surgery

Preliminary examination: ask the patient, relatives, physician *before* admission if the patient has symptoms of gastroenteritis. This is especially important in periods of epidemics of norovirus and rotavirus; especially autumn and winter.

If suspected/confirmed viral gastroenteritis, there are at least two options: (a) postpone admission to the patients infection status is resolved; (b) admit and isolate the patient until infection status is clarified.

54.4.2 Isolation and Other Preventive Measures [4–6]

- *Index patient* is contact isolated with own toilet/shower and preferably own decontaminator. Avoid cohort isolation due to repeated outbreaks. The patient cannot walk into the corridor or common patient rooms but can walk directly out of the hospital.
- *Patients exposed*—have been in the same room as the index patient with symptoms—are isolated separately from the index case during incubation time for a minimum of 2–3 days [1–7]. Treat as possible infected.
- *Personnel wear PPE* (gown, gloves, surgical mask/cap (air transmission, especially when vomiting) and room-bound shoes that can be disinfected or shoe covers). Follow routines for taking off infection control equipment. Carefully remove any shoe covers with gloves on, and wash hands after wearing gloves.

- *The use of PPE* must be properly implemented to prevent spread of infection. Taking on PPE is carried out in a defined clean area in the sluice of the isolate or on the corridor outside the patient room. *Only clean equipment must be on the hallway!*
  - Wash or disinfect hands before donning.
  - Gown (single use), long-sleeved cuff.
  - Gloves pulled over the gown's cuff.
  - Room-bound shoes (or disposable cover). Room-bound shoes should be machine-washed at 85 °C or autoclaved.
  - Surgical mask/cap.
- *Taking off the PPE* is carried out in the defined area of the isolate sluice or in the patient room at the exit door. *Never doff in the corridor outside the isolate!*
  - If using shoe covers, these must be removed first. Gloves are used when gently removing the overcoat shoe deposited in contaminated waste.
  - Remove the gloves; grab the left glove at the wrist (not higher up) and gently turn it inside out, and use the inverted glove as a cloth to grab through to remove (roll off) the remaining glove. Learn to remove gloves without contamination!
  - Hand hygiene.
  - The gown is taken off by opening behind the back (neck)—avoid touching the front and arms—pull the cuffs over the hands, and roll the gown gently along from the sides and from above downwards without touching the outer side. Place gently in the waste bag.
  - Hand hygiene.
  - Remove surgical mask/cap by loosening back on the head—not touching the front.
  - The hands are finally washed with soap and water.
  - Use eventually a "cloth" with chloramine 5% in the sluice for wiping off the shoes. Replace this for each shift.
- *Norovirus and other intestinal pathogenic viruses* attach easily to the skin [4, 8, 9] There may be a failure effect of both handwash and hand disinfection.
- *Handwash with soap and water* may work probably better than hand disinfection and is therefore used for norovirus [4–9]. Always wear gloves when there is suspected gastrointestinal infections, and perform hand hygiene before and after use of gloves!
- *Personnel* with symptoms report sickness and stay at home for at least 2 days after symptom freedom [1, 7].
- *Inform* all personnel and visitors.
- *Visitors* should follow procedures for using PPE and hand hygiene and should not stay in common rooms, corridors, etc. together with other patients/visitors. They may be infected with the same microbiological agent and spread the infection in the department. Visitors with symptoms should be at home until 2–3 days after freedom of symptoms (except for relatives of children and critically ill).
- *Limit general access*, and avoid thoroughfare.
- *Limit surveys/treatment* of the actual patients at other departments while the outbreak is going on.

54.4.3 Other Measures [4–6]

- *Exposed healthcare professionals* should not work at other healthcare institutions or other departments before the outbreak is over.
- *Hand hygiene is* reviewed and sharpened. Alcohols have limited effects on norovirus. Therefore, important with glove use.
- *Admission stop* is considered, depending on the isolation conditions. Admission should be stopped for 48–72 h after the last new case with gastroenteritis (diarrhoea and/or vomiting).
- *Discharge of patients* who can manage at home should be considered. Do not discharge to other healthcare institution from the unit before 48–72 h after symptom freedom.
- *Drinks and food service,* etc. *on the corridor are removed.* The ice maker machine is emptied, decontaminated and washed. Should not be used during outbreaks at the department. Do not use common coffee machines, etc. on the corridor. No self-service.
- *Report to infection control unit daily while the outbreak is going on.*
- *Closure and disinfection of wards.* Occasionally, the entire department must be closed, emptied and disinfected. Particularly important are common service rooms, equipment stores, clean textile rooms, kitchens, etc.

54.4.4 Sampling

Preferably, only aqueous, loose faeces samples if not epidemiological examination. Faeces from patients in the acute phase and preferably within the first 3 days (up to 7 days) after the disease starts. Take samples from all cases during the primary outbreak, including personnel with symptoms. If the outbreak continues, sampling is unnecessary if the virus is already detected. 5–10 g faeces (a spoon) is sampled in a sterile test tube and sent immediately or stored in a refrigerator until sent to the laboratory (no more than 2 days).

54.4.5 Disinfection of Rooms and Surfaces [4–7]

Environment and equipment around the patients may be heavily contaminated by norovirus or other intestinal pathogens [4–7, 10, 11]. Norovirus may survive for more than a year in the environment if not removed and if the transmission dose is very low: 10–100 virus particles [1, 4]. All decontamination should be carried out thoroughly. Proper use of effective disinfectants as 5% chloramine or 10% household bleaches (home) or peracetic acid is important [4, 7].

- *Daily disinfection* of all patient-related equipment and common touch points × 3 with alcoholic wipes (eventually, chloramine 5% or household bleach 10%).

- *Daily disinfection* with 5% chloramine; wipe over fixtures, door handles, off and on knots, the floor and all surfaces. Then use normal soap and water over the same surfaces immediately afterwards. See isolation regimens.
- *Terminal disinfection* of all rooms where the patient has stayed.
- *Hydrogen peroxide gas/aerosol* can be effective at terminal disinfection in an empty room [4, 12, 13].

54.4.6 Isolation Period, Readmission, Transfers [4–7]

- *The patient is isolated throughout the hospital stay* even after the diarrhoea/vomiting is stopped. Especially elderly can shed viruses for days to weeks after symptoms have disappeared, and up to 30% may be healthy virus carriers [1, 6, 14–17].
- *When transferring to another health institution*, inform about norovirus infection and also for patients exposed to infection.

54.5 Background Information

New and old entero-pathogenic viruses are increasing in the society and in the healthcare and may cause large, global outbreaks. The *Calicivirus* family (norovirus, sapovirus, astrovirus) and the *Reovirus* family (*rotavirus*) (especially infant, toddler and elderly) are the most common. More rarely may other viral types such as adenovirus (especially serotypes 40 and 41), bocavirus, parechovirus, enterovirus and a variety of other types (including sars) cause outbreaks [1–4]. In all types of gastroenteritis, infection prevention measures are performed as with norovirus [4–7].

54.6 Norovirus

Small, round virus with high infectivity; <10–100 virus particles are enough to start a gastroenteritis [1, 4]. Norovirus (former Norwalk virus) is the cause of "winter vomiting disease" inside and outside institutions, especially winter time (see Fig. 54.1). There is large amount of virus in vomit and faeces (10^{12} viruses/gram faeces) during acute disease, and it is rapidly transmitted via vomiting; drops/aerosols; contaminated equipment, textiles, faeces, food and water; etc. [1, 4, 7]. Epidemics are especially associated with certain genotypes with more virulent viruses that develop and change over years [1, 4].

Norovirus is heat resistant, survives 75 °C, and is also resistant to a variety of disinfectants, including chlorine in lower concentrations, and survives dry for days to months (>10 months) on equipment, textiles, food and water and otherwise in the environment [4, 7–11, 18].

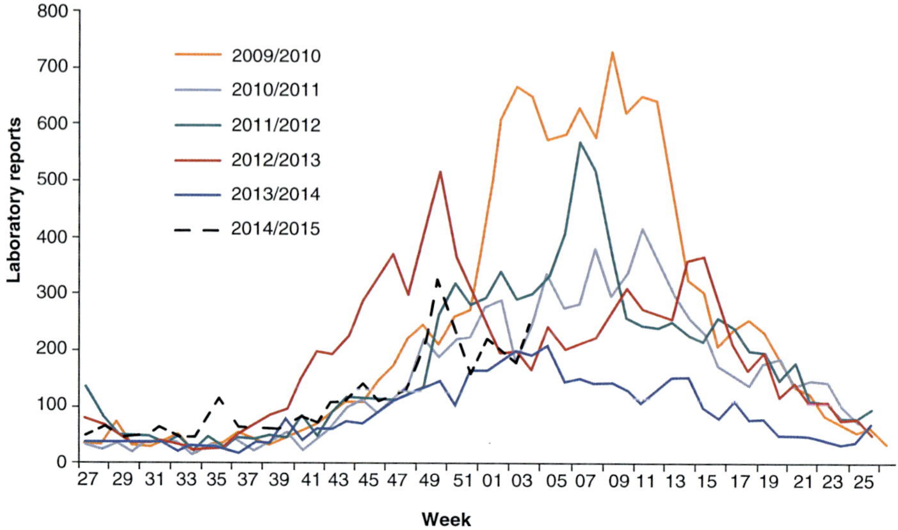

Fig. 54.1 Norovirus outbreaks causing closure of hospital wards in England: variation in seasons. In 2014, there were 690 outbreaks with closed wards in 640 cases. (Source: Public Health England. August 14, 2015) [23]

Mild disease symptoms occur in most patients, with short or no immunity, so repeated sickness may occur in the same patient, and there is no vaccine and no specific treatment. Up to 50% of a ward or department may start with symptoms approximately simultaneously (both patients and personnel) [4, 16].

Incubation time of 1/2–2 days may often start abruptly without any other symptoms other than vomiting.

Clinical symptoms: elderly and patients in a poor condition are more likely to have severe progression and longer diarrhoea and can shed viruses for a very long time [1, 4, 14, 17–19]. Symptoms include nausea, vomiting (2–3 days), diarrhoea (2–5 days), incontinence and fever 38–39 °C, of approximately 2–3 days duration.

Reinfections and subclinical infections are common.

54.6.1 Occurrence, Costs and Mortality

Global spread pattern since 1995 with more than 300 million cases a year and has become a year-round disease, although the winter frequency increases over 200-fold when people are closer together. The virus circulates in the environment and creates hyperendemic periods—especially in 2002, 2003, 2007 and 2010. In 2003, 23 million were sick of norovirus in the United States (12–13% of the population), and CDC (Centers for Disease Control and Protection) estimates that 1 in 14 people becomes ill each year [4]. Nowadays approximately 40% of all foodborne infections are caused by norovirus. It is observed as a large problem in connection with outbreaks in cruise ship traffic; up to six consecutive cruises with the same boat have led to major outbreaks [4, 20–22]. CDC register cruises with norovirus outbreaks, and Norwegian ships are often involved [21].

The major epidemic waves in the society, schools, kindergartens, colleges, universities, passenger ships, hotels, conferences, trains, military camps, sports (Olympic ski sport in 2018), etc. are steadily further entering hospitals, nursing homes and other health institutions, often with long-lasting outbreaks: 19 days in hospital at average, 16 days in nursing homes and 7 days outside the health service [4, 14–17, 20–22].

Healthcare institutions with norovirus outbreaks lead to closure of departments and even hospitals. England is continuously registering outbreaks in hospitals [23]. In 2014 there were 690 outbreaks that resulted in closure of departments/units in 640 of the cases! In the first 4 weeks of 2015, there were already 62 outbreaks that all resulted in closure of the ward [23].

Norway is experiencing larger and smaller outbreaks, especially related to food and drink, international food trade and cruise boats [20–22, 24–26]. Also hospitals and nursing homes are strongly exposed to the infection [27, 28].

Outbreaks described in Norway from the Norwegian Institute of Public Health:

- 2001: Eikedalen, Hordaland; alpine resort, 400 were sick from drinking water.
- 2003: Bergen; seminar for health professionals, > 50 were ill.
- 2005: Oslo; 2 major outbreaks, 138 soldiers (starting with the kitchen staff) and 33 cases participating in a seminar after eating food from a catering company.
- 2006: Asker and Bærum; 17 were sick from eating oysters from France—part of an international outbreak.
- 2007: Stavanger; 81 were sick in 6 different parties with food from the same catering company.
- 2008: Oslo; 70 were sick in 6 different parties been on the same restaurant. Oysters from Ireland.
- 2008: Hamar; 150 were sick after hotel stay, kitchen staff infected.
- 2008: Ullensaker; more than 200 were sick at an airport hotel. Sick kitchen workers.
- 2009: Passenger ship from Oslo to Copenhagen; 36 were ill from 5 different sport teams (orientation). Some of these were probably sick in advance.
- 2010: National outbreak; Lollo lettuce from Denmark. At least ten outbreaks.
- 2010: Cruise ship from Oslo; springtime, several hundred were sick in three different trips from Oslo with "Vision of the seas". Several returns during the cruise.
- 2012: Oslo; 41 sick at "Christmas dinner" at a hotel. Infected oysters [24, 25].
- 2015: Cruise ship, on the Norwegian Fjords, May–June; 300 or more were probably sick [22].
- In addition, outbreaks at several healthcare institutions with 40–100 people involved per outbreak, almost as many personnel as patients.

54.7 Rotavirus

The rotavirus is the most common cause of disease in small children and the elderly but can also cause epidemic outbreaks in the community and in healthcare institutions [3, 4]. 40–60% of infant gastroenteritis is caused by rotavirus. 80–90% has had rotavirus infection at 4 years of age.

Clinical symptoms: acute vomiting, followed after a few hours of heavy diarrhoea with rapid dehydration and rapid, cholera-like diarrhoea with development of dehydration and loss of electrolytes, especially in the smallest children. Sunken fontanelle in infants, hollow orbital cavity and standing skin folds are classic signs of severe dehydration in toddlers. Infants/toddlers are admitted to hospitals for observation and rehydration.

If no prompt administration and treatment with intravenous therapy, it may lead to shock and death. It is estimated that 450–750,000 children die of rotavirus infection each year, globally. Vaccine is available.

Incubation period: 1–3 days

See also references [1–4] for more information.

References

1. Dolin R, Treanor JJ. Noroviruses and sapoviruses. In: Mandell GL, Douglas RG, Bennett JE, editors. Principles and practice of infectious diseases. 8th ed. London: Elsevier Churchill Livingston; 2015. p. 2122–7.
2. Dolin R, Treanor JJ. Astrovirus and picobirnaviruses. In: Mandell GL, Douglas RG, Bennett JE, editors. Principles and practice of infectious diseases. 8th ed. London: Elsevier Churchill Livingston; 2015. p. 2128–30.
3. Dormitzer PR. Rotaviruses. In: Mandell GL, Douglas RG, Bennett JE, editors. Principles and practice of infectious diseases. 8th ed. London: Elsevier Churchill Livingston; 2015. p. 1854–64.
4. Andersen BM. Gastrointestinal virus infections. In: Handbook for hygiene and infection control for hospitals. Part 1: microbiology and infection protection. Fagbokforlaget; 2014. p. 248–54.
5. Andersen BM. Prevention of viral gastroenteritis norovirus and the like. In: Handbook for hygiene and infection control for hospitals. Ullevål University Hospital; 2008. p. 459–61.
6. Andersen BM. Prevention of viral gastroenteritis—norovirus and similar infections. In: Handbook for hygiene and infectious care for nursing homes, long-term institutions. Akademika forlag; 2013. p. 249–54.
7. CDC. Guideline for prevention and control of norovirus gastroenteritis outbreaks in healthcare settings. 2012. IX Appendices.
8. Kampf G, Grotheer D, Steinmann J. Effect of three ethanol-based hand rubs against feline calicivirus, a surrogate virus for norovirus. J Hosp Infect. 2005;60:144–9.
9. Tuladhar E, Hazeleger WC, Koopmans M, et al. Reducing viral contamination from finger pads: handwashing is more effective than alcohol-based disinfectants. J Hosp Infect. 2015;90:226–34.
10. Cheesbrough JS, Green J, Gallimore CI, Wright PA, Brown DW. Widespread environmental contamination with Norwalk-like viruses (NVL) detected in a prolonged hotel outbreak or gastroenteritis. Epidemiol Infect. 2000;125:93–8.

11. Lee N, Chan MCW, Wong B, et al. Fecal viral concentration and diarrhoea in norovirus gastroenteritis. Emerg Infect Dis. 2007;13:1399–401.
12. Andersen BM, Rasch M, Hochlin K, Jensen FH, Wismar P, Fredriksen JE. Decontamination of rooms, medical equipment and ambulances, using a dry fog or hydrogen peroxide disinfectant. J Hosp Infect. 2006;62:149–55.
13. Andersen BM, Hochlin K, Daling JP. Cleaning and decontamination of reusable medical devices, including the use of hydrogen peroxide gas decontamination. Microbiol Biochem Technol. 2012;4:57–62.
14. Gaspard P, Ambert-Balay K, Mosnier A, et al. Burden of gastroenteritis outbreaks: specific epidemiology in a cohort of institutions caring for dependent people. J Hosp Infect. 2015;91:19–27.
15. Thouillot F, Delhostal C, Edel C, et al. Gastroenteritis outbreaks in elderly homes in the east of France during winter 2009/10: aetiology research for a series of 37 outbreaks. Euro Surveill. 2012;17(9):pii: 20103.
16. Harris JP, Lopman BA, O'Bien SJ. Infection control measures for norovirus: a systematic review of outbreaks in semi-closed settings. J Hosp Infect. 2010;74:1–9.
17. Aoki Y, Suto A, Mizuta K, Ahiko T, Osaka K, Matsuzaki Y. Duration of norovirus excretion and the longitudinal course of viral load in norovirus-infected elderly patients. J Hosp Infect. 2010;75:42–6.
18. Barker J, Vipond IB, Bloomfield SF. Effects of cleaning and disinfection in reducing the spread of norovirus contamination via environmental surfaces. J Hosp Infect. 2004;58:42–9.
19. Gustavson L, Andersson LM, Lindh M, Westin J. Excess mortality following community-onset norovirus enteritis in the elderly. J Hosp Infect. 2011;79:27–31.
20. Vivancos R, Keenan A, Sopwith W, et al. Norovirus outbreak in a cruise ship sailing around the British Isles: investigation and multi-agency management of an international outbreak. J Infect. 2010;60:478–85.
21. Anonymous. Outbreak updates for international cruise ships. CDC 2015. 2015.
22. Mail on line. Passengers hit down by "horror" vomiting bug on Norwegian Fjords cruise vow never to go again "even if they paid us". 2015.
23. Anonymous. Suspected and laboratory-confirmed reported norovirus outbreaks in hospitals: outbreaks occurring in weeks 1–4. 2015. Public Health England. 2015.
24. Outbreak of norovirus infection in Norway. Institute of Public Health. 2009.
25. Steens A. Gastroenteritis outbreak during a "Christmas dinner" in a hotel in Oslo. December 2012. Public Health Institute. 2013.
26. Evanger N. Norwalk virus outbreak from marzipan cake. MSIS. 2002;30:32.
27. Andersen BM. Norovirus gastroenteritis—a challenge in and outside health institutions. Tidsskr Sykepleien. 2003;39.
28. Andersen BM, Størvold G, Vainio K. Norovirus gastroenteritis at Ullevål University Hospital. Tidsskr Nor Legeforen. 2003;123:1239.

Prion Diseases: Infection Protection

55

Abstract

Prion disease (Creutzfeldt-Jakobs disease (CJD), bovine spongiform encephalitis (BSE), "mad cow disease", etc.) is a slowly evolving degenerative disease caused by different types of "infected proteins" that can be found in all tissues and secretions from infected humans and animals (scrapie in sheep, chronic wasting disease of deer, moose, etc.). It is believed that the "infection" may also be associated with special neurodegenerative forms of dementia and other neurological diseases.

The following chapter is focused on practical measures to detect and prevent transmission of prion disease in healthcare institutions.

Keywords

Prion protein disease · Creutzfeldt-Jakobs disease · CJD · Bovine spongiform encephalitis · BSE · "Mad cow disease" · Scrapie · Prion protein scrapie (PrPsc) Chronic wasting disease · Dementia · Neurological disease · Information Screening · Isolation · PPE · Decontamination · Environment · Eradication Nosocomial infections · Infection control · Hygiene · Prevention

55.1 Purpose

- To prevent transfer of prion disease to patients, staff, visitors and environment in the hospital.
- The transmission is mainly via blood and tissue, but secretions and excretions from humans and animals may be contagious [1–16].

B. M. Andersen, *Prevention and Control of Infections in Hospitals*,
https://doi.org/10.1007/978-3-319-99921-0_55

55.2 Comprise

All patients, who are suspected of prion disease or unknown degenerative brain disease, having a rapid developing dementia. All equipment that has been used for such patients and been in contact with their tissues, secretes or mucous membranes. All patients and personnel who may be exposed to prion infection via transplants, transfusions, insecure sterilized/disinfected equipment from suspected prion cases, etc. [1–5, 17–23].

55.3 Responsibility

The hospital's management provides written procedures for diagnosing, isolating and treating patients with suspected prion disease and guidelines for how to treat potentially exposed equipment, patients and personnel.

The department management implements guidelines and reports to the Director concerning resource problems (personnel, expertise, isolation, disinfection methods) that may lead to infection risk for patients or personnel.

Employees follow routines and report if general and special preventive procedures are not followed.

55.4 Practical Measures [1–5, 17–23]

55.4.1 General Prophylaxis Against CJD and Other Prion Disease

- *Human biological material* should always be treated as potentially contagious, and procedures for this should be followed (gloves on direct contact with blood/tissue, surgical mask/screen at risk of blood/tissue spray).
- *Sterilization of instruments and equipment that penetrates skin/mucous membranes*: equipment should be autoclaved after thorough cleaning in the instrument washing machine/ultrasonic bath. Autoclaving often occurs at lower temperatures or shorter times than is necessary to remove prions!
- *Used instruments should be cleaned immediately after use*: do not let tissue/blood dry in on instruments! [3, 5, 24, 25] Instruments that dry in with protein residues are difficult to clean and can pose a risk. Prions stick strongly to steel and other metal (adhesive) [24, 25]. Therefore, instruments should be cleaned immediately (<1 min) after use; do not dry, but put into liquid.

55.4.2 Removal of Prions: General Recommendation

- Autoclaving at 134 °C for a minimum of 18 min in one pre-vacuum autoclave (no higher temperature) [1–4].
- Or at 132–134 °C for 60 min in gravity autoclave [1, 4].

This should be evaluated and used as a standard routine for autoclaving.

Note: the effect is not sure if much biological material is present, especially with variant CJD [26].

Note: formalin, ethylene oxide vapour or hydrogen peroxide has no effect on CJD!

Protein residues that are difficult to remove from instruments and equipment and are not removed or destroyed by autoclaving require new solutions today [1, 3, 5, 19–29]. Equipment like brushes and dental equipment like root canal instruments are difficult to clean between uses. In such cases disposable equipment is recommended [5, 27–29].

55.4.3 Special Prophylaxis on Suspicion or Detected CJD/Prion Disease

- *Blood contamination*: the patient is treated as "blood contamination"—infection transmitted by blood and tissue. See Chap. 17 isolation by blood-borne infection.
- *Human biological material* should always be treated as potentially contagious. Procedures should be followed: gown and double gloves on direct contact with blood/tissue and in addition surgical mask/cap/goggles/visor at risk of blood/tissue spray. All tissues/blood/secretions/mucosa from patients with suspected prion disease are considered to be infectious.
- *In case of accident*, clean the wound by 5% chloramine (or sodium hypochlorite) or 1N NaOH for 5–10 min, and then wash with soap and water. Mucous membranes exposed to possible infection: rinse with sterile saline for 5–10 min.
- *Skin contact with infectious material*: disinfect with 1N NaOH.
- *Spills mm*, start from the periphery and inwards: disinfect with 1N sodium hydroxide for 1 h.

55.4.4 Treatment of Patients with Suspected CJD/Prion Disease and Equipment Used

- Patients with suspected/proven CJD/prion disease should be treated as with blood/tissue infection.
- The patient is isolated on a single room.
- Use disposable equipment or equipment that can be disposed of (autoclaved and burned) following invasive procedures.
- In case of invasive procedures or spills, use disposal gown, double gloves, visor/goggles and cap/surgical mask.
- All equipment used for dressing is double-packed in the patient room/operating room, placed in thick yellow risk bag, labelled and sent to burn by a special transport.
- Used instruments and blood/tissue material are autoclaved/disinfected before burning (see below). Prions may survive high temperatures; therefore follow instructions carefully.

- After autoclaving/disinfection, the equipment is sent as a contaminant for burning.
- In case of uncertainty, questions, etc., contact an infection control personnel.

55.4.5 Sterilization of Instruments/Equipment Used in Examination/Treatment of Possible CJD/Prion Disease

- *Invasive equipment*: select disposable, single-use equipment or reusable equipment that can be disposed of after the actual use. Immediately after use, the equipment is immersed for 1 h in a risk container of 5% chloramine or with 1N NaOH (at room temperature) [3, 17]. Then it is autoclaved at 134 °C for 1 h, packaged as contamination and sent to burning. If prion disease is suspected retrospectively, previously used equipment is called back and subsequently processed and destroyed as above. The identity of the persons to which this equipment is used is noticed. All instruments used on patients with suspected prion disease should be detected, recorded and destroyed [3, 5, 17, 20].
- *Non-invasive* reusable equipment can either be autoclaved (as described above) or immersed in 1N NaOH (1 h) or chloramine 5% (1 h) with or without subsequent autoclaving.
- *See also* Chap. 59, *"Technical disinfection"*.

55.4.6 Disinfection of Surfaces/Environment

Follow regular routines: 5% chloramine for 1 h or 1N NaOH for 1 h.

55.5 Background Information

Prion disease (Creutzfeldt-Jakobs disease (CJD), bovine spongiform encephalitis (BSE)) is a slowly evolving degenerative disease caused by different types of "infected proteins" that can be found in all tissues and secretions from infected humans and animals (scrapie in sheep, chronic wasting disease of deer, moose, etc.) [1–15]. It is believed that the "infection" may also be associated with special neurodegenerative forms of dementia and other neurological diseases [1, 5].

Prions are infectious, modified cell proteins, atypically folded and tightly aggregated protein material of an original normal protein structure on the surface of all human and animal cells [1–3]. Prion protein scrapie (PrPsc), which causes sickness in sheep and goats, differs slightly from normal surface structure (PrPc) on human and animal cells [1–5]. A new nasal tissue test can provide a fast and reliable diagnosis [30].

Diseases in humans: kuru (cannibalism), Creutzfeldt-Jakobs disease (CJD), Gerstmann-Straussler-Scheinker (GSS, 1/40 million), fatal familial insomnia (FFI, 1 < 40 million) [1–5]. Prion disease occurs due to infection (kuru, CJD), protein mutation (CJD, GSS, FFI) and unknown (CJD). People may still be nosocomially infected; a patient developed CJD after potential surgical exposure in the United States [31]. Recently, two cases were reported in Salento (Puglia, Italy), an area with a high incidence of CJD, 4/million, against normal, 1/million [32].

Diseases in animals: scrape sickness is well known in sheep, goat, cattle and other animals. Bovine spongiform encephalitis (BSE) is also called "mad cow disease". Scrape sickness has been transferred to 1500 sheep through contaminated vaccine [5]. Otherwise, hundreds of thousands of sheep have earlier been destroyed after detection of the sickness in Norway and other countries. From 1988 to 1995 more than 160,000 cattle in the United Kingdom got bovine spongiform encephalitis (BSE) after ingestion of contaminated feed [5]. Monkeys (macaques) fed with high-dose brain material (>5 g) from cattle with BSE got—all 18 animals—prion disease after median incubation period of 4.5 years (up to 10 years) [15]. Incubation period varies for monkeys and probably also for humans. Prions can be detected in saliva from BSE-infected cattle 2 months before symptoms appear [13].

Occurrence of CJD in man: approximately 1/million people a year [1–5]. Nosocomial infections have been transmitted by coronary transplant, EEG electrodes, implantation of dura mater, human growth hormone, etc. [1–5, 18–23, 33–37]. In England there are over a hundred cases in later years of Creutzfeldt-Jakobs disease variant (vCJD): 1996–2012, 177 cases [4, 5]. These cases are infected by eating contaminated beef from cattle with bovine spongiform encephalitis (BSE). It is estimated that 1 in 2000 Britons is exposed to prion disease by vCJD. Several hundred are exposed to uncertainly cleaned instruments [4, 5, 37, 38]. It is assumed that only 1–3 Norwegians may have been infected during the relevant period (1986–1996) of infected meat in the United Kingdom or from imported meat to Norway [39]. Chronic wasting disease is recently detected among some flocks of reindeers in Norway. The infected flocks are taken out. However, there is a certain prevalence of prion disease (Fig. 55.1) [5].

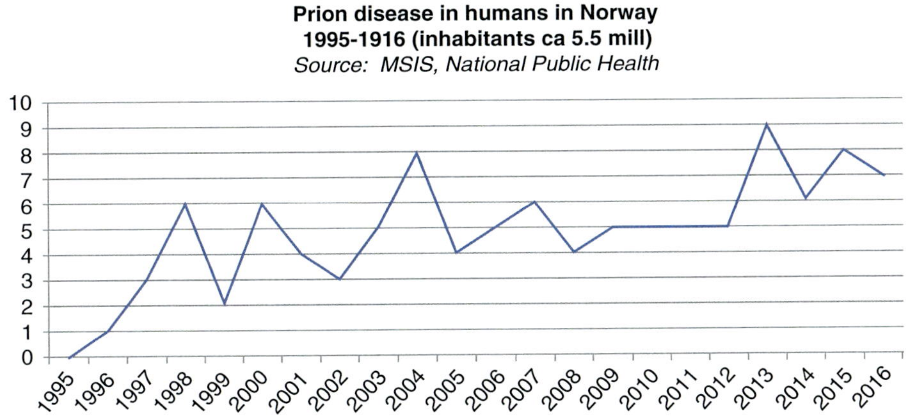

Fig. 55.1 Prion disease in humans in Norway 1995–1916 (inhabitants ca 5.5 million). *Source: MSIS, National Public Health*

The infection is widespread and consists of small cellular protein molecules that can be found in the blood, lymphoid tissue, tonsils, brain, spinal cord and fluid, appendix, kidney, spleen, lung, etc. [5].

Resistant infectious agents are resistant to high temperatures and chemical substances and have a very long survival in the environment. Therefore, it is important to follow special routines and measures in case of suspected or detected prion disease. Contaminated electrodes stored in ethanol and formalin for several years have been shown to induce CJD in chimpanzees. Four chemicals may reduce prions with >4 logs, of which chlorine (>10,000 ppm for 1 h) show the most consistent prion inactivation. One to 2N NaOH may have failing effect, and aldehydes may increase prion resistance (see also technical disinfection).

Incubation varies in relation to type of prion disease and transmission of infection—from 18 months (intracerebral instrumentation, corneal transplant) up to 40 years (human growth hormone, etc.).

Symptoms: subacute to chronic developing dementia in the ages 40–70 years, cerebellar symptoms, ataxia, insomnia and autonomic dysfunction.

Disease time to death: 4–12 months.

55.6 New Prion Diseases

New types and variations of prion diseases are detected as diagnostics is getting better. The last type is "Shy-Drager syndrome" (multiple system atrophy—MSA) that "raises the question of whether or not also Alzheimer's and Parkinsonism are contagious" [40]. This syndrome has also misfolding of prion protein (PrP) with accumulation of a substance (alpha-synuclein) in the brain [40]. "All chemicals that kill bacteria and viruses do not harm prions" [40].

References

1. Bosque PJ, Tyler KL. Prions and prion disease of the central nervous system (Transmissible neurodegenerative diseases). In: Mandell GL, Douglas RG, Bennetts JE, editors. Principles and practice of infectious diseases. 8th ed. London: Elsevier Churchill Livingston; 2015. p. 2142–53.
2. Prusiner SB. Prions of humans and animals. In: Mahy BWJ, Collier L, editors. Topley & Wilson. Virology. London: Arnold; 1998. p. 805–31.
3. Rutala WA, Weber DJ. Disinfection, sterilization, and control of hospital waste. In: Mandell GL, Douglas RG, Bennetts JE, editors. Principles and practice of infectious diseases. 8th ed. London: Elsevier Churchill Livingston; 2015. p. 3296–309. (3305).
4. Government, UK. Infection prevention and control of CJD, vCJD and other human prion diseases in healthcare and community settings. Transmissible spongiform encephalopathy agents: Safe working and the prevention of infection: Part 4. Revised and updated January 2014.
5. Andersen BM. Prion disease (Creutzfeldt-Jacob's disease-CJD, etc.). In: Handbook in hygiene and infection control for hospitals. Part 1: microbiology and infection protection. Fagbokforlaget; 2014. p. 351–5.

6. Gambetti P, Dong Yan J, et al. A novel human disease with abnormal prion protein sensitive to protease. Ann Neurol. 2008;63:697–708.
7. Promed mail January 12, 2005. Chronic wasting disease update 2006: USA.
8. Promed mail September 9, 2009. Chronic wasting disease, cervids—USA: disease spread. Healthy deer can spread prion disease through faeces.
9. Gregory L, Kovac's GG, Alexeeva I, Budka H, Rohwer RG. Excretion of transmissible spongiform encephalopathy infectivity in urine. Emerg Infect Dis. 2008;14:1406–12.
10. Gonzales-Romero D, Barria MA, Leon P, et al. Detection of infectious prions in urine. FEBS Letters, online. Promed mail August 12, 2008.
11. Douet JY, Zafar S, Perret-Liaudet A, et al. Detection of infectivity in blood of persons with variant and sporadic Creutzfeldt-Jacob's disease. Emerg Infect Dis. 2014;20:114–7.
12. Tamgney G, Miller MW, Wolfe LL, et al. Asymptomatic deer excrete infectious prions in faeces. Nature. 2009;461:529–32.
13. Okada H, Murayama Y, Shimozaki N, et al. Prion in saliva or bovine spongiform encephalopathy—infected cattle. Emerg Infect Dis. 2012;18:2091–2.
14. Bellworthy J, Dexter G, Stack M, et al. Natural transmission of BSE between sheep within an experimental flock. Vet Rec. 2005;157:206.
15. Holznagel E, Yutzy B, Schultz-Schaeffer W, et al. Foodborne transmission or bovine spongiform encephalopathy to nonhuman primates. Emerg Infect Dis. 2013;19:712–20.
16. Gill ON, Spencer Y, Richard-Loendt A, et al. Prevalent abnormal prion protein in human appendixes after bovine spongiform encephalopathy epizootic: large scale survey. BMJ. 2013;347:15675.
17. Andersen BM. Prevention of prion disease. In: Handbook in hygiene and infection control for hospitals. Ullevål University Hospital; 2008. p. 462–5.
18. Alcalde-Cabero E, Almazan-Isla J, Brandel JP, et al. Health professions and risk of sporadic Creutzfeldt-Jakob disease, 1965 to 2010. Eurosurveillance. 2012;17.
19. NHS. Patient safety and reduction of risk of transmission of Creutzfeldt-Jakob disease (CJD) via interventional procedures. Interventional procedure guidance 196. 2008.
20. Belay ED, Blase J, Schulster LM, Maddox RA, Sconberger LB. Management of neurosurgical instruments and patients exposed to Creutzfeldt-Jakob disease. Infect Control Hosp Epidemiol. 2013;34:1272–80.
21. McDonnel G, Dehan C, Perrin A, et al. Cleaning, disinfection and sterilization of surface prion contamination. J Hosp Infect. 2013;85:268–73.
22. Fishman M, Fort GG, Mikolich DJ. Prevention of Creutzfeldt-Jakob disease in health care workers: a case study. Am J Infect Control. 1998;26:74–9.
23. Herve R, Secker TJ, Keevil CW. Current risk of iatrogenic Creutzfeldt-Jakob disease in the UK: efficacy of available cleaning chemistries and reusability of neurosurgical instruments. J Hosp Infect. 2010;75:309–13.
24. Secker TJ, Herve R, Keevil CW. Adsorption of prion and tissue proteins to surgical stainless steel surfaces and the effectiveness of decontamination following dry and wet storage conditions. J Hosp Infect. 2011;78:251–5.
25. Lipscomb IP, Pinchin H, Collin R, Keevil CW. Effect of drying time, ambient temperature and pre-soaks on prion-infected tissue contamination levels on surgical stainless steel: concerns about prolonged transportation of instruments from theatre to central sterile service departments. J Hosp Infect. 2007;65:72–7.
26. Fernie K, Hamilton S, Somerville RA. Limited efficacy of steam sterilization to inactivate vCJD infectivity. J Hosp Infect. 2012;80:46–51.
27. Walker JT, Dickinson J, Sutton JM, Raven NDH, Marsh PD. Clean ability of dental instruments—implications of residual protein and risks from Creutzfeldt-Jakob disease. Br Dent J. 2007;203:395–401.
28. Walker JT, Budge C, Vassey M, et al. vCJD and the clean ability of endodontic files: a case for single use. Endo. 2009;3:115–20.

29. Spongiform Encephalopathy Advisory Committee (SEAC). VCJD and dentistery. 2007.
30. Promed mail August 6, 2014. Prion disease update: nasal tissue test.
31. Promed mail February 11, 2014. Creutzfeldt-Jakob's disease—USA, potential surgical exposure.
32. Promed mail August 11, 2015. Creutzfeldt-Jacob disease—Italy Puglia.
33. Brown P, Brandel JP, Sato T, et al. Iatrogenic Creutzfeldt-Jakob disease, final assessment. Emerg Infect Dis. 2012;18:901–7.
34. Appleby BS, Lu M, Bizzi A, et al. Iatrogenic Creutzfeldt-Jakob disease from commercial cadaveric human growth hormone. Emerg Infect Dis. 2013;19:682–4.
35. Promed mail February 9, 2006. CJD (new variant)—UK: 3 [RD] transfusion-related case.
36. Promed mail September 20, 2013. Creutzfeldt-Jakob disease—USA: transmission risk.
37. Promed mail November 27, 2013. Prion disease update 2013: instrument sterilization controversy.
38. Promed mail March 5, 2014. Prion disease update 2014: vCJD blood test verified.
39. Blystad H, Hareide B. Creutzfeldt-Jakob's disease in Norway. MSIS. 2001;29:25.
40. Promed mail 7 September 2015. Prion disease update: novel prion disease, Shy-Drager syndrome.

Tuberculosis: Control in Hospitals 56

Abstract

Tuberculosis (TB) has increased globally since 1975 and today is the most common cause of death worldwide, by communicable diseases. One out of 3–4 people in the world has been infected with TB, and about 10% of them get symptoms. Ten million new tuberculosis cases occur each year; 95% of these are in developing countries in Asia and Africa. More than 1000 new cases occur every hour of the year, more than 3.5 million patients are major spreaders of TB and more than three million die every year of tuberculosis. Most patients, 60–80%, have pulmonary tuberculosis. TB is caused by a slow-growing, robust bacterium, called *Mycobacterium tuberculosis*. A wide variety of *Mycobacteria* called the *Mycobacterium tuberculosis* complex are causing the same severe clinical course as TB. Vague symptoms like coughing, night sweats and weight loss may occur 1–2 years after exposed to infection in 10% of the cases. The disease is difficult to detect in previously poor and weakened patients in hospitals. Multidrug-resistant tuberculosis (MDR-TB), resistant to minimum rifampicin and isoniazid, is widely spread and occurs during incomplete therapy. MDR accounts for at least 3–6% of the cases in Europe. In areas with very high incidence of TB like in Mongolia, treatment may fail in one out of three cases, and MDR-TB occurs during relapses. In 2012, totally resistant TB bacteria were detected in India. Problems are all concerning how to detect, isolate and treat such cases. *Remember, cardinal* symptoms are persistent cough, weight loss and night sweats! Only one single TB bacterium can cause disease and may survive for up to 1 year in the environment! The following chapter is focused on practical measures to detect and prevent transmission of tuberculosis in healthcare institutions.

Keywords

Mycobacterium tuberculosis · *M. tuberculosis* complex · Tuberculosis · TB Pulmonary disease · Multidrug resistance · MDR · Information · Screening Isolation · PPE · Respirator · Airborne infection · Decontamination · Environment Eradication · Nosocomial infections · Infection control · Hygiene · Prevention

B. M. Andersen, *Prevention and Control of Infections in Hospitals*,
https://doi.org/10.1007/978-3-319-99921-0_56

56.1 Purpose

- To prevent transfer of TB to patients, staff, visitors and environment in the hospital.
- The transmission is mainly airborne, but secretions and excretions from humans and animals (bovine and other types of tuberculosis) may be contagious [1–16].

56.2 Comprise

Patients, personnel, visitors, equipment, medical equipment, textiles, rooms and surfaces and the complete environment exposed to TB.

56.3 Responsibility [2, 4–8]

The hospital's management is (according to law and regulation) responsible for written practices regarding training, proper preventive measures, isolation, control, contact tracing and information concerning TB infection. The management shall ensure satisfactory isolation and competent personal and adequate personal protective equipment (PPE).

Department management is responsible for implementing hospital routines, for training and information of personnel and patients and for informing hospital management in case of lack of capacity, expertise or infection control equipment.

The Occupational Safety and Health Department/Occupational Health Services should monitor exposed and infected persons and conduct environmental investigations in collaboration with lung medicine specialists, infection control units, specialist in infectious diseases and the tuberculosis coordinator.

Every employee has personal responsibility to report about suspected or detected TB. All personnel are required to inform if exposed to tuberculosis in or outside the hospital or after travelling/working in areas with high incidence of tuberculosis. In such cases there may be state control routines [5].

56.4 Practical Measures

56.4.1 Prevention of Tuberculosis in the Society [2, 4–10]

The level of infection control concerning tuberculosis has been reduced in many developed countries, like in Norway, during the last 15–20 years. It has always been a great variation concerning prevention of TB: vaccination and screening of the population. This is described for Norway as a special approximation to the problem. From the BCG vaccination of all children, tuberculin tests and lung X-ray screen surveys around the country, the Norwegian healthcare system has turned away from the problem. The general social control has disappeared together with the disappearance of vaccination, TB tests and X-ray control [5]. Only defined risk persons are examined and vaccinated [5]. This is in spite of a steady increase in tuberculosis and imports of more resistant bacteria [2, 3, 5].

Screen examination (lung X-ray) of risk groups is now only undertaken for asylum reception, suspicion of pulmonary tuberculosis and infection detection and screening of particularly vulnerable groups, like drug addicts. Also elderly with previous positive screenshots should be followed up for clinical suspicion of relapses, but this is not performed as a routine today in many countries, including Norway.

BCG vaccination was performed until 2009 in Norway, as a voluntary part of the childhood vaccination program, and was given at approximately 14 years of age. The BCG vaccination for all children was stopped in 2009. The protective effect of the vaccine has been considered to be up to 80% of the first 4 years after vaccination and later on a certain protection against military tuberculosis [1, 2]. Groups recommended for BCG vaccine *after* 2009 are in Norway:

- Tuberculin-negative persons without prior BCG vaccination, coming from risk areas and staying in Norway for more than 3 months.
- Unvaccinated persons in contact with (been in the same room as) detected cases of contagious lung tuberculosis
- Unvaccinated persons who are travelling to TB-risk areas.
- Children in whom one or both parents are from countries with high incidence of tuberculosis.
- Healthcare personnel.

Control of immigrants and others [5]:

- All persons who come from risk areas for tuberculosis and who stayed in Norway for more than 3 months are obliged to undergo tuberculin tests. X-ray thorax (screenshot) is required for all over 15 years.
- All persons who have been exposed to tuberculosis infection (been in the same room as) must be checked.
- Specific provisions are available regarding tuberculosis and later control of certain occupational groups: healthcare workers, military, teachers, childcare workers and workers on ships and oil platforms.

See Chap. 10. also the section on TB control of healthcare professionals.

56.4.2 Tuberculosis Prevention in the Hospital [2, 5, 11, 12]

56.4.2.1 Admission/Examination/Treatment/Outpatient Clinic in Hospital

- If known or suspected tuberculosis, directly admit in isolate for airborne disease with the use of PPE, including respiratory protection P3 mask. No more contact tracing if proper infection control has been completed, including transport by ambulance.

- If unknown or suspected tuberculosis—without correct use of contraceptive measures—see below.

56.4.2.2 Unknown/Suspected Tuberculosis Detected After Admission in the Hospital

The department management determines the patient's infection status in cooperation with infection control personnel and sends a report to the Occupational Health Department/Corporate Health Service with the following information:

- Name of the department, name of the infectious patient, date of birth and address.
- The period the patient was admitted in the department.
- Name and date of birth of staff who have been in close contact with the patient (cared for, examined, treated, been in the same room as, etc.) and total exposure time.
- Occupational health department/corporate health service, etc. conducts tbc tests and follow-up of employees exposed to infection, in collaboration with infection control unit/lung specialist.
- The department management at the relevant department where infection was detected is responsible for informing patients on the same room as the index patient, relatives and other close contact persons and referred to investigation. Contact the TB coordinator in primary healthcare for proven tuberculosis.

56.4.2.3 Follow-Up of Superinfected (BCG-Vaccinated), Infected (Tuberculin Positive, Not BCG-Vaccinated) and TB-Disease Among the Staff

Registration is done by the occupational health department/company health service in cooperation with lung specialist/infection control. Overview of site of infection, number of infected persons and time of infection should be included in the annual report from the occupational health department/company health service.

56.4.2.4 Measures for Patients with Infectious Tuberculosis, Not Isolated from Admission

- The department's responsible physician is informed immediately. Patients with infectious pulmonary tuberculosis should be placed directly in isolation for airborne diseases.
- The patient is placed in a single room if no isolate is available immediately, and the procedure for air isolation should be followed with gloves, protective gown, cap and respiratory protective device, P3 mask. See Chap. 18 on airborne/droplet infection isolation.
- During transport, the patient should use a surgical mask or respirator. The staff should be informed of suspected TB and use adequate PPE (gloves, own, cap and respiratory protection, P3 mask). The ambulance is subsequently disinfected with chloramine 5%.

- The department management records personnel (including ambulance staff) and patients who may have been exposed to infection, i.e. have *not* used adequate infection protection equipment. This is important for the tracing of TB in cooperation with the occupational health services.
- Room disinfection with chloramine 5% is carried out on the patient's room and toilet/bath and other rooms where the patient has stayed. See procedures for disinfection.
- In the case of detected pulmonary tuberculosis, medical devices used in the patient's room should be considered as a possible risk in use for other patients. If the equipment draws air from the room for cooling of the inside engine / electrical parts and cannot be disinfected in a safe way with regard to TB, it should not be used by other patients. Disposed as infectious waste after use.

56.4.3 Contact Tracing of Exposed or Infected Cases

Contact tracing is required among all contacts of a TB-infected patient with infectious lung tuberculosis. Contact tracing is also done for all newly infected cases, superinfected (BCG-vaccinated with a large tuberculin response) and infected (tuberculin highly positive, not BCG-vaccinated)—with and without symptoms. All exposed to infection, patients, visitors, and anyone who has been in the same room as an infectious TB patient, should be followed up.

The department management, in cooperation with the infection control unit/corporate health service, is responsible for infection detection/information in the hospital, as well as information to other healthcare institutions that have had contact with the patient. The local authority/tuberculosis coordinator is responsible for contact tracing outside the hospital (nursing home, healthcare centre, home nursing, etc.).

56.4.3.1 Infectious Lung Tuberculosis

- Patients in the same room as the index patient, visitors to the room, staff who have been in contact with or treated the index patient, and cleaners and other service personnel who have been in the patient's room should—*regardless of length of contact time with the patient*—be tested first [1, 2].
- Tuberculin samples must be made of relevant persons who have been in close contact—in the same room—as the infectious person.
- Tuberculin test should be repeated after 8 weeks in tuberculin-negative and in BCG-vaccinated subjects without significant increases from previous tuberculin tests.
- Screenshot (X-ray) is not applicable initially since early changes cannot be observed by this method.
- In case of suspected findings in personnel or persons with superinfection/infection, refer to the pulmonary clinic/diagnostic station.
- In case of positive findings, TB infection, in a person in the environment around the index patient, the second person's contacts should be investigated further.
- BCG vaccination of tuberculin-negative persons in the TB patient's immediate environment should be considered and is usually recommended.

56.4.3.2 Newly Infected (Tuberculin Test Positive, No BCG Vaccination)

- The purpose is to find the source of infection, i.e. a person with infectious pulmonary tuberculosis.
- In addition to anamnesis (family and person history), lung X-ray examination of close contacts is the most important investigation.
- Tuberculin samples of people in the local contact area.

56.4.4 Special Occupational Groups

When infectious tuberculosis is detected in a person belonging to specific occupational groups like healthcare professionals, sickness leave is provided as long as the disease is considered contagious. The assessment is carried out in collaboration with diagnostic stations and specialists in infectious medicine/pulmonary medicine.

56.4.4.1 Reports and Information [4, 5, 8]

- Tuberculosis is a nominative mandatory (group A disease) to the National Public Health.
- Physicians who detect or suspect tuberculosis should report this to the local authority, the tuberculosis coordinator and the National Public Health Institute. A copy of the message must be kept in the patient's journal.
- Also send a message to the hospital's infection control unit in cases where an infectious person is to be hospitalized or recently been hospitalized or been in other institutions.
- Use the report form.
- Healthcare institutions, policlinics, laboratories and healthcare centres are also responsible for reporting tuberculosis.
- Nurses, midwives and health sisters who, in their professional practice, suspect that a patient has a contagious tuberculosis are obliged to immediately in writing and orally notify the local medical authority/infection control doctor in the community where the person is staying [4, 5, 8].

56.5 Background Information

Tuberculosis (TB) has increased again since 1975 and is the most common cause of death worldwide caused by communicable disease [1, 2, 13, 17]. One out of 3–4 people in the world have been infected with TB, and about 10% develop the disease [1, 2]. Ten million new tuberculosis cases occur each year; 95% of these are in developing countries in Asia and Africa. More than 1000 new cases occur every hour of the year, more than 3.5 million patients are major spreaders of TB and more than three million die every year of tuberculosis.

Most patients, 60–80%, have pulmonary tuberculosis. TB is caused by a slow-growing, robust bacterium, called *Mycobacterium tuberculosis*. A wide variety of

Mycobacteria called the *Mycobacterium tuberculosis* complex are causing the same severe clinical course as TB [1]. Vague symptoms like coughing, night sweats and weight loss may occur 1–2 years after being exposed to infection in 10% of the cases. The disease is difficult to detect in previously poor and weakened patients in hospitals.

56.5.1 Definitions

- *Tuberculin* positive: person with positive reaction in the tuberculin test (Mantoux). In unvaccinated persons, a positive test may be a sign that the person is infected with TB.
- *Mantoux method*: replaces *Piquet* testing from July 2004 (Norway) and is performed by inserting 0.1 mL tuberculin intracutaneously in the left forearm. Reading will take place after 72 h (3 days). Positive test is induration of 6 mm or more.
- *A newly infected person is* defined differently depending on whether the person is BCG-vaccinated or not.
- *Natural positive*: previously tuberculin-negative, unvaccinated person who has become tuberculin *positive* due to infection.
- *Superinfected person*: enhanced tuberculin reaction as a result of TB infection in a former BCG-vaccinated person.
- *Person with infectious tuberculosis*: a person with clinical signs of tuberculous pulmonary disease or other tuberculous disease that may be contagious. Tuberculosis in other organs other than the lungs is infrequently infectious. Exceptions are tuberculosis in skin and during operative treatment with incision in tuberculous tissue.
- *Vaccinated person*: a person who is vaccinated (BCG) against tuberculosis and after which has a scar in the skin as a result of the vaccination.
- *The BCG vaccine*: probably protects against tuberculosis from the first 4 years after vaccination and may perhaps have a suppressing effect on later disease development [1]. But BCG vaccination does not prevent superinfection, i.e. infection with tuberculosis bacteria and development of primary complex. A number of countries do not use the BCG vaccine but follow up health professionals with regular/annual tuberculin tests. There have been many voices for and against the BCG vaccine, but historically it seems that it has worked in Norway, along with other measures [1, 2]. Due to increased incidence and resistance development, the author recommends the BCG vaccine until a better vaccine is available.
- *MDR-TB* (*multidrug-resistant tuberculosis*): resistant to rifampicin and isoniazid as a minimum is widely spread, both in developing countries and in industrialized countries such as Norway, and occurs during incomplete therapy [1, 2, 18–25]. MDR accounts for at least 3–6% of the cases in Europe. In areas with very high incidence of TB, like in Mongolia, treatment may fail in one out of three cases, and MDR-TB occurs during relapses [24].

- *XDR-TB* (*extensively drug-resistant tuberculosis*): a rare type of MDR-TB which is also resistant to fluoroquinolones and against one or more of second-line medications against TB [2].
- *Total resistance*: in 2012, totally resistant TB bacteria were detected in India [2, 20]. There are major problems related to how to detect, isolate and treat such cases [1, 2].

In Norway, 300–400 people are diagnosed with tuberculosis each year (5.5–7.3 per 100,000 inhabitants), hence about 2/3 with lung tuberculosis [1, 2], mostly younger immigrants or older Norwegians. In 2014, 327 cases of the *M. tuberculosis* complex were detected against 401 cases in 2013 [3]. Of these, 175 were born in Africa, 98 in Asia, 29 in Europe outside Norway, 2 in America and only 23 in Norway [3]. Nearly 13% of isolates tested were resistant to isoniazid, 3.8% against rifampicin, 2.6% against ethambutol, 10.6% against streptomycin, 7.2% against pyrazinamide and 3.8% were MDR-TB. One case had extended resistance, XDR-TB, against a variety of good medicaments [3].

56.5.2 Risk in Hospitals

In hospitals, an accumulation of patients with undiagnosed tuberculosis may lead to transmission to the environment and to patients, personnel and visitors that are infected (previously not BCG-vaccinated) or superinfected (previously BCG-vaccinated). Many patients with reduced infection defences due to poor general condition may increase the risk of TB spread and development.

Nosocomial infection is not uncommon and is caused by a number of factors such as lack of isolation, improper use of personal protective equipment, improper room ventilation, delayed or lack of diagnosis, extrapulmonary forms of TB, lack of monitoring and follow-up of close contacts and inadequate treatment and control [1, 2, 13–16, 23, 24, 26–35].

TB is a lurking, chronic respiratory disease with cough, night sweats and weight loss. Therefore, the disease is difficult to detect if not thought about.

56.5.3 Transmission

Tuberculosis is transmitted primarily through air (airborne) from a patient with pulmonary tuberculosis and with large amounts of bacteria in the sputum. Transmission can also occur via contact, food, water, milk, waste, etc. In water, atypical mycobacteria are often the most important for patients with reduced infection defences.

Mycobacterium tuberculosis can under favourable conditions live in the environment for up to 1 year, and only one single bacterium is enough to cause infection [1, 2]. An index case with lung tuberculosis can infect about 20 other people, and 10% of them get symptoms, usually within 1–2 years [1, 2]. The other 90% may have a primary complex, usually in the lungs, with live, inactive bacteria, which rarely may be reactivated later in life, especially in patients with severely impaired immune defence.

Reservoir is mainly infected humans, but some animals (pigs, cattle) may also be TB infected; a former very important way of transmission [1, 2]. The bacterium survives in a dry state without access to sunlight (kills the bacterium) and can stay alive outside the human body, for example, in dried sputum, in handkerchiefs, on floors, etc. When a person suffering from infectious pulmonary tuberculosis coughs, sneezes, talks, laughs, etc., small bacteria-containing aerosols of droplets and droplet nuclei are spread in the air; may re-aerosolize via particles, skin cells, dust, etc.; and can stay in the room for a long time. The smallest droplets can reach the alveoli in the lungs after inhalation. In rare cases, infection can be transmitted through basil-containing dust that is inhaled. Tuberculosis in other organs other than the lungs and in the skin is usually not contagious (OBS surgery, rupture of tuberculosis abscesses and the like). *Mycobacterium bovis* may infect through unpasteurized milk. *Mycobacteria* are relatively resistant to a variety of disinfectants but are killed by chloramine 5% for 1 h [1, 2].

56.5.4 Symptoms/Development

- Development from infection to increased tuberculin reaction takes 4–8 weeks, i.e. natural infected or superinfected, but usually not ill. After about 3 months, changes in the lungs can sometimes be seen by X-rays. Ca.10 % develop tuberculosis after 1-2 years, but TB may also develop many years after the time of infection. The risk of getting sick decreases over the years but is present for the rest of life [1, 2].
- Early stage of active pulmonary tuberculosis may proceed without symptoms.
- *Main symptoms of lung tuberculosis* are *persistent cough* (with or without purulent expectorate), *emaciation and night sweats.* Presence of slackness, fever, chest pain (pleural pain), etc. may vary.
- Tuberculosis can later attack many organs in the body outside the lungs, for example, the lymph nodes, bones, joints, kidneys, bowel, skin, pleura and meninges. The symptoms of extrapulmonary tuberculosis depend on the affected organ. In poor general condition, prolonged fever can be the only symptom of tuberculosis, both pulmonary and extrapulmonary.

56.5.5 Diagnosis

X-ray examination, tuberculin test (Mantoux), blood tests and detection of tuberculosis bacteria by direct microscopy and culture of expectorate, bronchial fluid, urine, faeces, pus or tissue biopsies. Cultivation takes 2–6 weeks, but faster diagnostics are performed using genetic technology.

- Suspected pulmonary tuberculosis: at least three expectorate samples, one sample each day for 3 consecutive days.

- Samples are taken from the first sputum in the morning before the patient eats. The patient has to cough up deeply from the chest, preferably promoted by physical therapy.
- The samples are taken on a sterile plastic container without addition and placed in a refrigerator for shipment to the laboratory.
- Pencil samples may also be taken from larynx or via bronchoscopy and aspirate from abscesses.

56.5.6 Airborne Isolation and Treatment

- In case of drug-sensitive pulmonary tuberculosis, airborne isolation regime for the first 3 weeks of treatment and for drug-resistant TB for 8 weeks or more. Infectious pulmonary tuberculosis must be isolated as long as TB is detected in respiratory samples.
- Combination treatment with multiple medications (usually four) is given, and the duration of the treatment is at least 6 months. Further treatment is conducted as DOT treatment, i.e. directly observed therapy.
- For MDR-TB, treatment lasts for at least 18 months with up to eight different tuberculosis drugs. There are at least 1500 MDR cases detected in the European region each year, especially the eastern part [36]. The treatment effect is poor; half of the cases dies or has treatment failures.
- XDR-TB bacteria are highly resistant, also against one or more second-line drugs against tuberculosis. A total of 10–15% of the approximately 1500 MDR cases are XDR-TB [36]. Only one in four carries out successful treatment, and many die.
- The expenses for treatment are usually covered by the State.

56.5.7 Tracing Tuberculous Infection in Primary Care [5, 10]

The coordinator for TB and local authority/district physician are responsible for tracing infections in the index patient's family and contacts (work, school, institutions, etc.). Tracing of infection is required when detecting contagious lung tuberculosis or newly infected cases.

56.5.7.1 Infectious Lung Tuberculosis

- Find newly infected among contacts of the index case.
- The nearest contacts are tested first (family, friends, work-colleagues).
- Tuberculin test of relevant persons is carried out.
- Tuberculin test should be repeated after 8 weeks in tuberculin-negative and in BCG-vaccinated subjects without significant increase from previous tuberculin results.
- Natural infected cases or persons with TB superinfection are referred to the pulmonary clinic/infectious disease department for further diagnosis.

- If the person around the index patient has a positive finding, new investigation of this person's immediate contacts is needed.
- BCG vaccination of tuberculin-negative persons in the index patients' immediate environment should be considered.

56.5.7.2 Newly Infected Persons

- The source of infection may be a person with infectious pulmonary tuberculosis.
- Information, X-ray and examination of close contacts.
- Tuberculin tests of close contacts.

56.5.7.3 Professional Groups

If infectious tuberculosis is detected in a person belonging to specific occupational groups, e.g. healthcare personnel and other caregivers, teacher, food producers, military, etc., sick leave must be approved as long as the local authority considers the disease to be infectious. Evaluation is done in cooperation with specialists in infectious medicine/lung medicine.

56.5.8 Today's Situation and the Future

Tuberculosis should be eliminated as a serious fatal disease, already 40 years ago. However, today the disease is still increasing worldwide, and the bacteria are becoming increasingly resistant. The situation has been compared to the early twentieth century, before antituberculous drugs were invented.

The ECDC (European Centre for Disease Prevention and Control) reported in 2015 that 360,000 Europeans developed tuberculosis in 2013: 1000 people every day! [36] There has been a certain decline in new cases in the West of Europe, while there may be an increase in East Europe from 2013 to 2015; see charts from ECDC (Fig. 56.1) [36, 37]. The low endemic countries in the European region report less than 20 TB cases per 100,000 inhabitants per year. North, Western and Southern Europe are included in this group.

ECDC and WHO have defined 18 high-risk countries for tuberculosis in the European region:

"Armenia, Azerbaijan, Belarus, Bulgaria, Estonia, Georgia, Kazakhstan, Kyrgyzstan, Latvia, Lithuania, Moldova, Romania, Russia, Tajikistan, Turkey, Turkmenistan, Ukraine and Uzbekistan" [36]. These 18 generate 85% of all new TB cases in the European region and also had the most deaths of the 38,000 TB-related deaths in 2013 [36].

56.5.9 MDR-TB

Still, there are in Europe a high number of patients infected with multidrug-resistant tuberculosis; about 1500 cases or more are reported each year, but there may be some reduction from 2013 to 2015; see Figs. 56.2 and 56.3 [36, 37]. In Western Europe, including Norway, MDR-TB is largely linked to immigration [36].

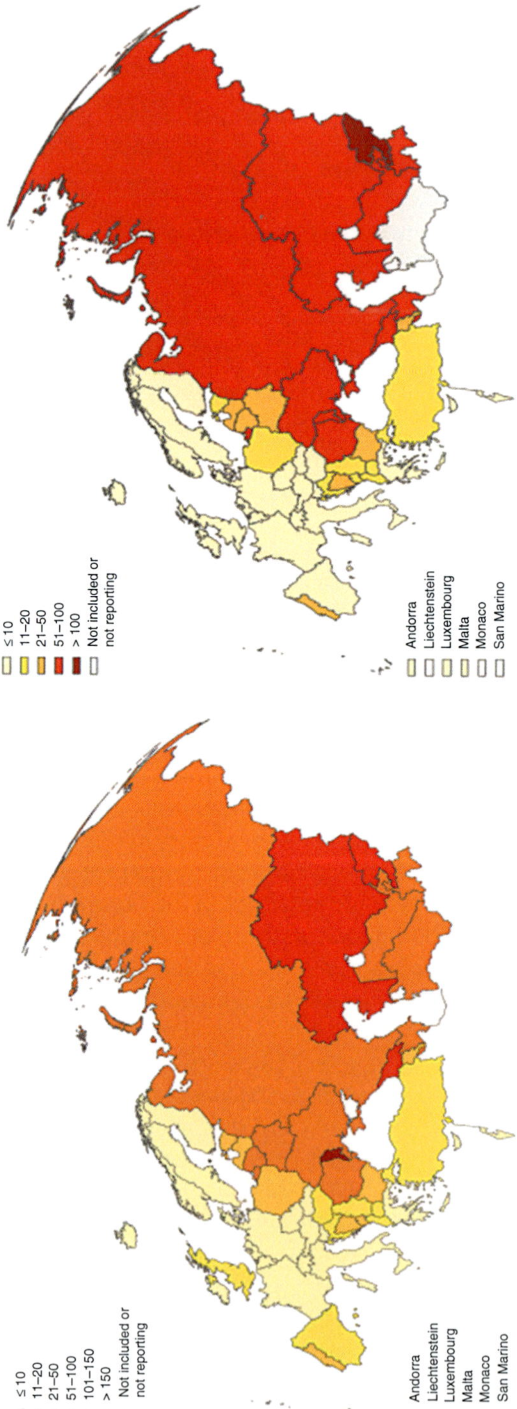

Fig. 56.1 **(a, b)** Tuberculosis incidence per 100 000 inhabitants, European region, 2013 (left) and 2015 (right). Source: ECDC 2015 and 2017 [36, 37]

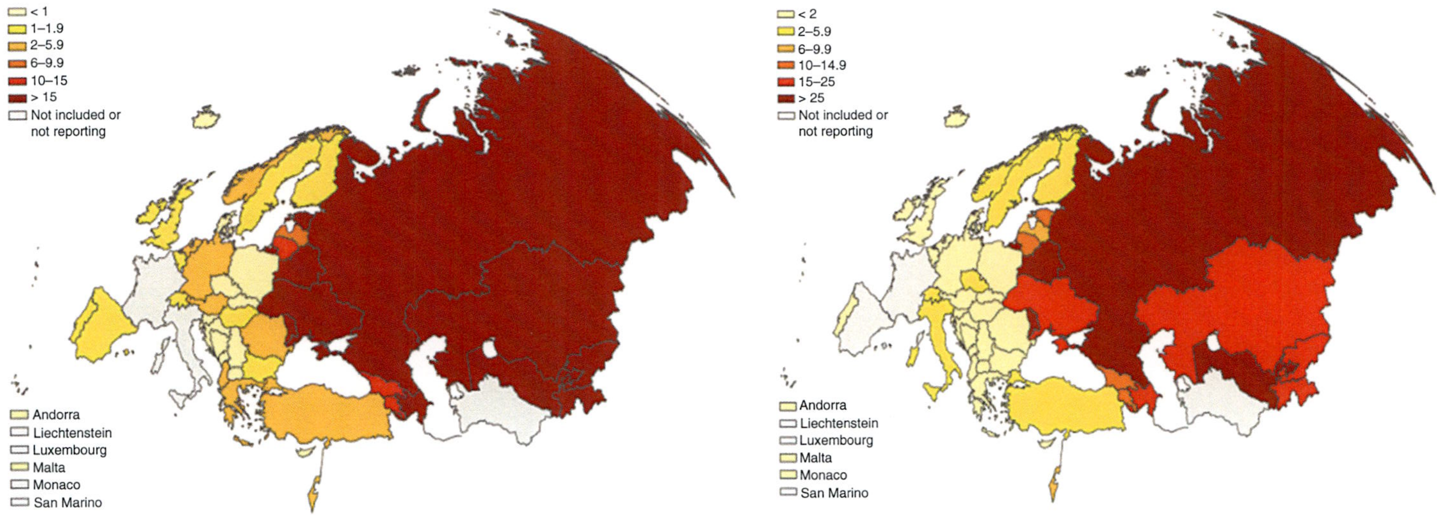

Fig. 56.2 (**a**, **b**) Percentage of multidrug-resistant (MDR) cases of tuberculosis among new pulmonary TB cases, European region, 2013 (left) and 2015 (right). Note high incidence in Eastern Europe. Source: ECDC 2015 and 2017 [36, 37]

56.5.10 Increase in Developed Countries Like Norway

In contrast to the general trend in Europe, Norway has some increase in tuberculosis, mostly imported (Fig. 56.4) from ECDC [37]. There is a trend towards failure of treatment, less overview and deaths in cases of tuberculosis in Norway (Fig. 56.4) [36].

With increasing immigration in Europe, the problem will be enhanced if good health control and follow-up are not carried out for new immigrants. Increased travel activity to countries with high levels of resistant TB is a challenge that should be treated with greater attention than today. Hospitals and healthcare in general must be upgraded concerning infection control to prevent further increase of tuberculosis in Europe.

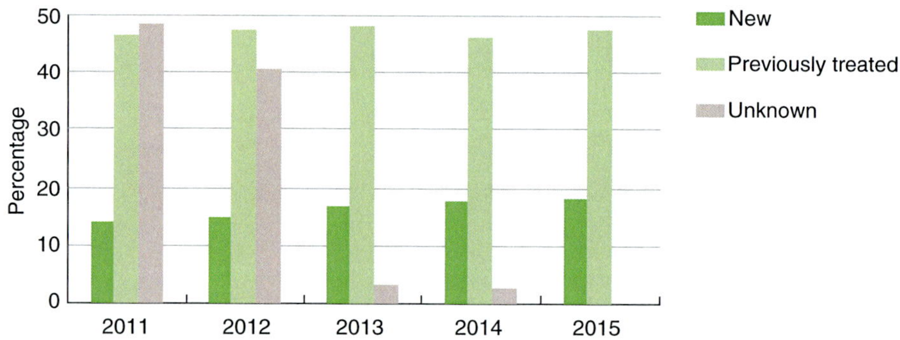

Fig. 56.3 Percentage of multidrug-resistant (MDR) cases of tuberculosis among new pulmonary TB cases, European region, 2015. Note some increase in new cases. Source: ECDC 2017 [37]

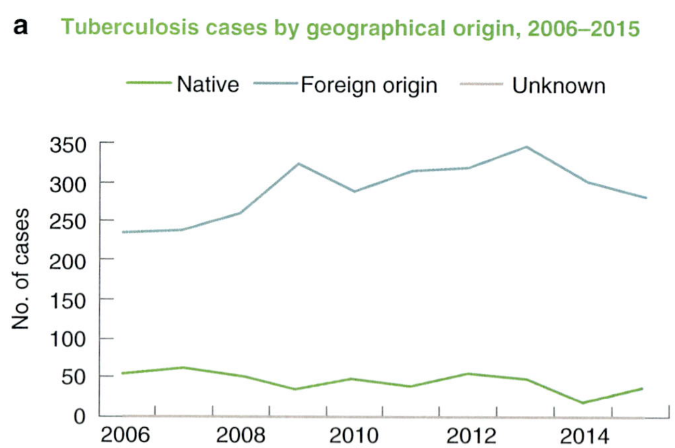

Fig. 56.4 (**a**, **b**) Development of tuberculosis in Norway, geographic origin, failure of treatment success and MDR-TB. Source: ECDC 2017 [37]

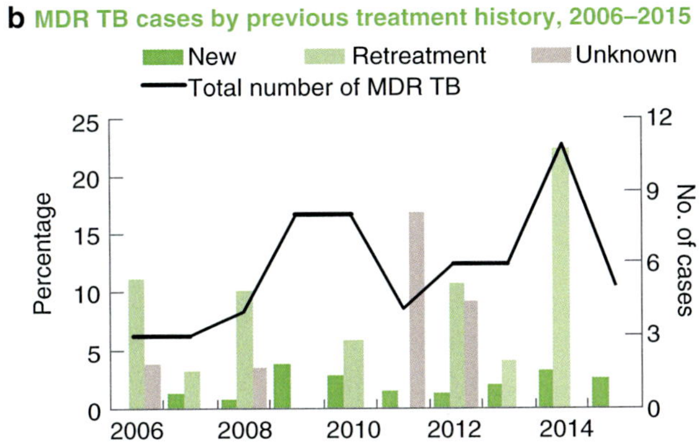

Fig. 56.4 (continued)

References

1. Andersen BM. Mycobacterium tuberculosis. In: Bakterier og sykdom. Epidemiologi, infeksjoner og smittevern. Oslo: Gyldendal Akademisk. Gyldendal Norsk Forlag; 2005. p. 409–28.
2. Andersen BM. Mycobacteria. In: Handbook in hygiene and infection control for hospitals. Part 1: microbiology and infection protection. Bergen: Fagbokforlaget; 2014. p. 135–43.
3. Anonyme. Mycobacterium tuberculosis. NORM-NORM-VET. 2014: 97.
4. Ministry of Social Affairs and Health. Regulation on tuberculosis control, 2001, 2002.
5. Norwegian Board of Health. Tuberculosis guideline. 07/04/2010.
6. The Directorate of Labour Inspection. Regulations for protection against exposure to biological agents (bacteria, viruses, fungi, etc.) in the workplace, FOR Oslo: 1997-12-19 nr.1322.
7. European-Council Directive 2000/54/EC of 18 September 2000 on the protection of workers from the risks related to exposure to biological agents at work.
8. Norwegian Board of Health. Regulation on pre-examination of workers in healthcare-antibiotic resistant bacteria IK-36/1996.
9. Bjartveit K. Control of tuberculosis. In: Handbook for primary healthcare. Oslo: Norwegian Board of Health; 1996.
10. Andersen BM. Prevention and control of tuberculosis. In: Handbook in hygiene and infection control for nursing homes. Oslo: Akademika Forlag; 2013. p. 323–33.
11. Andersen BM, Rasch M. Control when detected tuberculosis. In: Handbook in hygiene and infection control for hospitals. Oslo: Ullevål University Hospital; 2008. p. 475–81.
12. CDC. Guidelines for preventing the transmission of *Mycobacterium tuberculosis* in healthcare facilities, 1994; Notice federalregister. 59.
13. WHO. Definitions and reporting framework for tuberculosis—2013 revision. WHO/HTM/TB/3013.2.
14. WHO. Tuberculosis (TB) WHO monitoring of Xpert MTB/RIF roll-out, 2013.
15. WHO. The global plan to stop TB 2011-2015. www.stoptb.org.
16. WHO Report 2011: Global tuberculosis control.
17. WHO Stop TB Department. Drug-resistant tuberculosis. 26 January 2012.
18. ECDC. Tuberculosis surveillance and monitoring in Europe 2012. www.ecdc.europa.eu.
19. Pai M, Kalantri A, Aggarwal AN, Menzies D, Blumberg HM. Nosocomial tuberculosis in India. Emerg Infect Dis. 2006;12:1311–8.

20. Udwadia ZF, Amale RA, Ajbani KK, et al. Totally drug-resistant tuberculosis in India. Clin Infect Dis. 2012;54:579–81.
21. European Concerted Action. Beijing/W genotype *Mycobacterium tuberculosis* and drug resistance. Emerg Infect Dis. 2006;12:736–43.
22. Falzon D, Belghiti R, et al. Tuberculosis: still a concern for all countries in Europe. Eurosurveillance. 2007;12:77–9.
23. Golesi F, Brignatz J, Bellenfant M, Raoult D, Drancourt M. *Mycobacterium tuberculosis* Beijing outbreak in a school in Marseille, France, 2012. Eurosurveillance. 2013;18(2):pii: 20354.
24. Dobler CC, Korver S, Batbayar O, et al. Multidrug-resistant tuberculosis in patients from whom first-line treatment failed, Mongolia, 2010-2011. Emerg Infect Dis. 2015;21:1451–7.
25. Dahle UR. Total resistant tuberculosis? Tidsskr Nor Legeforen. 2012;132:634.
26. Jonson J, Kan B, Berggren I, Bruchfeld J. Extensive nosocomial transmission of tuberculosis in a low-incidence county. J Hosp Infect. 2013;83:321–6.
27. Lambert LA, Pratt RH, Armstrong LR, Haddad MR. Tuberculosis among healthcare workers, United States, 1995–2007. Infect Control Hosp Epidemiol. 2012;33:1126–32.
28. Augustynowicz-Kopec E, Jagielski T, Kozinska M, et al. Transmission of tuberculosis within family-households. J Infect. 2012;64:596–608.
29. Hubad B, Lapanje A. Inadequate hospital ventilation system increases the risk of nosocomial *Mycobacterium tuberculosis*. J Hosp Infect. 2012;80:88–91.
30. Harstad I, Jacobsen GW. Failure in following-up after screening for tuberculosis. Tidsskr Nor Legeforen. 2012;132:14–5.
31. Pugliese G, Tapper ML. Tuberculosis control in health care. Infect Control Hosp Epidemiol. 1996;17:819–27.
32. Storla D. Are we taking tuberculosis seriously? Tidsskr Nor Legeforen. 2012;132:6.
33. Brunvatne R, Strand Jenssen M, Al-Ani R, Furulund Borg E. Tuberculosis in asylants in Norwegian official reception camp. Tidsskr Nor Legeforen. 2012;132:14–5.
34. Van der Werf MJ, Sprenger M. Joint efforts needed to stop transmission of tuberculosis in Europe. Eurosurveilllance. 2013;18(12):pii: 20435.
35. Sandgren A, Hollo V, van der Werf MJ. Extrapulmonalry tuberculosis in the European Union and European Economic Area, 2002–2011. Eurosurveillance. 2013;18(12):pii: 20431.
36. ECDC and WHO. Surveillance Report. Tuberculosis surveillance and monitoring in Europe 2015. Surveillance Report. www.ecdc.europa.eu; www.euro.who.int.
37. ECDC and WHO. Surveillance Report. Tuberculosis surveillance and monitoring in Europe 2017. Surveillance Report. www.ecdc.europa.eu; www.euro.who.int.

Scabies: Control in Hospitals 57

Abstract
A little skin mite—*Sarcoptes scabiei*—runs on humans and animals and can cause irritable itching, dermatitis and eczema, especially on the hands. Scabies mite is invisible to the eye, cannot fly but has a high speed on warm skin (2.5 cm in 1 min) and may come over from one hand to the next within a few minutes. Outbreaks of scabies may often be large and persisting in institutions, day-care centres, schools, families and long-term institutions as nursing homes. Hospitals are occasionally exposed to infection, and both patients and personnel are infected. The following chapter is focused on practical measures to detect and prevent transmission of scabies in healthcare institutions.

Keywords
Sarcoptes scabiei · Scabies · *Norwegian scabies* · Mite · Itching · Dermatitis Eczema · Hands · Outbreaks in institutions, day care centres, schools, families, long-term institutions, hospitals · Contact infection · Information · Screening Isolation · Decontamination · Environment · Eradication · Nosocomial infections Infection control · Hygiene · Prevention

57.1 Purpose

- To prevent transfer of scabies/mite to patients, staff, visitors and environment in the hospital.
- The transmission is mainly contact-borne, but biologic materials from humans and animals may be contagious for a period.

B. M. Andersen, *Prevention and Control of Infections in Hospitals*,
https://doi.org/10.1007/978-3-319-99921-0_57

57.2 Comprise

- Patients, personnel, visitors, equipment, medical equipment, textiles, rooms and surfaces and the complete environment exposed to scabies.
- All direct contacts of patients with scabies/suspected scabies and with clothing and equipment used by patients with scabies.

57.3 Responsibility

The hospital's management is responsible for the existence of written procedures for the proper control of scabies.

The department's management is responsible for following procedures for infection control and tracing in cooperation with the infection control unit, occupational health services or working environment during outbreaks of scabies.

Personnel are responsible for following current routines and preventive measures and for participating in sanitation/disinfection.

57.4 Practical Measures [1–4]

57.4.1 Inpatient/Outpatient Clinic

- *If known or suspiciously scabies*—directly in contact isolation. No more tracing of scabies in the hospital if proper infection protection has been carried out from the start, including transport in the ambulance.
- *If unknown at the admission/outpatient clinic*—preventive measures; see below.

57.4.2 Scabies: Discovered in Hospitals

The department management cooperates with the infection control unit and the occupational health services/working environment.

- *Contact isolation of the patient for* up to 2–3 days after application of the scab medicament. After treatment for scabies, the patient should have clean clothes, clean bed linen and be placed in a clean room. Personal caring for the patient with scabies is using gloves and disposable gown with long sleeves and cuffs. Room-bound shoes or shoe covers (wear gloves when shoe covers are carefully removed) is applicable. Wash hands after wearing gloves. Use the infectious waste bag in the room.
- *Make sure the diagnosis is correct.* Clinical diagnosis is often easier than microscopic. Itching and itching marks, mite tunnels in the skin, mites, eggs or faeces from mites may be seen [1, 2]. Microscopic detection should be conducted on a minimum of three to five people and preferably all if there are many involved and

many are "itching". Microscopy may be negative in early stages and by psoriasis-like rashes (*Norwegian scabies*) [1, 2].

- *Disinfection of the room* is applicable during ongoing treatment (floor and horizontal surfaces) and as end disinfection after completion of treatment. This is especially accomplished because scabies dermatitis often is infected with *Staphylococcus aureus* and/or group A streptococci.
- *Furniture with textiles* should be removed from the room, packed in plastic for 10 days (or placed in freezer containers), placed outside if cold weather and replaced with washable furniture.
- *Clothing and laundry* which is used before treatment should be washed at least at 50 °C for 10 min to kill the mites and eggs. Bedding (pillow, quilt, mattress, etc.) may be placed in a freezer (or out in the cold in winter).
- *Shoes and other goods* that cannot be cleaned can be put in a plastic bag for 10 days or placed in a freezer to kill the mite (or out in the cold in winter).
- These measures will be implemented until test samples have shown negative findings for 3 consecutive days.
- *Personnel, relatives and others* who have been in contact with a patient with scabies—before treatment—should be registered and treated, preferably at the same time (avoid reinfection in the environment).
- *Personnel* resumes work after treatment. Personnel who have had symptoms should wear gloves for the first 2–3 days after they return to work after full treatment.

57.4.3 Exposed Patients, Personnel and Visitors

Set up a list of all exposed to the index patient last month and inform about treatment.

The patient, other patients in the same room and anyone with direct (skin) contact to the patient (personnel, visitors, etc.) should be followed up for treatment and control. Remember stand-in personnel, extra staff, priests, service units and others who have been in direct contact with the patient.

Everyone is treated at the same time to avoid reinfection. Make sure that everyone understands that they must follow the treatment to the point. Even those who have not been studied for scabies but have been in contact with the index patient during the last month must be treated.

57.5 Background Information

A little skin mite—Sarcoptes scabiei—runs on humans and animals and can cause irritable itching, dermatitis and eczema, especially on the hands [1]. Mite is invisible to the eye, cannot fly but has a high speed on warm skin (2.5 cm in 1 min) and may come over from one hand to the next within a few minutes [1]. Outbreaks of scabies often have a large extent in institutions, day-care centres, schools, families and long-term institutions as nursing homes [1–3]. Hospitals are occasionally exposed to infection, and both patients and personnel are infected [1, 2, 4].

57.5.1 Scabies

Sarcoptes scabiei variant *hominis* is a little skin mite that may cause irritable itching, dermatitis and eczema, especially on the hands [1]. The mite is invisible to the eye, cannot fly but has a high speed on warm skin (2.5 cm in 1 min) and may come over from one hand to the next within a few minutes [1]. Outbreaks of scabies often have a large extent in institutions, day care centres, schools, families and long-term institutions as nursing homes [1–3]. Hospitals are occasionally exposed to infection, and both patients and personnel are infected [1, 2, 4].

A clinically significant variant of the mite causing widespread infection is called *Norwegian scabies* (*Scabies norvegicus*) [1]. This form is the most common cause of scabies outbreaks of long-term infusions since it produces significant amounts of mites. The infection is highly contagious. The skin lesions of the Norwegian clinical variant can be widespread and in part resemble dermatitis or psoriasis and are often misdiagnosed. Also nail beds can be affixed with loss of nails. Atypical courses of scabies are observed relatively often.

57.5.2 Incidence

Every year, about 300 million people get scabies, mostly in developing countries, but scabies is also increasing in industrialized countries, linked to major travel activities, immigrants, poor hygiene in refugee camps, hospitals, etc. [1]. Scabies is a known problem in modern schools, kindergarten, prison and health institutions—especially long-term institutions where there is much contact between patients and between patients and healthcare professionals/relatives [1, 2, 5–14].

Over a year, 17% of 725 long-term institutions in Michigan had proven scabies [5]. In 2015, Kentucky (Federal Government) used fines for at least 20 nursing homes that had problems with scabies and allowed it to spread in several months before anything was done [10]. At last, 45% of patients were infected! [10] Among the five worst nursing homes, the fines were up to 900,000 $ [10].

Sometimes, scabies may spread in hospitals from infected patients admitted from home, abroad, school, kindergarten, prison, etc., and even from nursing homes/retirement homes. Scabies can often last for a while in the hospital before it is detected as cause of itching and "eczema" between fingers, and such outbreaks can thus be very extensive in hospitals [1, 6, 14–21]. Kidney patients, transplanted patients and others with severe reduced infection defences have usually more widespread scabies than others and serious infections can occur by secondary infection in scabies skin eruptions [21].

- In 2009, 1659 people were exposed to scabies at an intensive care and rehabilitation centre [7]. All exposed persons were screened by a dermatologist, and 1640 was treated, including the household of healthcare personnel. The index patient had HIV and incrustation wounds of Norwegian scabies. The attack rate among health professionals who cared for the index patient was 26–32%. During 7 months, 19 cases were diagnosed, of which 6 were children. Failure to treat, relapse and reinfection in families were linked to too restrictive definition of individuals "at risk", lack of treatment and limited drug effects [7].

- In 2011, approximately 900 employees at a hospital in the United States were treated after detected scabies in an emergency patient [19]. At least one dozen healthcare personnel who had had close contact with the patient, clothes or equipment were sent home for immediate treatment, and about the same number of persons was infected [19].
- A kidney transplant patient was admitted three times at a hospital in the United States in 2010 before the finding that he had scabies [13]. Many patients and personnel had been exposed to the patient who had been hospitalized by two departments. Rapid infection detection revealed five employees and two patients with scabies. A massive prophylactic treatment was initiated for all at the two departments. One more case was found, and 6 weeks later, the outbreak was declared terminated. The total cost was $20,000 [13].
- A transplanted patient infected 37 nurses at a cardiovascular intensive department in Halifax in 2014 [20]. The patient was treated there for 2 months. The outbreak led to the cancellation of several operations due to a lack of nurses [20].
- In July 2015 a major outbreak was reported at an intensive department in Alabama, with 19 patients and 99 staff with scabs, of which 46 had pruritus and rash [16].
- In Canada, there was an outbreak of scabies in July 2015 at a childhood hospital in Alberta [21]. Index patients had crustated scabies and approximately 100 people were exposed to infection. All employees, patients and visitors, including their family, were recommended for scab-prophylactic treatment [21].

57.5.3 The Mite's Lifetime and Survival

The scabies mite is—during a period of 30 days—producing eggs, 2–3 eggs a day, while digging a skin tunnel. The eggs develop into larvae within 3–4 days, move on to the skin surface and develop into adult mites within 10–17 days. Most patients who have scabies have at least 10–15 mites who dig a tunnel and lay eggs. Within 2–4 months, the mite society is built up before the actual large skin itching starts [1].

The usual incubation period is approximately 1 month and 1–2 weeks if infected again.

Transfer via *direct and indirect contact.* The close contact patient/healthcare staff, especially at long-term institutions, is responsible for prolonged outbreaks of scabies if no preventive activity is introduced. In the case of one patient with a scab, up to 50% of other patients and healthcare professionals at the same department can be infected. In case of direct contact with a scab patient, it only takes 2 min for transmission of infection. Personnel working with scab patients who have sores/ itching marks between the fingers have 40–70% chance of being infected. In families, approximately 40% of other family members are infected when one of the members have scabies symptoms. Scabies skin rash that causes skin peeling/eczema/crusts (especially the Norwegian clinical variant) has led to large amounts of mites in the environment of the patient—up to 7600 mites in 2 days is calculated. Mites are living a minimum of 36 h outside the body [1].

Linen, other clothes and equipment in the patient's room may be highly contaminated of mites. Infections may also be transmitted via infected skin creams, etc. and via infected laundry to laundry workers [1].

57.5.4 Diagnosis on Suspicion of Scabies

Scabies diagnosis is: maculo-papular, nodular and/or itchy rashes (especially between fingers) *and* the physician's diagnosis *or* laboratory-confirmed diagnosis (microscopy of skin scraping, mite, egg, faeces). The sensitivity of the laboratory examination is unfortunately only 10–60% and must be repeated to confirm the diagnosis. It is recommended to contact dermatologic department if scabies is suspected (Fig. 57.1).

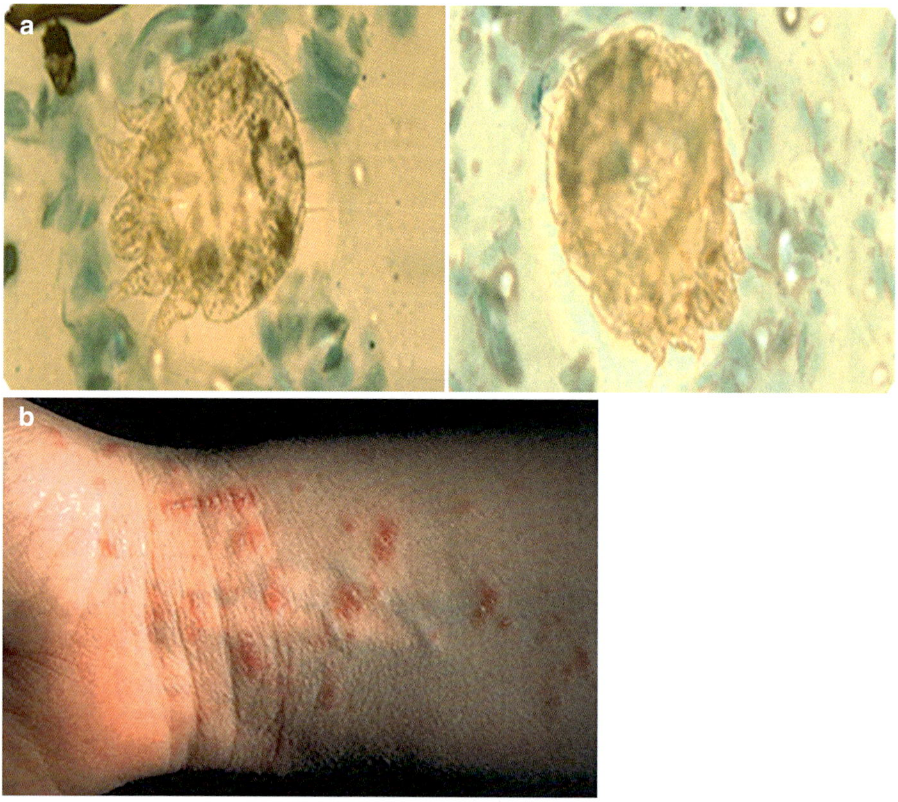

Fig. 57.1 (**a**, **b**) *Sarcoptes scabiei* in adult, seen in microscope, and itching marks and tunnels in the skin. Illustration (**a**) from CDC

References

1. Andersen BM. Scabies. In: Handbook in hygiene and infection control. Microbiology and prevention. Part 1. Bergen: Fagbokforlaget; 2014. p. 388–92.
2. Andersen BM, Haugen H, Rasch M, Heldal Haugen A, Tageson A. Outbreak of scabies in Norwegian nursing homes and home care patients: control and prevention. J Hosp Infect. 2000;45:160–4.
3. Centers for Disease Control and Prevention. Scabies in health care facilities- Iowa. MMWR Morb Mortal Wkly Rep. 1988;37:178–9.
4. Centers for Disease Control and Prevention. Scabies. Epidemiology and risk factors. Scabies in institutions. Atlanta, GA: CDC; 2010.
5. Andersen BM, Rasch M. Scabies in hospitals; tracing and control. In: Handbook in hygiene and infection control for hospitals. Oslo: Ullevål University Hospital; 2008. p. 482–4.
6. Andersen BM. Scabies. In: Handbook in hygiene and infection control for nursing homes. Trondheim: Akademika; 2013. p. 367–70.
7. Buehlmann M, Beltraminelli H, Strub C, et al. Scabies outbreak in an intensive care unit with 1,659 exposed individuals—key factors for controlling the outbreak. Infect Control Hosp Epidemiol. 2009;30:354–60.
8. Tjioe M, Vissers WH. Scabies outbreaks in nursing homes for the elderly: recognition, treatment options and control of reinfestation. Drugs Aging. 2008;25:299–306.
9. Vorou R, Remoudaki HD, Maltezou HC. Nosocomial scabies. J Hosp Infect. 2007;65:9–14.
10. Anonymous. Nursing home fined for scabies. Kentucky.com. 2 Aug 2015.
11. Gooch JJ, Strasius ST, Bearmer B, Reiter MD, Correll GW. Nosocomial outbreak of scabies. Arch Dermatol. 1978;114:897–8.
12. Scheinfeld N. Controlling scabies in institutional settings: a review of medications, treatment models, and implementation. Am J Clin Dermatol. 2004;5:31–7.
13. Bouvresse S, Chosidow O. Scabies in healthcare settings. Curr Opin Infect Dis. 2010;23:111–8.
14. Kahn A, O'Grady S, Muller MP. Rapid control of a scabies outbreak at a tertiary care hospital without ward closure. Am J Infect Control. 2012;40:451–5.
15. Tollitt J, Duncan A, Woywodt A. Of mites and men: scabies in patients with kidney disease. Clin Kidney. 2013;6:125–7.
16. Anonymous. A scabies outbreak associated with a hospital's intensive care unit in Jefferson County, AL–July, 2015 (AL1507SCB-37a).
17. Anonymous. Scabies outbreak in Dane Co. jail. 24 Aug 2015.
18. Hope M. Scabies outbreak in Texas middle school. 3 Apr 2005.
19. Davis D. Hospital treats patients for scabies outbreak. 8 Dec 2011.
20. Anonymous. Scabies outbreak spreads a Halifax hospital as 37 nurses are diagnosed. 29 Apr 2014.
21. Booth L. Alberta Children's hospital on alert for scabies. CDC. 1 Aug 2015.

Part XI

Disinfection, Sterilization, Cleaning, Control

58 Disinfection of Skin and Mucous Membranes

Abstract

The skin has rich, permanent and temporary (transient) normal flora of largely harmless bacteria. Mucous membranes in upper airways and gastrointestinal tracts have an even richer and more variable normal flora. A small stick through the skin or mucous membranes is usually harmless and is healed quickly if the wound does not go deeper. In sterile tissue cavities, almost any harmless microbe can multiply and create infection. If a foreign body is placed through poorly disinfected skin or mucous membranes, bacteria may rapidly multiply and become the starting point for a more serious infection. Especially vulnerable are people who have prosthetic or other foreign matters in the body. Skin and mucous membrane disinfection may prevent invasion of microbes and/or contamination of specimens and samples taken. Some disinfectants have better and longer-lasting effect than others. The following chapter is focused on practical measures to disinfect the skin and mucous membranes in healthcare institutions.

Keywords

Disinfection · Skin flora · Mucous membranes · Infection control · Hygiene Prevention

58.1 Purpose

- To reduce microbes on the patient's skin and mucous membranes and thereby the risk of introducing microbes into deeper tissue
- To reduce contamination of samples taken from the skin, tissue or mucous membranes

B. M. Andersen, *Prevention and Control of Infections in Hospitals*,
https://doi.org/10.1007/978-3-319-99921-0_58

58.2 Comprise

- All punctures or injections through the skin and mucous membranes

58.3 Responsibility

Hospital management provides written guidelines for disinfection of the skin and mucous membranes before punctures, injections and operations and is responsible for the hospital's infection control guidelines.

Department management implements routines and reports to the Director if lack of resources (capacity, expertise, infection protection equipment, etc.) may result in infection risk for patients, personnel or visitors.

Staff follows routines. Stick injuries, uncontrollable spill of infected blood/tissue or severe contamination of the skin/mucous membranes upon surgery must be reported to the department management.

58.4 Practical Measures [1–7]

Hand hygiene: Wash or disinfect hands before and after wearing gloves.

Unsterile gloves: Unsterile gloves may be contaminated if taken from an open glove box. Note that in sterile procedures, only sterile gloves are used.

Sterile gloves are used for sterile procedures and as part of sterile clothing.

Sterile gloves, sterile gown, surgical mask and cap and sterile equipment should be used, preferably in an operating room/clean room when performing the following procedures:

(a) Insertion of:
  - Central intravascular catheter (CVC)
  - Epidural catheter
  - Peritoneal catheter
  - Arteriovenous shunt
  - Venous access port and the like

(b) Punctures for -scopy and other local investigations:
  - Organ punctures
  - Arthroscopy
  - Myelography, etc.
  - Angiography, etc.
  - Operative treatment—always in an operating room

1. Disinfection before regular blood sampling:
   - Chlorhexidine alcohol (70% alcohol with chlorhexidine 2–5 mg/mL)
   - Or 70% alcohol
   - Or *wet* liquor compresses with disinfectants (alcohols)

  - Working time: 60 s.
  - Do not touch the area afterwards.
2. Disinfection before injections (intramuscular or subcutaneous):
   - Chlorhexidine alcohol (70% alcohol with chlorhexidine 2–5 mg/mL)
   - Or 70% alcohol
   - Or *wet* liquor compresses with disinfectants (alcohols)
     - Working time: 60 s.
     - Do not touch the area afterwards.
3. Disinfection before puncture in connection with special investigations/treatment:
   - Blood culture, blood to blood bank
   - Insertion of intravascular catheter, central and peripheral
   - Lumbar puncture
   - Punctures of other cavities
   - Organ punctures
   - Introduction of foreign body/fluids
   - Plexus anaesthesia, etc.
     - Chlorhexidine alcohol (70% alcohol with chlorhexidine 2–5 mg/mL).
     - Sterile compresses/gauze pads.
     - Sterile disinfection sets.
     - Working time: 60 s.
     - Repeat disinfection, start centrally and wash within the first area.
     - Working time: 60 s.
     - The skin should be dry between the two applications and before the perforation of the skin.
     - Do not touch the area afterwards.
4. Disinfection of mucous membranes (upper respiratory tract, genitalia, anus) [1]:
   - Chlorhexidine 0.5–1 mg/mL in aqueous solution.
   - Sterile gauze pads/compresses.
   - Short shelf life for chlorhexidine in aqueous solution—1 week. Check date.
   - *Chlorhexidine must not be used in the ear!*
5. Disinfection of the skin preoperatively:
   There are many methods of disinfection described (time used, number of applications of disinfectant, etc.): however, they are not well documented [1–3]. Most common methods used are described below:
   - Sterile dress for the person that is doing disinfection.
   - Sterile wash kit with sterile forceps and gauze pads/compresses, chlorhexidine alcohol 5 mg/mL.
   - Wash the field thoroughly with plenty of disinfectant, a total of at least five times.
   - A border is first created around the area of operation.
   - The field that is disinfected should be at least 10 cm larger than sterile cover in every direction.
   - The field within the frame must be disinfected.
   - Start centrally and disinfect outwards.

- Allow the disinfectant to work for 1 min each time.
- New application that starts centrally in the operating field. Do not wash as far as last time (contamination from non-disinfected skin).
- Let the disinfectant work for at least 1 min at the end so that the skin is air dried.
- The skin must be dry when covering.
- Do not contaminate when covering the operation area.

See Chap. 35.

58.5 Background Information

The skin has a rich, permanent and temporary (transient) normal flora of largely harmless bacteria such as coagulase-negative staphylococci, diphtheroids and anaerobic bacteria. Gram-negative intestinal bacteria are present around the anus and on the lower part of the body. Bedridden patients have after some days in hospital more gram-negative rods also on upper part of the body, including the face and head, especially after use of antibiotics.

A small break of the skin or mucosa is usually harmless and is healed quickly if the wound does not go deeper, for example, to sterile cavities. In sterile tissue, many skin microbes may multiply and create infection. If a foreign body is placed through poorly disinfected skin or mucous membranes, bacteria introduced may rapidly multiply and become the starting point for a more serious infection, see chapters on intravascular (Chap. 40) and urinary (Chap. 43) catheters, and operative infections (Chaps. 33–35). Especially vulnerable are people who have prosthetic or other foreign matters in the body. Skin and mucous membrane antisepsis removes superficial flora and prevents contamination of specimens and samples taken, which is undesirable by examination of tissue fluid or blood.

By sampling of blood or tissue for examinations, the specimen may be contaminated by normal skin or mucous flora, which is undesirable by examination of tissue or blood. Disinfection removes such superficial flora. However, disinfectants may have varying effects, some short- and other long-term effect [1–4, 6, 7]. At long-lasting operations in sterile tissues, this may be of importance because of the rapid recolonization of bacteria in areas where disinfectants deteriorate and lose effects [8].

Disinfectant is most often chlorhexidine alcohol combinations or different other types of alcohols [1–4, 6–9]. Iodine solutions like povidone-iodine can easily be contaminated with microbes after the vial is broken (use only single use packages). Iodine can cause an allergic reaction to some people.

References

1. Dumville JC, McFarlane E, Edwards P, Lipp A, Holmes A, Liu Z. Preoperative skin antiseptic for prevention of surgical wound infections after clean surgery. Cochrane Database Syst Rev. 2015;(4):CD003949.

2. Young HL, Reese S, Knepper B, Miller A, Mauffrey C. The effect of preoperative skin preparation products on surgical site infection. Infect Control Hosp Epidemiol. 2014;35:1535–8.
3. Wood A, Conner R. Guideline for preoperative patient skin antisepsis. AORN November 6, 2014. Updated 2015.
4. Rutala WA, Weber DJ. Disinfection and sterilization: an overview. Am J Infect Control. 2013;41:2–5.
5. Øgrey T, Rasch M, Andersen BM. Disinfection of skin and mucous membranes. Handbook in hygiene and infection control for hospitals. Ullevål University Hospital; 2008. p. 485–8.
6. Andersen BM. T1.18. Disinfection. Norwegian medicines guide for personnel; 2013. p. 100–5.
7. Andersen BM. L1.9 Disinfectants. Norwegian medicines guide for personnel; 2013. p. 776–84.
8. Johnston DH, Fairclough JA, Brown EM, Morris R. Rate of bacterial re-colonization of the skin after preparation: four methods compared. Br J Surg. 1987;74(1):64.
9. Chemical disinfectants for technical use in health and nursing. Oslo: The Norwegian Medicines Agency. December 2012, updated 2015.

Disinfection of Instruments and Equipment

59

Abstract

Disinfection is "destruction or removal of all organisms capable of causing infection" and "in practice leads to the removal of all microbes except spores—that is, an approximate sterilization process." In the healthcare system, instruments and equipment are disinfected with heat, chemical fluids, chemical vapours or gases. Prions are contagious protein sequences that are treated in a special way. Instruments from prion-sick cases are never reused on other patients.

Keywords

Disinfection · Instruments · Reusable equipment · Infection control · Hygiene Prevention

59.1 Purpose

- To remove pathogenic agents, bacteria, viruses, fungi and parasites, from instruments and equipment [1–8].
- To prevent transmission of infection from patients to other patients, staff, visitors or the environment through instruments, technical equipment, fixtures and rooms [1–11].

59.2 Comprise

- All equipment that has been in contact with biological materials.
- All equipment that will come in contact with mucous membranes, skin, secretions, excretions and/or other human biological materials.
- All other equipment/fixtures that may have been exposed to contamination of infectious agents that can cause disease (see isolation regimes, Chap. 14).

B. M. Andersen, *Prevention and Control of Infections in Hospitals*,
https://doi.org/10.1007/978-3-319-99921-0_59

- All instruments/equipment disinfected/cleaned before sterilization.
- *Note!* Equipment/instruments which come into contact with normally sterile sites (mucous tissue, cavities) should be *sterile.*
- Equipment that comes into contact with (not penetrating) unsterile mucosa (oral cavity, bowel, etc.) should at least be disinfected and preferably sterile. After disinfection, scopes and the like should be *sterilized* because they often may cause lesions of the mucosa. See Chap. 60 on sterilization and disinfection of endoscopes.

59.3 Responsibility

Hospital management provides written procedures for cleaning and disinfection of instruments and equipment and ensures enough resources, mechanical equipment and competence for proper disinfection.

Department management implements routines, ensures that machine equipment (temperature, detergents, etc.) used is controlled regarding use and disinfection and makes hygienic demands versus equipment manufacturers.

Personnel follow procedures and notify suspected failure of the disinfection process or risk of recontamination of disinfected equipment.

59.4 Practical Measures

Practical measures are based on international and national studies and recommendations concerning use of disinfectants, methods, special treatment of infectious agents, infectious waste and disinfection problems [1–20]. For instance, in Norway, the Norwegian Medicines Control Agency has approved defined disinfectants and methods for technical use in health care in almost 30 years [12, 19].

59.4.1 Removal of Infectious Agents [14–16]

Bacteria, viruses, fungi, etc. are removed in whole or in part by the following methods:

- Cleaning with soap and water: for example, floors and surfaces—environment—fabrics—textiles—cups and vessels. Organic matter, dust and dirt are removed along with most bacteria and other contaminants. The result depends initially on the pollution and cleaning methods.
- Disinfection with chemicals or heat. Machines with fully automatic disinfection cycles remove dirt and organic matter, as well as almost all microbes.
- Sterilization with heat and damp pressure: all common microbes are killed, see separate Chap. 61. All organic matter and dirt must be removed prior to sterilization.

(Autoclaving is also used in the treatment of infectious waste, e.g., from laboratories or in connection with infection isolates.)

59.4.2 Contaminated Equipment and Instruments [14–16, 21, 22]

All equipment contaminated with organic matter should be treated immediately. If transported to a separate treatment area, equipment must be treated as potential contaminated.

- During the cleaning process, most of the organic material is removed. If it dries onto the equipment, it is more difficult to clean, and important contaminants can be left, like prions.
- Bedpans with dried organic materials before the disinfection process may still have residues of biological material on it after washing or disinfection in the decontaminator.
- Operation instruments with dried blood and tissue residues are more difficult to clean in the instrument washing machine than well-rinsed instruments.
- *Machine tools* with internal machine components and electrical wires that cannot be opened and disinfected in liquid or heat are treated according to separate guidelines [9, 11].

59.4.3 Manual Cleaning of Equipment and Instruments [14–16]

- All manual cleaning should be done after disinfection of the instruments, to reduce personnel for exposure to infectious agents. But this process may sometimes be necessary before disinfection, for example, by complicated, combined, fragile instruments and scopes.
- Manual cleaning (regardless of whether the equipment is disinfected beforehand) must take place in defined, well-equipped and ventilated washroom under negative pressure compared to operating rooms and other clean rooms. The entire washing process should take place under the liquid surface, with great care, in a quiet environment to prevent spread of spills or aerosol in the room. There should be plenty of areal for "clean and unclean side," good light and access to inspect the equipment with magnifying glass.
- PPE: Single-use gown with waterproof front and sleeves, long cuff gloves and surgical mask/cap/eye protection should be used. In case of accident during procedures, infectious agents may spread.
- Brushes for brushing and rinsing narrow lumens, long canals and cavities in the instrument, etc. are recommended as disposable since they are difficult to clean for protein residues.
- All other equipment in the cleaning process itself should be decontaminated after use in the instrument washing machine.

- PPE is placed after use in contaminated waste, with the exception of glasses, etc., which may be decontaminated in the instrument washing machine.
- Washbasins and areas around are afterwards cleaned with soap and water. Finally rinse the washbasin (avoid splashing) with hot water (75 °C).

59.4.4 Disinfection [14–16]

- Disinfection is usually carried out before cleaning to protect staff and prevent spread of contaminants.
- Disinfect equipment as soon as possible. The effect reduces if organic materials are left to dry.
- Possible contagious equipment is packaged and labelled.
- Disinfect by moist heat or by chemical disinfectants.
- Heat disinfection is used for all heat-resistant equipment.
- Heat disinfection: boiling in water (100 °C) or mechanical heat disinfection in the decontaminator or instrument washing machine.

59.4.5 Boiling (Cooking at ≥100 °C) (Usually Not Used Anymore)

Boiling is a simple and safe disinfection method that is checked by inspection.

1. Boiling: in alkaline water, pH > 11 in 5–10 min is an excellent cleaning and disinfection method. Equipment and instruments should not be cleaned in advance.
2. When boiling, the equipment must be completely covered with water.
3. A suitable detergent (alkaline) is added by boiling to prevent adhesive combustion of organic material to instruments.
4. The boiling should take place at 100 °C for 5–10 min.

59.4.6 Heat Disinfection by Automatic Machine Systems [14–16]

- Decontaminator is a disinfection machine that use hot water at a temperature of at least 85 °C or higher for a certain period of time as part of an *automatic* washing process where organic matter and dirt are removed prior to disinfection.
- *Washing decontaminator* is used to drain the waste, flush and clean equipment with water and soap, and disinfect with a final hot water phase of at least 85°C in more than over one minute. This machine type is intended for urine bottles, bedpans, suction bottles, washbasin, flower vases, saliva cups and the like. Some machines also have a basket for instruments.
- *Instrument washing machine* is used for cleaning and disinfecting of equipment and instruments. There are special instrument washers for cleaning and disinfecting surgical instruments, drainage vials, different scope washing machines, special machines for ventilator equipment, laboratory equipment, etc. First step in the process is a thorough washing process adapted to the special equipment, then rinsing and thermal disinfection at least 85 °C for 3–10 min depending on

the machine type/wash program. The heat disinfection lasts for more than 3 min when the disinfection cycle occurs after the cleaning phase and 10 min when disinfection occurs during the cleaning phase.
- *Check* temperature, filter sand soap according to written procedures and documentation, and check the purity of equipment (blood, tissue, faeces, etc.) before storage.

59.4.7 Chemical Disinfection

Chemical disinfection is only used for equipment that does not withstand heat.

1. Use chemicals approved by the State Medicines Agency [12, 19, 20].
2. Follow the information given on the package about the effect range, preparation, working time and shelf life.
3. Always wear gloves, disposable liquid-proof protective gown, surgical mask/cap and possibly eye protection in direct work.
4. Chemical disinfection must be carried out in good ventilation in a suitable room with a negative pressure and with a separate outlet for chemical vapour.
5. Use suitable disinfectant vessel with a tight lid.
6. Compound equipment is separated as much as possible.
7. The items must be in total below the liquid level in the recommended time.
8. After disinfection, clean the equipment with soap and water adapted to the equipment, and then rinse all objects well under running water (see manual disinfection).
9. The equipment is dried well under clean conditions, stored in clean storage, or continued for inspection, packing and sterilization; see the Chap. 61 on sterilization. This process will not introduce new microbes from the environment.
10. Wash the work area with soap and water—brushes for hollow objects, etc. are used as disposable single use for each instrument, and disinfection vessels are drained, decontaminated and stored clean afterwards.
11. *Check* for disinfectant, durability, use, storage and accident.

Storage space for disinfected equipment must be clean and dry with written routines for storage and cleaning. Storage space should not be an office or a wet room with aerosol formation.

59.4.8 Disinfectants (Tables 59.1 and 59.2)

- Glutaraldehyde 2% has an effect on vegetative bacteria, mycobacteria, viruses and fungi. The room must have a separate outlet for chemical vapour that is toxic. The disinfectant is inactivated by a high yield of organic material.
- "Virkon," oxidative agent containing pentapotassium bis(peroxymonosulfate) bis(sulfate), has an effect on vegetative bacteria, viruses and fungi. It is not approved for use against tubercle bacteria and bacterial spores and is inactivated with a lot of organic material. The ppm values for effect against microbes are missing and it is a less stable agent.

Table 59.1 Chemical disinfectant in liquid form

Disinfectant	Effect on	Use concentration	Time min[a]	Shelf life[a] concentrate
ALDEHYDE: for equipment and instruments; effect on most microbes				
Glutaraldehyde	Virus	2%	30	1–2 years
	Bacteria	2%	30	
	Fungi	2%	30	
	Mycobacteria	2%	60	
CHLORINS: for equipment and surfaces; effect on most microbes			Effect time varies	
*Chloramine (12,500 ppm) ready for use.		5%	20–60	2 years
*Chloricide (Sodium hypochlorite, 4.5% active chlorine, 45,000 ppm, in concentrate and diluted 25%- ca 11,000 ppm)		25%[b]	30–60	1 year
*Household bleach (Sodium hypochlorite 5.25-6.15%, 52,000-61,000 ppm, in concentrate), can be used diluted at home		used in 1:10 to 1:100 dilution	30–60	
FENOLE: equipment and surfaces (usually not use)				
Effects on most bacteria, including TBC, but not virus		2%	60	3 years
ETHANOL (alcohols) (Uncertain effect on microbes)		70–85%	2–10	Chlorhexidine-alcohol: 1 week after open
Only for disinfection of clean equipment, surfaces, etc. Do not stand open and evaporate!				
OKSYDATIV disinfectants: for equipment and surfaces				
*Virkon; effect on most bacteria, not TBC and not well documented for virus (Potassium persulfate 50%, sulfamic acid 5%)		1%	30	3 years
*Peracetic acid/hydrogen peroxide (bacteria, spores, viruses)		0.26%	12	24 h
Used in special washers for endoscopes in combination with heat[c]				
*PeraSafe—peracetic acid; effect on most microbes, sodium percarborate 40–60%		16.2%		2 years
	Cleaned equipment	0.26%	10	
	Mycobacteria		30	

[a]Read the instructions on the bottle/jar. After use, solutions must be discarded. Effect time may vary

[b]% of concentrate

[c]Special washing machine with chemical-thermal disinfection

Table 59.2 Disinfectants for technical disinfection: medical equipment, surfaces, fixtures, etc. [5, 8, 16]

Disinfectant	Microbiological effect	Benefits	Disadvantage
Alcohols 70–90%	May affect some bacteria, viruses and fungi, but *not* all microbes, usually not *Clostridium difficile*, norovirus and spores	Fast-acting, environmentally friendly. Higher concentrations have better effect	Only on cleaned surfaces. No penetration of protein-rich material. Non-spore killing effect. Evaporates fast, uncertain effect
Glutaraldehyde 2% or more	Very good at right concentration and effect time. Bacteria, mycobacteria, viruses, fungi and spores	All kinds of materials, metals, rubber etc. Well documented. Cheap	Glutaraldehyde vapour irritates respiratory tract. Irritating smell, allergy. Slow effect on mycobacteria: 60 min. Coagulates and fixes tissue to equipment. Observe biofilm formation by poor cleaning of scopes and the like
Ortho-phthalaldehyde-Cidex	Effect of glutaraldehyde/ formaldehyde	Quickly acting, very effective. No activation. No irritation. Good material compatibility. Does not coagulate blood and does not fix tissue	Colours on skin, clothing, equipment. Limited experience. More expensive than glutaraldehyde. Eye irritation upon contact. Slow effect on spores. Note anaphylactic reaction in bladder cancer patients
Phenols—used a little today	Gram-positive and gram-negative bacteria, mycobacteria and fungi. Uncertain effect on viruses, especially lipid-free viruses. No effect on bacterial spores	Long shelf life of concentrate	Uncertain effect on viruses, no effect on spores. Slow-acting. Cannot be used on plastic or rubber material. Irritating to skin and mucous membranes and may be absorbed by direct contact. Unfortunate environmental effect. Unstable concentration by inaccurate dilution

(continued)

Table 59.2 (continued)

Disinfectant	Microbiological effect	Benefits	Disadvantage
Peracetic acid	Very good effect and not inhibited by organic/inorganic material. Bacteria, mycobacteria, viruses, fungi and spores	Quick cycle 30–45 min. Environmental friendly end products. Low temperature: 50–55 °C. Fully automated machines. Single-standardized doses. Standardized cycle. Increases removal of organic material. Increases the removal of endotoxin. Most materials tolerate the treatment. Does not coagulate blood and does not fix tissue. The disinfectant fluid passes through narrow canals. Quickly kills spores. Standardization of procedures	Unfortunate for materials like aluminium. Can corrode copper, brass, etc. Only for instruments that can be treated with liquid. Biological monitoring uncertain. Small capacity. Expensive. Eye and skin damage when contacted with concentrated solution. Not suitable for storage of sterile equipment. Unstable in diluted form
Peroxyacetic acid/ hydrogen peroxide combination	Good and fast effect. Bacteria, mycobacteria, viruses, fungi, slow effect on spores	No activation. Not irritating	Material incompatibility: lead, brass, copper, zinc. Limited experience. Eye and skin injuries by accident
Chloramine 5% (undiluted: 12,500 ppm) **Sodium hypochlorite** (chloricide undiluted: 45,000 ppm)	Very good effect. May be inactivated by much organic materials. Effect on bacteria, mycobacteria, viruses, fungi and spores	Well documented. Environmentally friendly. Cheap. Quick effect on dry areas. Effect on biofilm and dried microbes	Inactivated by blood. Material incompatibility: some metals, but not plastic or glass. Irritating vapours
Superoxidized water Hypochloric acid from electrolysed saline and chlorine	Effect like chloramine/chlorine	Depending on the amount of free chlorine. Environmentally friendly. Cheap. Quickly acting, very effective, <2 min	Inactivated by blood. Limited experience. Depending on good concentration of free chlorine >144 mg/L and time
Hydrogen peroxide 6.5–7% liquid substance	Very good effect and little effect of organic/inorganic material. Bacteria, mycobacteria, viruses, fungi and spores	No activation. Increases removal of organic matter. Not irritating. Does not coagulate blood and does not fix tissue. Inactivates *Cryptosporidium*	Material incompatibility in liquid form: brass, zinc, copper, nickel, silver. Eye damage when contacted

Table 59.2 (continued)

Disinfectant	Microbiological effect	Benefits	Disadvantage
Hydrogen peroxide (HPV) gas/aerosol (5–35%); with (35%) and without water vapour (5%)	Effect on bacteria, viruses and spores. No certain effect on mycobacteria. Increasing documentation regarding antimicrobial effect	Convert to oxygen and water. Effect time: 3–5 h. Suitable for robot disinfection of rooms, surfaces and medical equipment for infection outbreaks and terminal disinfection. Advantage of spore control and ppm control for disinfection effect documentation	Material damage is dependent on concentration of water vapour (35%). For dry HPV gas/ aerosol 5%, no material damage to medical devices has been detected. Concentration: ppm <1 before entering the room
Pentapotassium bis (peroxymonosulfate) bis (sulfate 50%—Virkon	Good effect on vegetative bacteria, some viruses, fungi. Uncertain effect on mycobacteria, spores and some viruses	Environmentally friendly. Low toxicity	Corrodes some metals
Sodium percarborate 40–60%—PeraSafe	Very good effect. Bacteria, mycobacteria, viruses, fungi and spores	Environmentally friendly. Low toxicity	Inactivated by organic materials

From: References [5, 8, 18]

- "PeraSafe," peracetic acid (from sodium per carbonate and tetra acetyl ethylene diamine), has an effect on vegetative bacteria, viruses, fungi and mycobacteria. It is inactivated with a high yield of organic material. The ppm values for effect are missing. It is used on cleaned equipment, working time 10 min and for *Mycobacterium tuberculosis* 30 min.
- Chloramine 5% and other chlorine compounds such as household chlorine 10% has an effect on bacteria, including tubercle bacteria, fungi and viruses, including hepatitis virus, HIV and norovirus. Chlorine compounds are inactivated by a high yield of organic material and cannot be used on aluminium.
- Hydrogen peroxide 5%, aerosol/dust with defined amount of silver ions, has an effect on vegetative bacteria, spores, viruses and fungi, but not mycobacteria and can be used on all types of metals. Define and monitor ppm values during the process and use spore tests for verification of effect.
- Alcohols (ethanol, isopropanol and disinfectant alcohols) have an uncertain and short-term effect on microorganisms. Alcohol has little ability to penetrate organic material and is therefore only suitable for disinfection of cleaned surfaces.

- Chlorhexidine has limited effect and is only approved for disinfection of cleaned equipment when heat disinfection, other approved chemical disinfectant or liquor cannot be used. It is not recommended as a disinfectant for technical disinfection.
- Several other chemical agents are approved for use in Norway as in other countries [19, 20].

Choice of disinfectant. The hospital should choose one or two clearly defined and documented disinfectants that are easy to handle, easy to understand and easy to throw away after use. The chemicals should not trigger allergies or other illnesses. Chloramine 5% or peracetic acid is recommended in countries with a long tradition of use, especially of chloramine. Hydrogen peroxide dry aerosol can be used for infection outbreaks and as terminal disinfection of isolates after infections with effect on surfaces, air and inner parts of mechanical equipment. No really good documented effect *on Mycobacterium tuberculosis*. By all disinfections using chemical aerosols, the room should be empty of people and checked afterwards for rest gas.

Single-use chemicals. Chemical disinfectants in liquid form should be changed after each use.

Hazardous waste. Small quantities of used chemical liquids can be further diluted with water and discharged into drains under running water. Larger amounts are treated as special waste.

Storage. Concentrates and solutions are stored in enclosed containers in locked cabinets.

59.4.9 Remarks for Chemical Disinfectants

- Follow the recommendation on the product's label regarding durability, range, working time, etc.
- All containers with disinfectant must be covered with a tight lid. Small liquid surface gives less evaporation to the environment.
- Good ventilation.
- Glutaraldehyde steam should be checked with dosimeter and not exceed 0.05 ppm when people are present in the room [8]. Separate exhaust.
- Poor cleaning of instruments can lead to biofilm residues and residues of chemicals.
- Critical symptoms in patients due to glutaraldehyde residues have been observed [8].
- The equipment must be dismantled at maximum, all cavities must be filled, and the equipment must be completely below the liquid level.
- The cleaner the surfaces/equipment, the better effect of chemical disinfection.
- Solutions in use are changed after each use, and the disinfection vial is washed and heat disinfected (decontaminator).
- Brushes for small and narrow instrument canals and cavities are difficult to clean for protein residues; therefore single use.

- These disinfection methods are not effective enough against prions (see under prions).
- Chemical disinfection agents approved by the Norwegian Medicines Agency; see Table 59.1.

59.4.10 Chemical: Thermal Disinfection for Scopes, Etc.

Used for equipment that does not withstand high temperatures. The treatment is done with a combination of disinfectant such as glutaraldehyde or PeraSafe and temperatures up to 60 °C [14–16, 21, 22].

See Chap. 60 on disinfection of endoscopes and other special equipment.

59.4.11 Gas Disinfection with 5% Hydrogen Peroxide, Dry Aerosol [8–11, 23–25]

Medical technical equipment. When cleaning internal parts of medical devices that cannot be immersed in disinfectant fluid, gas disinfection with hydrogen peroxide (5% H_2O_2) may be used. Hydrogen peroxide breaks down to water and oxygen. The disinfection room should be sealed so that gas does not leak out to other rooms while disinfection is in progress. Mechanical equipment is started up, runs and draws the disinfectant gas into the inner parts of the equipment, and the disinfection starts. Nobody should stay in the room during this process. Limit time to stay in a room with H_2O_2 aerosol/gas is <1 ppm in air or up to 15 min at less than 8 ppm.

The gas must be dry so that sensitive parts of internal instruments do not corrode. There are routines for this at special centres for medical technical equipment at hospitals or otherwise decided. Most often, gas disinfection occurs in combination with technical opening for removing dirt, dust and organic matter, which is often abundant in internal parts of the equipment [11]. Always use a spore test and a ppm meter to check the procedure!

Currently there is no gas agent that takes *Mycobacterium tuberculosis* [10, 26]. Therefore, medical devices that have been used in patients with infectious tuberculosis are treated as infectious waste.

Outbreaks and disinfection of rooms. Hydrogen peroxide dry gas (aerosol) can also be used as an alternative or in addition to disinfection with chemical liquid upon outbreak of MRSA, *Clostridium difficile*, multidrug-resistant bacteria, norovirus and other infections. Hydrogen peroxide gas is used for disinfection of rooms, store rooms with disposable equipment that cannot be disinfected with liquid disinfection and which would otherwise be thrown away, textiles that cannot be washed or are difficult to disinfect, and other rooms with storage of a lot of equipment. Afterwards, thorough cleaning of all surfaces and contact points is carried out. The disinfection method with 5% dry hydrogen peroxide gas includes three defined disinfection cycles! Otherwise, the equipment will not be properly disinfected. Spore test placed in the room and on equipment is an important control of effect, together with a ppm—measurer to control the concentration and the procedure.

59.4.12 Surface and Spot Disinfection

See Chap. 65 concerning cleaning of the wards.

59.4.13 Protective Measures

All chemical disinfectants release vapours that may cause health risks (skin and respiratory system, mucous membrane irritation, respiratory distress with asthma, allergy). Avoid skin contact, especially with chemical concentrates. Work in good ventilation and exhaustion (air extraction) and do not inhale! Gasses may be checked by measuring ppm in the air.

59.4.14 After Checking and Storage of Disinfected Equipment

Bedpans, urine bottles, instruments and other equipment must be checked for visual purity and handled with sterile gloves (at least clean) in order not to be recontaminated and are stored or further processed according to their intended use.

Disinfected equipment not further processed for sterilization should be packaged/stored in clean conditions in a clean cabinet with glass door. Cabinets must have regular cleaning procedures.

59.5 Prion Inactivation: Prion Diseases

(Creutzfeldt-Jakob's disease, CJD; variant CJD, vCJD; bovine spongiform encephalitis, BSE; and others—see Chap. 55 on prion disease)

Instruments and equipment cannot be disinfected or sterilized after contamination with prions and should not be reused [4, 27–36]. Contact infection control personnel.

The following decontamination methods are not effective:

- *Chemical disinfectants*: alcohol, formalin, glutaraldehyde, hydrogen peroxide, peracetic acid, iodophores, phenols, chlorine dioxide, and HCl.
- *Chemical gases*: ethylene oxide, formaldehyde vapour, hydrogen peroxide vapour, etc.
- *Physical methods*: boiling, dry heat, UVC, ionised radiation, and ordinary steam autoclaving.

The following decontamination method may have effect, *but not 100% sure*!

- *Chemical disinfectants*: NaOH 1 N for 1 h, sodium hypochlorite 20,000 ppm free chlorine in 1 h or formic acid 96% for 1 h (for histopathology).
- *Physical methods*: burning after autoclaving at 134–137 °C in 18–60 min.

59.5.1 Sterilization of Instruments/Equipment Used in Examination/Treatment of Possible CJD

In particular, BSE/vCJD has thermostable (−resistant) variants—sterilization is not completely effective.

- *Invasive equipment. Use disposable equipment or reusable equipment that can be destructed as infectious waste after use.*
  - Immediately after use, the equipment is immersed for 1 h in a hazardous container with sodium hypochlorite (household chlorine) 20,000 ppm free chlorine for 1 h.
  - 1 N NaOH (40 g NaOH in 1 L of water) for 1 h at room temperature
  - Autoclaving at 134–137 °C for 1 h, packaged as contamination and sent for burning.
- *Non-invasive* multiple-use equipment should preferably be treated as invasive equipment (as described above) or immersed in 1 N NaOH (1 h) or sodium hypochlorite 20,000 ppm for 1 h.
- *Tracking equipment used for CJD.* If, in retrospect, CJD is suspected, previously used equipment will be recalled which will then be processed and destroyed as above. The identity of people associated with this equipment is ensured.

59.5.2 Disinfection of Surfaces/Environment

Surfaces, benches, etc.: Spot disinfected with sodium hypochlorite 10,000 ppm or 1 N NaOH for 1 h and finish with normal disinfection; 5% chloramine (12,500 ppm) for 1 h or 1 N NaOH for 1 h.

59.6 Background Information

Disinfection is "destruction or removal of all organisms capable of causing infection" and "in practice, leads to the removal of all microbes except spores - that is, an approximate sterilization process" [1–8]. In the healthcare system, instruments and equipment are disinfected with heat, chemical fluids, vapours or gases [1–11]. Prions are contagious protein sequences that may be destructed after special methods [4].

"Disinfection" in the form of preventing contamination of food by smoking, salting, drying, etc. has probably been used for several thousand years. Disinfectants as such have been studied since the 1750s. In the nineteenth century, hypochlorite and other chlorine agents have been effective for their special use, first documented by Semmelweis in 1847 and later by Lister who combined hypochlorite with carbolic acid in operative activity.

Many disinfectants have an uncertain effect. Chemical disinfectants are usually less effective if much dirt and organic material are present; some disinfectants may not kill bacterial spores, fungi, virus and parasites; and others are ineffective against mycobacteria [2, 3, 5, 8–11]. Disinfectants and methods for use are changing in every greater tempo, for increasingly more complex equipment and instruments [1–8]. At the same time, knowledge increases of contagiousness, persistence and survival in the environment; of robust resistance to inactivation by heat, chemicals, UVC and other agents; and of a disturbing development of resistance, both against disinfectants and antibiotics [4, 8, 27–40].

Resistance to disinfectants. Bacteria with a long life in the environment (like MRSA, VRE, ESBL-stains, *Pseudomonas*, *Clostridium difficile*, etc.) are often associated with resistance to antibiotics, infectivity, low infection dose, virulence and resistance to disinfectants [37, 38, 41–44]. *An effective disinfection removes* most common human pathogenic bacteria and viruses, while some heat stable and/or chemically stable microbes survive [1–8]. The most resistant are spore-forming, usually harmless (with exception of *C. difficile*) "dust bacteria" without pathogen significance for others than for patients with reduced infection defence.

- Enterococci may survive in environment for several years and are heat resistant (up to 100 °C in organic materials) and have varying resistance to chemical disinfectants [45].
- Mycobacteria (TB, etc.) may survive in the environment for up to 1 year and are relatively resistant to chemical disinfectants [1–8, 10].
- Norovirus and special pathogenic viruses are robust survivors in the environment—for months—and are often resistant to many disinfectants.
- Hepatitis B and hepatitis E viruses are highly heat resistant, the same with adenovirus, parvovirus and a variety of other virus types.
- Unusually resistant are also certain rare, partially unknown viruses, virus-like particles and infectious proteins; prions (Creutzfeld-Jakobs, bovine spongiform encephalitis (BSE), and other prion diseases). New types and variations of prion disease still occur. The last type is "Shy-Drager syndrome" (multiple system atrophy—MSA) that "raises the question of whether or not also alzheimer and parkinsonism is contagious" [36]. "All chemicals that kill bacteria and viruses do not harm prions" [36].
- Fungal spores and microsporidia are often resistant to chemical disinfectant and high temperatures.
- Parasites like coccidia are highly resistant to chemical disinfectants, as are cysts from *Giardia lamblia, Cryptosporidia* and other protozoans [3, 8]. Trophozoites (not cyst form of protozoa) are more sensitive to chemical substances.

Thermal disinfection with moist heat (damp) is in most cases a safe and environmentally sound method of cleaning and disinfection of instruments and equipment.

59.6.1 Chemical Disinfection in Liquid Form

Chemical disinfectants are an environmental stress and can often be both expensive and uncertain. Therefore, chemical disinfection should only be used where heat disinfection cannot be carried out [8, 41, 45, 46].

Chloramine 5% has effects on spores (cortex), bacteria (peptidoglycan/cell wall), viruses (capsid, nucleic acid RNA/DNA, capsule, thiol groups) and fungi (intracellular amino groups)—with varying working time [38]. Effective part: HOCL, free chlorine, can be inactivated with much organic material present.

Chloramine 5% (12.5 g active chlorine)	12,500 ppm
Chloricid undiluted	45,000 ppm
Chloricid diluted 25%	11,000 ppm
Household chlorine (bleach), 5.25%	52,500 ppm
Household chlorine 1:10 dilution	5000 ppm

Inactivating effect on microbes

Hepatitis B/HIV virus in blood spills	5000 ppm
Mycobacteria/TB—60 min	1000–10,000 ppm
Spores >100 ppm kills 99.9% *B. subtilis*	100–1000 ppm
Other bacteria and viruses	200–1000 ppm
Fungi—varying killing effect	
Cysts—varying killing effect	
Prions—some effect—60 min	20,000 ppm

Glutaraldehyde 2–3% has an effect on spores (core), bacteria (cytoplasmic), viruses (capsid, thiol groups) and fungi (cell wall)—with varying effect time [38]. Proper use of disinfectant dilution and effect time are important. Observe time for durability and check glutaraldehyde vapour in the room with dosimeter: <0.05 ppm.

Alcohol can have bactericidal effects. Effect on hepatitis B virus and HIV, possibly after 2–10 min. Uncertain effect of alcohols, due to rapid evaporation and poor penetration ability in organic materials. Therefore it is used only on clean surfaces and clean equipment. A good virus-killing effect may be achieved by the alcohol mixture 80% ethanol and 5% isopropanol.

Hydrogen peroxide 3–6% in liquid and similar disinfectants are effective for most microorganisms. Six percent or higher concentration has an effect on *Cryptosporidium parvum* and working time of 20 min.

Peracetic acid has good general microbial effect in denaturing proteins: bacteria, spores, viruses and fungi and is used in combination with hydrogen peroxide.

Potassium persulfate ("Virkon") is effective against most microbes except for mycobacteria and does not have a good effect on spores and is not very well documented against viruses.

Sodium perborate ("PeraSafe") is effective against most microbes, including mycobacteria.

59.6.2 Chemical Disinfection in Gas:Steam-Aerosol Fogging Form

For more than 100 years, different chemical gases have been used to inactivate microbes, including formaldehyde, ethylene oxide vapour, ozone, peracetic acid vapour, chloricide vapour, etc. Formaldehyde steam and ozone are not active against spores.

Chlorine dioxide gas of 40 mg/L for 30 min at relative humidity 70–75% kills anthrax spores.

Formaldehyde gas moisture "fumigation" is used in poultry production, safety cabinets and laboratories. The effect is >8 log reduction of anthrax spores.

Formaldehyde gas + high humidity (used in ambulances) has no effect on spore tests (author, personal studies).

Ethylene oxide chamber—100% of anthrax spores killed.

Hydrogen peroxide gas/aerosol/vapour/fogging (HPV) is used for disinfection of rooms, surfaces, mechanical equipment, etc. It is well documented for most infectious agents (except for mycobacteria and prions) used correctly and with control of ppm, test spores, leaks and methods and caution with medical technical and other vulnerable equipment [9–11, 23–26]. Wet HPV gas may corrode metal, while dry gas/aerosol does not [9, 11].

Several HPV systems used today may lack control and documentation of efficacy. Disinfection with HPV necessitates control, ppm measurements and spore tests to avoid development of resistance, biofilm formation, adaptation, tolerance or other microbial "adaptations" to biocides [38, 41–44].

Some studies after 2006 are shown below: [9–11, 23–25, 47–59].

- HPV (Bioquell) 30%, effective against environmental contamination with MRSA [23].
- HPV dry aerosol ("mist") 5% had spore effect but no effect on *Mycobacterium tuberculosis* [9, 11].
- HPV dry aerosol 5%—effect on environmental pollution with MRSA [47].
- HPV effectively against *Clostridium difficile* [24, 48].
- HPV (Bioquell) 30% was compared with VPH (Steris—UK) 31% dry aerosol against bacteriophage. Not properly implemented but effect on a cycle [49].
- HPV (Bioquell) effectively in England against *C. difficile* outbreaks [50].
- HPV (Bioquell) 30% hydrogen peroxide in damp form can be considered more effective than a Sterinis system 5% with silver ions <50 ppm and orthophosphoric acid <50 ppm, from Johnson & Johnson [51].
- Automatic "no-touch" system including HPV can be useful for infection control in hospitals [52].
- VPH (Steris—UK) 35% hydrogen peroxide in steam form—effective in combination with other measures against multidrug-resistant *Acinetobacter baumannii* [53].

- VPH (Steris—UK) 35% hydrogen peroxide in steam form; not completely effective against MRSA—a cycle [54].
- VPH (Steris—UK) 35% compared to Ecasol and Citrox aerosols—VPH's widest effective spectre [55].
- HPV (Bioquell) decontamination and terminal-disinfection intervention: significant reduction of *C. difficile* [56].
- HPV (Bioquell) used in conjunction with standard cleaning reduced risk of MDRO (multidrug-resistant organisms) infection [57].
- HPV (Bioquell) decontamination of sterile packaged equipment [58].
- HPV dry aerosol (mist) and HPV (Bioquell) were both used in the epidemic of multidrug-resistant *Acinetobacter baumannii* in 84 secondary intensive cases infected from patients with intercontinental transmission in a French hospital [59].
- HPV dry aerosol (mist) are proven as effective as active chlorine disinfectant to disinfect rooms and surfaces [60].

59.6.3 Radiation

- UV radiation is effective if the object is not covered [40]. Up to 90% of anthrax spores are killed.
- Gamma radiation; anthrax spores—100% killed.

59.6.4 May Single-Use, Disposable Equipment Be the Future?

Prion-like diseases and new resistant agents like microsporidia and other resistant agents may cause that the focus may be put on disposable rather than reusable, disinfected equipment. This applies especially for devices that come in contact with mucous membranes in the respiratory, oesophageal-gastro-intestinal, urinary and genital areas and which cannot be sterilized [36].

References

1. Rutala WA. Selection and use of disinfectants in health care. In: Mayhall CG, editor. Hospital epidemiology and infection control. London: William and Wilkins; 1996. p. 913–36.
2. Weber DJ, Barbee SL, Sobsey MD, Rutala WA. The effect of blood on the antiviral activity of sodium hypochlorite, a phenolic, and a quaternary ammonium compound. Infect Control Hosp Epidemiol. 1999;20:821–7.
3. Weber DJ, Rutala WA. The emerging nosocomial pathogens *Cryptosporidium, Escherichia coli* O157: H7, *Helicobacter pylori*, and hepatitis C: epidemiology, environmental survival, efficacy of disinfection, and control measures. Infect Control Hosp Epidemiol. 2001;22:306–15.
4. Rutala WA, Weber DJ. Creutzfeldt-Jakob disease: recommendations for disinfection and sterilization. Clin Infect Dis. 2001;32:1348–56.
5. Rutala WA, Weber DJ, et al. CDC guideline for disinfection and sterilization in healthcare facilities, 2008. CDC; 2008.

6. Weber DJ, Brown V, Huslage K, Sickbert-Bennett E, Rutala WA. Device-related infections in home health care and hospice: infection rates, 1998-2008. Infect Control Hosp Epidemiol. 2009;30:1022–4.
7. Rutala WA, Weber DJ. Disinfection and sterilization: an overview. Am J Infect Control. 2013;41:2–5.
8. Rutala WA, Weber DJ. Disinfection, sterilization, and control of hospital waste. In: Bennett JE, Dolin R, Blaser MJ, editors. Mandell, Douglas, and Bennets principles and practice of infectious diseases, vol. 2. 8th ed. Philadelphia: Elsevier; 2015. p. 3294–309.
9. Andersen BM, Rasch M, Hochlin K, Jensen FH, Wismar P, Fredriksen JE. Decontamination of rooms, medical equipment and ambulances, using a dry fog or hydrogen peroxide disinfectant. J Hosp Infect. 2006;62:149–55.
10. Andersen BM, Syversen G, Thoresen H, Rasch M, Hochlin K, Seljordslia B, Snevold I, Berg E. Failure of dry fog or hydrogen peroxide 5% to kill *Mycobacterium tuberculosis*. J Hosp Infect. 2010;76:80–3.
11. Andersen BM, Hochlin K, Daling JP. Cleaning and decontamination of reusable medical devices, including the use of hydrogen peroxide dry-fog gas decontamination. J Microbiol Biochem Technol. 2012;4:57–62.
12. Fossum K, Baksaas I, editors. Disinfection and sterilization in the health service. Oslo: Norwegian Medicines Control, Department of Pharmacotherapy; 1988.
13. Hauff Ulvestad K, Hagen ST. Sterilforsyning i sykehus. Oslo: Universitetsforlaget; 1998.
14. Andersen BM, Levy F. Technical disinfection of instruments and equipment. In: Handbook for hygiene and infection control for hospitals. Oslo: Ullevål Hospital; 1996. p. 185–90.
15. Andersen BM, Hochlin K, Solheim N, Rasch M, Levy F. Technical disinfection of instruments and equipment. In: Handbook for hygiene and infection control for hospitals. Oslo: Ullevål University Hospital; 2008. p. 347–55.
16. Andersen BM. Technical disinfection and sterilization. In: Handbook for hygiene and infectious care for nursing homes, long-term institutions. Oslo: Akademika Forlag; 2013. p. 467–76.
17. Andersen BM. T1.18. Disinfection. Norwegian medicines guide for personnel; 2013. p. 100–5. Same chapter in 2004, 2007 and 2010.
18. Andersen BM. L1.9 Disinfectants. Norwegian medicines guide for personnel 2013. p. 776–84. Same chapter in 2004, 2007 and 2010.
19. Anonymous. Approval of disinfectant. Norwegian Medicines Agency. 4 September 2015.
20. Anonymous. Chemical disinfectants for technical use in health and nursing. Norwegian Medicines Agency. Updated June 2015.
21. Andersen BM, Norman BI, Røed RT, Solheim N. Spirometry and lung function. Disinfection and cleaning methods. Ullevål Hospital, Lovisenberg Diakonale Hospital; 1998.
22. Røed RT, Gullord TP, Norman BIS, Andersen BM. Flexible endoscope. Prevention of infections, 2002. Oslo: Occupational Committee, Division for Infection Control, Health Region East and Ullevål University Hospital; 2002.
23. French GL, Otter JA, Shannon KP, Adams NMT, Watling D, Parks MJ. Tackling contamination of the hospital environment by methicillin-resistant *Staphylococcus aureus* (MRSA): a comparison between conventional terminal cleaning and hydrogen peroxide vapor decontamination. J Hosp Infect. 2004;57:31–7.
24. Boyce JM, Havill NL, Otter JA, et al. Impact of hydrogen peroxide vapor chamber decontamination on *Clostridium difficile* environmental contamination and transmission in a healthcare setting. Infect Control Hosp Epidemiol. 2008;29:723–9.
25. Chan FT, White P, Sheorey H, Cocks J, Waters MJ. Evaluation of biological efficacy of hydrogen peroxide vapour decontamination in wards of Australian hospitals. J Hosp Infect. 2011;79:125–8.
26. Andersen BM. Does "airborne" hydrogen peroxide kill *Mycobacterium tuberculosis*? J Hosp Infect. 2011;77(1):81–3; Letter
27. Spencer RC, Ridgway GL, vCJD Consensus Group. Sterilization issues in vCJD-towards a consensus. J Hosp Infect. 2002;51:168–74.

28. Bosque PJ, Tyler KL. Prions and prion disease of the central nervous system (Transmissible neurodegenerative diseases). In: Bennett JE, Dolin R, Blaser MJ, editors. Mandell, Douglas, Bennetts principles and practice of infectious diseases. 8th ed. London: Elsevier Churchill Livingston; 2015. p. 2142–53.
29. Government, UK. Infection prevention and control of CJD, vCJD and other human prion diseases in healthcare and community settings. Transmissible spongiform encephalopathy agents: safe working and the prevention of infection: Part 4. Revised and updated January 2014.
30. Andersen BM. Prion disease (Creutzfeldt-Jacob's disease-CJD, etc.). In: Handbook for hygiene and infection control for hospitals. Part 1: microbiology and infection protection. Bergen: Fagbokforlaget; 2014. p. 351–5.
31. Belay ED, Blase J, Schulster LM, Maddox RA, Sconberger LB. Management of neurosurgical instruments and patients exposed to Creutzfeldt-Jakob disease. Infect Control Hosp Epidemiol. 2013;34:1272–80.
32. McDonnel G, Dehan C, Perrin A, et al. Cleaning, disinfection and sterilization of surface prion contamination. J Hosp Infect. 2013;85:268–73.
33. Secker TJ, Herve R, Keevil CW. Adsorption of prion and tissue proteins to surgical stainless steel surfaces and the effectiveness of decontamination following dry and wet storage conditions. J Hosp Infect. 2011;78:251–5.
34. Lipscomb IP, Pinchin H, Collin R, Keevil CW. Effect of drying time, ambient temperature and pre-soaks on prion-infected tissue contamination levels on surgical stainless steel: concerns about prolonged transportation of instruments from theater to central sterile service departments. J Hosp Infect. 2007;65:72–7.
35. Fernie K, Hamilton S, Somerville RA. Limited efficacy of steam sterilization to inactivate vCJD infectivity. J Hosp Infect. 2012;80:46–51.
36. Promed Mail September 7, 2015. Prion disease update: novel prion disease, Shy-carrier syndrome.
37. Kramer A, Schebke I, Kampf G. How long do nosocomial pathogens persist on the surfaces? A systematic review. BMC Infect Dis. 2006;6:130–8.
38. Russel AD, Furr JR, Maillard JY. Microbial susceptibility and resistance to biocides. AMS News. 1997;63:481–7.
39. Sagripanti JL, Bonifacino A. Comparative sporicidal effect of liquid chemical germicides on three medical devices contaminated with spores of *Bacillus subtilis*. Am J Infect Control. 1996;24:364–71.
40. Andersen BM, Bånrud H, Bøe E, Bjordal O, Drangsholt F. Comparison of UVC light and chemicals for disinfection of surfaces in hospital isolation units. Infect Control Hosp Epidemiol. 2006;27:729–35.
41. McDonnel G, Russell AD. Antiseptics and disinfectants: activity, action and resistance. Clin Microbiol Rev. 1999;12:147–97.
42. Maillard JY. Bacterial target sites for biocidal action. J Appl Microbiol Suppl. 2002;92:16–27.
43. Russell AD. Mechanisms of antimicrobial action of antiseptics and disinfectants: an increasingly important area of investigation. J Antimicrob Chemother. 2002;49:597–9.
44. EU Directorate-General for Health and Consumers. Scientific Committee on emerging and newly identified health risks. Beoordeling van de antibiotische resistentie effecten van biociden. SCENIHR; 2009.
45. Renner P, Peters J. Resistance to enterococci to heat and chemical agents. Zentralbl Hyg Umweltmed. 1999;202:41–50.
46. US Food and Drug Administration. Device evaluation information. FDA-cleared sterilants and high level disinfectants with general claims for processing reusable medical and dental devices. 2009. www.fda.gov/cdrh/ode/germlab.html.
47. Bartels MD, Kristoffersen K, Slotsbjerg T, Rohde SM, Lundgren B, Westh H. Environmental methicillin-resistant *Staphylococcus aureus* (MRSA) disinfection using dry-mist-generated hydrogen peroxide. J Hosp Infect. 2008;70:35–40.
48. Boyce JM. New approaches to decontamination of rooms after patients are discharged. Infect Control Hosp Epidemiol. 2009;30:515–7.

49. Pottage T, Richardson C, Parks S, Walker JT, Bennett AM. Evaluation of hydrogen peroxide gas disinfection systems to decontaminate viruses. J Hosp Infect. 2010;74:55–61.
50. Cooper T, O'Leary M, Yezli S, Otter JA. Impact of environmental decontamination using hydrogen peroxide vapour on the incidence of *Clostridium difficile* infection in one hospital Trust. J Hosp Infect. 2011;78:238–40.
51. Fu TY, Ghent P, Kumar V. Efficacy, efficiency and safety aspects of hydrogen peroxide vapor and aerosolized hydrogen peroxide cream disinfection systems. J Hosp Infect. 2012;80:199–205.
52. Otter JA, Yezli S, Perl TM, Barbut F, French GL. The role of "no-touch" automated room disinfection systems in infection prevention and control. J Hosp Infect. 2012;83(1):1–13.
53. Chmielarczyk A, Higgins PG, Wojkowska-Mach J, et al. Control of an outbreak of *Acinetobacter baumannii* infections using vaporized hydrogen peroxide. J Hosp Infect. 2012;81:239–45.
54. Pottage T, Macken S, Walker JT, Bennett AM. Methicillin-resistant *Staphylococcus aureus* is more resistant to vaporized hydrogen peroxide than commercial *Geobacillus stearothermophilus* biological indicators. J Hosp Infect. 2012;80:41–5.
55. Galvin S, Boyle M, Russell RJ, et al. Evaluation of vaporized hydrogen peroxide, Citrox and pH neutral Ecasol for decontamination of an enclosed area: a pilot study. J Hosp Infect. 2012;80:67–70.
56. Manian FA, Griesnauer S, Bryant A. Implementation of hospital-wide enhanced terminal cleaning of targeted patient rooms and its impact on endemic *Clostridium difficile* infection rates. Am J Infect Control. 2013;41(6):537–41.
57. Otter JA, Nowakowski E, Salkeld JAG, et al. Saving costs through the decontamination of the packaging of unused medical supplies using hydrogen peroxide vapor. Infect Control Hosp Epidemiol. 2013;34:472–8.
58. Passaretti C, Otter JA, Reich NG, et al. An evaluation of environmental decontamination with hydrogen peroxide vapor for reducing the risk of patient acquisition of multi-drug resistant organisms. Clin Infect Dis. 2013;56:27–35.
59. Landelle C, Legrand P, Lesprit P, et al. Protracted outbreak of multidrug-resistant *Acinetobacter baumannii* after intercontinental transfer of colonized patients. Infect Control Hosp Epidemiol. 2013;34:119–24.
60. Ferrari M, Bocconi A, Anesi A. Evaluation of the effectiveness of environmental disinfection by no-touch hydrogen peroxide technology against MDR bacteria contamination and comparison with active chlorine disinfectant. Antimicrob Resist Infect Control. 2015;4(Suppl):P43.

Endoscopes and Other Special Equipment

60

Abstract

Endoscopic procedures are increasingly used in medicine both diagnostic and therapeutic. Complications and infections are rare, 1 per 1.8 million procedures, but there are no other instruments that are associated with as many infections as endoscopes. This is due to lack of routines, not following routines or lack of competence. An analysis of published exogenous endoscopy-related infections, pseudo-infections and toxic reactions between 1974 and 2004 showed 140 outbreaks where more than 94% of the cases could be prevented by improved decontamination of instruments. Endoscopes are often very complex composed equipment that is difficult to sterilize. They may have combined parts that can be sterilized (high hygienic level) and parts that may only be disinfected (lower hygienic level). In addition, scopes may often have long, narrow lumens, are flexible and may be difficult to clean for organic materials. Still there may be great problems concerning certain endoscopes and other equipment that are difficult to decontaminate. The following chapter is focused on practical measures to disinfect, sterilize and control endoscopes and other special equipment in healthcare institutions.

Keywords

Endoscopes · Heat-sensible instruments · Reusable equipment · Disinfection Sterilization · Infection control · Hygiene · Prevention

60.1 Purpose

- To ensure that all products that undergo a disinfection or sterilization process are disinfected or sterile afterwards [1–4].
- To remove pathogenic agents: bacteria, viruses, fungi, parasites, spores, from endoscopes and other heat-sensitive equipment.

B. M. Andersen, *Prevention and Control of Infections in Hospitals*,
https://doi.org/10.1007/978-3-319-99921-0_60

- To prevent transmission of infection from patients to other patients, staff, visitors or the environment through instruments, technical equipment.

60.2 Comprise

- Endoscope and the like that undergoes disinfection (“high level”) and/or sterilization.
- All equipment, including endoscopes that have been in contact with biological materials.
- All equipment that will come in contact with mucous membranes, skin, secretions, excretions, and/or other human biological materials.
- Endoscopes which come into contact with normally sterile sites (mucous tissue, cavities) should be *sterile.*
- Endoscopes and other equipment that come into contact with (*not penetrating*) unsterile mucosa (oral cavity, bowel, etc.) should at least be disinfected and preferably sterilized.

60.3 Responsibility

The hospital management should ensure enough resources and written routines for modern disinfection and sterilization procedures.

Department management implements routines to ensure that endoscopes and other special equipment are pre-treated, controlled, packed, transported, sterilized, re-controlled and stored in a safe manner. Lack of resources and accidents that constitute a risk of infection for patients or personnel are reported to the Director immediately.

Personnel follow hospital procedures for processing disinfected and sterile goods.

Preparedness in connection with deficiencies/failure (machine shutdown, flood, etc.) regarding sterilization and disinfection capacity must be ensured by planned cooperation with other hospitals and sterilization centres.

60.4 Practical Measures [1–4]

60.4.1 Personal Protection

The personnel working on endoscopy/processing of endoscopes should follow routines for the use of protective equipment for the treatment of patients and unclean equipment. For manual treatment of unclean endoscopes, like washing, drying, etc., it is important to protect the person with the use of gloves, gown (preferably waterproof), cap, eye protection and respiratory protection.

Treatment of *clean equipment* should be done in clean environment/clean room, with clean gown, surgical mask/cap and gloves.

60.4.2 Choice of Purity Level on Endoscope

60.4.2.1 High-Risk Endoscopy: Critical Concerning Sterility of the Scope

- Invasive endoscopes in sterile tissues and sterile mucous membranes
- All instrumentation with risk of lesions in mucous membranes (biopsies, etc.) regardless of sterile or unsterile mucosa

60.4.2.2 Intermediate-Risk Endoscopy: Semi-critical—Concerning Sterility of the Scope

- Endoscope use in unsterile areas like colon. No planned perforation of "unsterile normal mucous membranes"

Invasive endoscopes must be sterile, and all endoscopy procedures should take place in an operating room, with the same requirements for quality of hygiene and infection protection as for surgery.

- *All heat-sensitive endoscopes* like GIT endoscopes, bronchoscopes and nasopharyngoscopes must be thoroughly cleaned and at least undergo a "high-level" disinfection program between each patient [1, 4].
  - *High-level disinfection* destroys most microbes, but there is no good effect on spores, free-living amoebas and *Mycobacterium chelonae* [1–5].
  - There may also be an uncertain effect on *M. tuberculosis*, *M. avium intracellulare*, other mycobacteria and other microbes.
  - Lack of effect may be discovered by biofilm formation, failures in automatic endoscopy disinfection machines and using too short exposure time [1–7].
  - *There is no effect on prions of high-level disinfection.*

60.4.3 Risk Areas in General

- Biofilm formation—in endoscope channels and channels for disinfection machines [1–4, 7, 8].
- Water sources—sterile and non-sterile. Filtered water is not enough [1, 4].
- Other attached equipment—lack of sterilization.
- Disinfectants that fix microbes and organic material to the instrument [1, 4].
- Prion diseases, water amoebas, fungi, enterococci, spores, microsporidies, mycobacteria, *Pseudomonas* and other infectious agents that can survive disinfection process.
- Brush reuse: organic residual material and reuse of damaged brushes that destroy inner scope parts [1, 4].
- Lack of protection of patients and personnel.

60.4.4 Recommendations from CDC [1, 2, 4]:

- IA = A strong recommendation supported by high- to moderate-quality evidence suggesting net clinical benefits or harms.
- IB = A strong recommendation supported by low-quality evidence suggesting net clinical benefits or harms or an accepted practice (e.g. aseptic technique), supported by low- to very low-quality evidence.
- IC = A strong recommendation required by state or federal regulation.
- II = A weak recommendation supported by any quality evidence suggesting trade-offs between clinical benefits and harms.

- *Annual control* of the knowledge and implementation of the endoscope disinfection/sterilization process is recommended: **IA**
- *Protection* of patients and personnel. **IA**
- *Pre-cleaning* of the equipment—immediate cleaning and wiping off most of organic materials—the instrument should not dry up: **IB**
- *Transport*—directly to the laundry room/disinfection room—in a closed container before the rest of the organic material dries in: **II**
- *Pressure leak test* after each use—follow guidelines: **IB**
- *Before manual or automatic disinfection*: cleaning of the entire endoscope and divided into every small component and brushed through and rinsed in all channels and surfaces (disposable sponge)—all under liquid level. Note flaps of the scope that may be difficult to rinse. Check that proper soap/enzyme (detergent) is used. **IB**
- *Use brushes* adapted to channel width, connectors and openings. Means for use during the washing process (brushes, sponges, cloths, etc.) should be disposable (or thoroughly cleaned before disinfection/sterilization between use) and **II** Should only be used one time (author).
- *Discard enzymatic detergents* every time after use. **IB**
- *Biopsy instruments* that perforate/damage mucous membranes are cleaned, disinfected and sterilized as common surgical instruments. **IA**
- *Ultrasonic cleaning* can be used for problem instruments. **II**
- *Endoscopes in contact with all types of mucous membranes should at least undergo high-level disinfection between each use.* **IA**
- *High-level disinfection systems* for endoscopes must be approved for the current use. **IA**
- *Exposure and time* depend on disinfectant and scope. For example, it is required for use of glutaraldehyde *more than* 2% (2.4%) at 25 °C from 20 to 90 min (FDA). **IA**
- *Use technology* that is consistent with the quality of the scope/manufacturer. **IB**
- *New technology and resources*—ensure approval. **II**
- *The entire endoscope should be* immersed under the liquid surface in the washing process. If this is not done, the scope must not be used. **IB**

- *Automatic endoscope re-processors (AERs) may fail*—must be checked and used in a defined manner relative to machine, disinfectant and scope. **IB**
- *If AER is used*, check connectors and follow the manual so that all internal parts are disinfected. **IB**
- *If the AER process is interrupted*, everything must be reversed. **II**
- *Infection control personnel* should check AER system against manuals and use. **II**
- *After disinfection*, rinse all channels and rinse the endoscope outside with sterile water—the water is removed after each cycle. Finally rinse with 70–90% alcohol and dry with *clean* compressed air. **IA**
- *Inspect the cleanliness* through the process and destruct or send to repair damaged scope. **II**
- *Store the scope vertically* for drying (see producer manual). The scope must be protected from contamination. **II**
- *Disinfect the scope before use* if uncertain storage—storage time maximum 10 days. Undefined
- *The water bottle and hose mounted in the suction/flushing system* are at risk and should be washed and sterilized between each use. Only sterile water should be used. **IB**
- *Note name, date, time and scope number* if it needs tracing. **II**
- *Routine testing of the disinfectant* should be performed daily or more often with chemical indicator. **IA**
- *Use disinfectant only once* and follow the manual if this is not done. **IB**
- *Areas for endoscopy and cleaning/disinfection* should provide a safe environment for patients and personnel. Good ventilation and control of chemical gases. **IB and IC**
- *Personnel* who work with scopes must be approved also for the use of chemical substances. Only competent personnel shall participate in the work. **IA** and **IC**
- *Personal protective equipment, gloves, gown, eye protection, respiratory protection and cap* should be readily available and should be used by all when exposed to blood, tissues and chemical substances. **IC**
- *The endoscope* should be marked for when and where the disinfection process was completed. **II**
- *Microbiological testing of scope and environment*—undefined, but should be done for scopes. Is conducted internationally in many places today.
- *Microbiological testing shall in that case* be made with standard tests. **II**
- *The scope equipment—follow recommendations.* **II**
- *In case of infection outbreak—suspect scope infection or toxic substance*—carry out environmental and scope sampling according to the standard. **IA**
- *Endoscope-related infections must be reported* in the hospital's routines and to relevant health authorities, etc. **IB and IC**

After the outbreak of multidrug-resistant, gram-negative infections associated with endoscopes, CDC recently (March 2015) has tightened the routines for cleaning and inspection—especially of the ERCP endoscope [9, 10].

- The CDC recommends that the following steps should be taken when reprocessing duodenoscopes [9]:
- *Inspection and manual cleaning*: Ensure that the elevator mechanism located at the distal tip of the duodenoscope is thoroughly cleaned and free of all visible debris. The visible inspection is to be done with the elevator in the “open/raised” position as well as with the elevator in the “closed/lowered” position to ensure there is no visible debris above or below the elevator mechanism. Consider to use a magnifying glass (e.g. 10×) to improve detection of residual debris around the elevator mechanism.
- *Drying*: Ensure that the channels of the duodenoscope and elevator mechanism are *thoroughly dried* prior to storage. This should include an alcohol flush followed by forced air drying if these procedures are compatible with the duodenoscope as per the manufacturer’s instructions. If canals and the elevator are not completely dry, bacterial growth can occur, forming a biofilm that is difficult to remove and could result in persistent contamination [9].

60.4.5 Short Version

60.4.5.1 After Pressure Leak Test, Proceed as Follows [1–4]

1. Clean the equipment mechanically—outer and inner surfaces—and brush thorough channels and rinse all channels with water and an enzymatic soap.
2. Disinfect either:
   (a) Automatic disinfection machine, using glutaraldehyde 2.4% or peracetic acid, perasafe, etc.
   (b) Manual immersed in disinfectant, flushing with disinfectant in all channels for a defined time
3. Clean: The endoscope and all channels with sterile water—filtered water are not good enough.
4. Dry: Clean/rinse tubes and canals with alcohol and dry with clean pressure air.
5. Store: Protected against re-contamination, vertically or arcuate in a ventilated, clean cabinet [3].
6. This procedure will completely remove *one test* of 10 [5, 6] *Mycobacterium tuberculosis* bacteria in organic matter dried into the endoscope, in a difficult place and in the absence of cleaning [1, 2, 4]. It is documented that this can be done with 2.4% glutaraldehyde, disinfection time 45 min at 25 °C [4].

60.4.6 Problems

Automated endoscope reprocessors (AER) have been used for many years also in Norway [3]. They have great advantages in reducing exposure to organic materials and disinfectants. However, used according to international guidelines, there have been a number of infections and bacterial colonization. This may be due to not following the procedures or that the procedures are not good enough. There have been problems with cleaning, not enough water or not using sterile rinsing water, connectors, micro-organisms and organic materials left in places like elevator wire channel in ERCP, etc. [4, 9–19].

Automatic endoscope machines and use of detergents. There are significant differences with regard to types of detergents—enzymatic and non-enzymatic soaps—both in terms of visible purity and microbiological purity (reduction factor), compared with water control [11]. The requirement is, among other things, that cleaning alone should reduce the bioburden with a $\log_{10}$ reduction of 4. Use defined enzymatic soaps for defined scopes and machines.

Sterile water for rinsing after terminal disinfection is important to avoid recontamination. This should be controlled by routines for microbial sampling [12, 13].

Coupling error for suction duct where the disinfectant does not pass the scope lumen has been reported in connection with outbreak of imipenem-resistant *Pseudomonas aeruginosa* [14]. Coupling systems may be misunderstood by unauthorized personnel.

Biofilm formation in automatic scope machines is a problem that can lead to growth of various resistant microbes, which are very difficult to eradicate [6, 7, 15, 16].

Risk of contamination is present for the light source, knots, hoses, manoeuvres head, biopsy channel, air channel, suction, ocular, etc. The inside of the suction duct, 2.8 mm in diameter, may be contaminated with biofilm formation, etc. and are often instrument design problems [1–4, 9, 10].

In contrast to the CDC guidelines, other countries have used other routines and different types of scope machines. Four main types of endoscope machines have been used in Norway, three of which have a disinfection temperature of about 60 °C and do not reuse disinfectant (glutaraldehyde and peracetic acid/hydrogen peroxide) and one with disinfection temperature of 20 °C and reuse of disinfectant (Table 60.1) [3]. There have been few problems associated with endoscopic use in Norway.

Table 60.1 Disinfection machines for flexible endoscopes used in Norway in 2002, ref. [3]

Machine types	A	B	C	D
Cleaning phase	Yes	Yes	No	Depending on the product
Leak test	Yes	Yes	Yes	Some types
Disinfectant	Glutaraldehyde	Glutaraldehyde	Peroxyacetic acid/hydrogen peroxide	Glutaraldehyde
Drains out the washing water	Program I: no Program II: yes	Yes	No cleaning phase	Yes
Direct connection to endoscope channels	Yes	No	Yes	Yes
Disinfecting time	5–10 min	Decide for yourself	12 min	10 min and 60 min by TBC
Reuse of disinfectant	No	No	No	Yes
Disinfection temperature	60 °C	60 °C	58 °C	20 °C
Disinfection of rinse water	UVC irradiation	>85 °C	Sterile filtration	Someone has sterile filtration

Røed R et al. Flexible endoscope p. 2002 ref. [3]

60.4.7 Cause of Infections

- More long, narrow channels—hard to clean.
- Moist or wet scope—increases microbe growth.
- The scope does not tolerate temperatures >65 °C—do not tolerate heat sterilization.
- Worn out, destroyed scopes with holes in suction ducts, etc.
- Couplings—weaknesses—malfunction of hoses, suction, etc.
- Non-smooth surfaces, sharp angles, "dead ends", absorbent materials, pits in the material, etc.
- Often few, expensive instruments.
- Manoeuvre head not properly disinfected.
- Lack of disinfection of workplace, light source, etc.
- Too short time for cleaning and disinfection—before new use.
- Contaminated scope washing machines, especially water inlet (*Pseudomonas aeruginosa* and other gram-negative), air intake, soap intake.
- Thick biofilms in scope and in scope washing machine with gram-negative bacteria.
- *Brushes with residues of organic material transferred from scope to next scope! Damaged brushes can damage internal parts of the scope.*
- Wrong detergent.
- Lack of visual control with magnifying glass.
- Lack of microbiological control at the end of treatment.
- Recontamination during storage of endoscopes in separate ventilated, clean cabinet. After 24 h the scope should be 100% clean inside, and after 7 days this may be reduced to 90% clean [4, 9, 10].
- Contaminated environment, poor hygiene and cleaning between patients and terminal cleaning and disinfection.
- Poor hand hygiene, personal hygiene and attire of personnel working with the patient.

60.4.8 Control: Visual and Microbiological

- By evaluating reprocessing of 89 GIT endoscopes and 3 automatic scope reprocessors in the period 2006–2014 at a hospital in France, 846 samples were taken for microbial growth [17]. French guidelines for treating scopes were followed in 86% of cases, varying with type of scope and seasons. A total of 118 of 846 samples (14%) showed growth of indicator microbes like *Pseudomonas aeruginosa*, *Stenotrophomonas maltophilia*, *Enterobacteriaceae* and *Candida* sp. The result was not satisfactory [17].
- Therefore, microbiological monitoring of automatic scope washers is important for maintaining good practice and for detecting endoscopes that need technical improvement or need to be discarded [11, 17, 18].

60.5 Background Information

Endoscopic procedures are used in a large number, diagnostic and therapeutic, and experience lasts at least 50 years back. Complications and infections are rare, 1 per 1.8 million procedures, but there are no other instruments that are associated with as many infections as endoscopes [1, 2, 4]. An analysis of endoscopy-related infections, pseudo-infections and toxic reactions, 1974–2004, documented 140 outbreaks where more than 94% of the cases could be prevented by improved decontamination of scopes [19].

60.5.1 Cleaning

A proper and thoroughly performed washing processes and selection of enzymatic detergents are central. All organic material must be removed. The disinfection processes does not inactivate prions which is a growing problem. There may also be bacteria, spores and biofilm that is difficult to remove [1–4, 9, 10, 20].

60.5.2 Disinfectant

All disinfectants are inactivated by a lot of organic materials and dirt. Therefore, the instrument must be cleaned for all organic material before disinfection. Do not use endoscopes that cannot completely be immersed in disinfectants. Spores can be detected from all types of disinfection methods.

Glutaraldehyde is widely used, 2% alkaline glutaraldehyde. It is effective, but higher concentrations like 3.3% have some better effect [21]. Concentration decreases over time in disinfection vessels [22]. Glutaraldehyde is well documented, destroys not instruments, is non-corrosive and is relatively inexpensive to use. The downside is slow inactivating effect on mycobacteria, no effect on spores, fixes and coagulates tissue and blood to the metal, must be activated to be effective enough, emits allergenic gases and requires control and protection for users. The smell of glutaraldehyde in the room indicates too high concentration of the disinfectant.

Other disinfectants that can be used are ortho-phthalaldehyde (OPA), hydrogen peroxide, peracetic acid/hydrogen peroxide, chlorine dioxide and PeraSafe.

Do not use these! Iodophores, alcohol, chlorhexidine gluconate, quaternary ammonium solutions, glutaraldehyde (0.13%) with phenol, benzalkonium chloride and hexachlorophene.

60.5.3 Brushes, Sponges and Cloths

All brushes are used once and discarded after use. They can be hardly cleaned for organic matter. Brushes that are damaged at the end can tear up internal parts of the scope. Biopsy elevator (ERCP) must be cleaned with a soft brush [3] (Fig. 60.1).

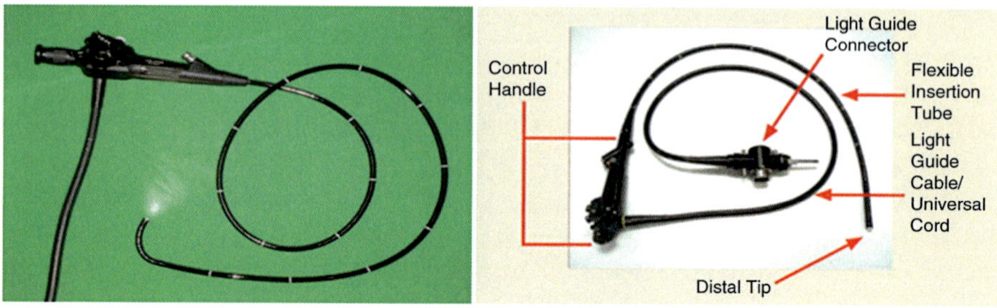

Fig. 60.1 Endoscope. Source: Kebomed.no

60.5.4 Transmission of Microbes

60.5.4.1 Bronchoscope

- Transfer of infection via bronchoscope is well known [15, 19, 23, 24].
- Until 2007, there were >50 outbreaks with more than 2000 patients exposed to infection and more than 750 patients infected. Dominant agents were *Mycobacterium tuberculosis*, atypical mycobacteria and *Pseudomonas aeruginosa* [19].
- Disinfection of bronchoscope should be at the highest level, really full sterilization. Main problems are inadequate disinfectant, concentration, working time, punctured suction channels, inadequate cleaning, lack of sterilization of biopsy equipment, non-customized duct links, biofilm formation when channels are not well cleaned before disinfection, etc. [8, 15].

60.5.4.2 Gastrointestinal Endoscopy: GIT

- In 1974, 240,000 gastrointestinal (GIT) endoscopies were studied retrospectively, including oesophageal-gastro-duodenoscopy (EGD) and colonoscopy. In all, 24 infections were recorded; two deaths of cholangitis, two deaths of pancreatitis, and it was estimated one infection per 10,000 endoscopies and one death of infection per 60,000 scopies [25]. In 1993, there were 377 published infections following GIT endoscopy or bronchoscopy.
- In 1992, 71 used GIT endoscopes were studied: 23% of inner channels had >100,000 bacteria after full disinfection/sterilization [26]. Unauthorized disinfectants had been used for several of the scopes.
- Bacterial contamination of duodenoscopes is associated with problems with disinfection of "Albarran level". This is avoided by following validated procedures for recycling processes [27].
- In 2007, >70 outbreaks were reported, and more than 6000 patients were exposed, and more than 400 patients were infected [19]. A total of 70% were caused by *Salmonella* sp. and *Pseudomonas aeruginosa*. The clinical range varied from colonization to death (4%) [19].

60.5.4.3 Endoscopic Retrograde Cholangiopancreatography (ERCP)

- In 1978, complications from ERCP were recorded in totally 1.3% of the cases and 0.7% infections (sepsis, cholangitis), and 1 in 4 died of the infection [28].
- In 1976 was infection associated to ERCP present in 1.1% of the cases; 97/10,425, and 13.4% of infected patients died [29].
- In Canada, 37 hospitals were asked about the reuse and reprocessing of ECRP, as well as microbial sampling form 119 scopes [30]. Microbial growth was found in 7% of cases, and only 43% followed the national guideline cleaning and disinfection. There was a greater amount of protein, carbohydrates and endotoxin with ERCP scopes disinfected with glutaraldehyde than with peracetic acid [30]. There was a lack of immersion of scopes under water for manual cleaning, large enough volume for cleaning, adequate drying before storage and separation of "ERCP valves" from scopes during storage [30].
- In 2015, some failure with ERCP from Olympus in the United States was reported. At least 16 patients were infected with multidrug-resistant carbapenem-resistant *Pseudomonas* bacteria at several hospitals [31]. Resistant *E coli* (ESBL) outbreaks were reported from other hospitals. More than 500 people are checked for infection, and several patients died due to infections. The problem was not reported to the Food and Drug Administration—FDA—until 2015. The FDA inspected four companies that had Olympus scope in the United States and Japan. The infections came despite the manufacturer's instructions for cleaning were followed [31]. The scopes had been modified by Olympus with camera and other equipment inserted into the scope—in such a way that it could not be cleaned well enough. The bacteria adhered to inner parts together with residues of organic materials and fluids from other patients, the FDA concluded. The scope modifications were not reported to the FDA. A minimum of 500,000 procedures are performed in the United States in recent years. At some hospitals, the endoscope has been discontinued, and some use ethylene oxide gas sterilization, which results in an additional period of aeration to prevent patients from toxic products [31].
- An outbreak of multidrug-resistant, carbapenem- and cephalosporin-resistant (CR) *E. coli* infection in seven patients in the United States, 2012–2013, was associated with ERCP and non-satisfactory *guideline* for reprocessing of scopes [18]. Among the 35 cases consistent with casus definition, 30-day mortality was 16% and for patients with CR infection 56%. Bacteria were detected in scopes after disinfection (2/8), while environmental samples were negative. Recommended scope product guide was not satisfactory [18].

60.5.4.4 Colonoscopy

Hepatitis C infection is transmitted by colonoscopy [32]. Genetic identical HCV was transferred from a patient to two others being examined by colonoscopy the same day. The source of infection had a high yield—3.5 million genome equivalents—of HCV per ml of blood. The biopsy suction duct had never been sterilized [32].

60.5.5 Types of Infections That Usually Are Transmitted

60.5.5.1 Endogenous Infection

- Microbes may occur in blood (bacteraemia) like enterococci, gram-negative rods, anaerobic bacteria, etc. during the scopy process. For instance, during sigmoideum scopy ca.10% of the cases may have bacteraemia lasting for about 15 min—obs risk of endocarditis/heart affection.

60.5.5.2 Exogenous Infection

- Gram-negative rod bacteria grow in "wet areas" in the endoscope after 14–18 h. *Pseudomonas aeruginosa* growth after ERCP. Other bacteria are *Klebsiella*, *Enterobacter*, *Serratia marcescens*, *E coli*, *Helicobacter pylori* (patient to patient infection), Whipples's disease (patient to patient infection), salmonella (EGD colonoscopy, patient to patient infection), etc.
- *Mycobacterium tuberculosis*. Patient for patient infection. Culture-positive bronchoscope is detected after 30 min disinfection with povidone-iodine solution. Note especially the suction channel. Other mycobacteria are even more difficult to remove by disinfection, like *M. chelonei*.
- *Clostridium difficile*. Probable patient to patient transmission—by small doses of spores.

60.5.6 Other Microbes More Seldom Transmitted

Fungi: Trichosporon beigelii, and others, microsporon

Parasites: Pneumocystis carinii, Cryptosporidies, Strongyloides (Oesophagitis epidemic)

Virus: Hepatitis A, B, C, D (at B carrier), E, HIV, etc. can be transmitted by contaminated scopes.

Recent studies suggest that the infection rates after colonoscopy and endoscopy may be "far higher than expected" [33]. This may partly be due to a not effective drying method [34].

References

1. Rutala WA, Weber DJ. Disinfection, sterilization, and control of hospital waste. In: Mandell, Douglas, and Bennets principles and practice of infectious diseases. 8th ed. vol. 2. Philadelphia: Elsevier Churchill Livingstone; 2015. p. 3294–309.
2. Petersen BT, Chennat J, Cohen J, et al. Multisociety guideline on reprocessing flexible GI endoscopes: 2011. ASGE-SHEA guideline. Infect Control Hosp Epidemiol. 2011;32:527–37.
3. Røed RT, Gullord TP, Norman BIS, Andersen BM. Flexible endoscope. Prevention of infections, 2002. Oslo: Occupational Committee, Division for Infection Control, Health Region East and Ullevål University Hospital; 2002.
4. CDC. Disinfection of healthcare equipment. Concerns about implementing the Spaulding scheme. In: Guideline for disinfection and sterilization in healthcare facilities, 2008; 2009.

5. Greub G, Raoult D. Biocides currently used for bronchoscope decontamination are poorly effective against free-living amoebae. Infect Control Hosp Epidemiol. 2003;24:784–6.
6. Kressel AB, Kidd F. Pseudo-outbreak of *Mycobacterium chelonae* and *Methylobacterium mesophilicum* caused by contamination of an automated endoscopy washer. Infect Control Hosp Epidemiol. 2001;22:414–8.
7. Davidson WM, Pitts B, Stewart PS. Spatial and temporal patterns of biocidal action against *Staphylococcus epidermidis* biofilms. Antimicrob Agents Chemother. 2010;54:2920–7.
8. Marion K, Freney J, James G, et al. Using an efficient biofilm detaching agent: an essential step for the improvement of endoscope reprocessing protocols. J Hosp Infect. 2006;64:136–42.
9. CDC. Interim duodenoscope surveillance protocol. Interim protocol for healthcare facilities regarding surveillance for bacterial contamination of duodenoscopes after reprocessing. CDC; 2015.
10. Meyer GW, Salzman JR, Travis AC. Endoscope disinfection. UpToDate; 2015.
11. Zuhlsdorf B, Floss H, Martiny H. Efficacy of 10 different cleaning processes in a washer disinfector for flexible endoscopes. J Hosp Infect. 2004;56:305–11.
12. Marek A, Smith A, Peat M, et al. Endoscopy supply water and final rinse testing: five years of experience. J Hosp Infect. 2014;88:207–12.
13. Working party report. Rinse water for heat labile endoscopy equipment. J Hosp Infect. 2002;51:7–16.
14. Sorin M, Segal-Maurer S, Mariano N, et al. Nosocomial transmission or imipenem-resistant *Pseudomonas aeruginosa* following bronchoscopy associated with improper connection to the Steris system 1 processor. Infect Control Hosp Epidemiol. 2001;22:409–13.
15. Weber DJ, Rutala WA. Lessons from outbreaks associated with bronchoscopy. Infect Control Hosp Epidemiol. 2001;22:403–8.
16. MacKay WG, Leanord AT, Williams CL. Water, water everywhere nor any a sterile drop to rinse your endoscope. J Hosp Infect. 2002;51:256–61.
17. Saviuc P, Picot-Gueraud R, Sing JSC, et al. Evaluation of the quality of reprocessing of gastrointestinal endoscopes. Infect Control Hosp Epidemiol. 2015;36:1017–23.
18. Wendorf KA, Meagan K, Baliga C, et al. Endoscopic retrograde cholangiopancreatography-associated AmpC *Escherichia coli* outbreak. Infect Control Hosp Epidemiol. 2015;36:634–42.
19. Seoane-Vazquez E, Rodriguez-Mongiuio R, Visaria J, Carlson A. Endoscopy-related infections and toxic reactions: an international comparison. Endoscopy. 2007;39:742–78.
20. La Scola B, Rolain JM, Maurin M, Raoult D. Can Whipple's disease be transmitted by gastroscopes? Infect Control Hosp Epidemiol. 2003;24:191–4.
21. Akamatsu T, Tabata K, Hironaga M, Uyeda M. Evaluation of the efficacy of a 3.2% glutaraldehyde product for disinfection of fibreoptic endoscopes with an automated machine. J Hosp Infect. 1997;35:47–57.
22. Meester HHM, van Loenen AC, de Goede PNFC, Koeleman JGM. Glutaraldehyde: current status and uses. Infect Control Hosp Epidemiol. 1995;16:621–2.
23. Wendt C, Kampf B. Evidence-based spectrum of antimicrobial activity for disinfection of bronchoscopes. J Hosp Infect. 2008;70:60–80.
24. Bou R, Aguilar A, Perpinan J, et al. Nosocomial outbreak of *Pseudomonas aeruginosa* infections related to a flexible bronchoscope. J Hosp Infect. 2006;64:129–35.
25. Silvis SE, Nebel O, Rogers G, et al. Endoscopic complications: results of the 1974 American Society for Gastrointestinal Endoscopy Surgery. JAMA. 1976;235:928–30.
26. Kaczmarek RG, Moore RM, McCrohan J, et al. Multistate investigation of the actual disinfection/sterilization of endoscopes in healthcare facilities. Am J Infect Control. 1993;21:75.
27. Paula H, Presteri E, Tribl B, Diab-Elshahawi M. Microbial surveillance of duodenoscope reprocessing at the Vienna University Hospital from November 2004 through March 2015. Infect Control Hosp Epidemiol. 2015;36:1233–5.
28. Colin-Jones DG, Cockel R, Schiller KF. Current endoscopic practice in the United Kingdom. Clin Gastroenterol. 1978;7:775–86.
29. Bilbao MK, Dotter CT, Lee TG. Complications of endoscopic retrograde cholangiopancreatography (ERCP). A study of 10,000 cases. Gastroenterology. 1976;70:314–20.

30. Alfa MJ, Olson N, DeGagne P, Jackson M. A survey of reprocessing methods, residual viable bioburden, and soil levels in patient-ready endoscopic retrograde cholangiopancreatography duodenoscopes used in Canadian centers. Infect Control Hosp Epidemiol. 2002;23:198–206.
31. Promed Mail March 4, 2015. Antibiotic-resistant *Enterobacteriaceae*—USA. (California, Connecticut) ERCP endoscopes.
32. Bronowicki JP, Botte C, Monhoven N, et al. Patient-to-patient transmission or hepatitis C virus during colonoscopy. N Engl J Med. 1997;337:237–40.
33. Hutfless S. Infection rates after colonoscopy, endoscopy at ASCs are far higher than expected. John Hopkins Medicine. Infection control today. 2018.
34. Ofstead CL, Heyman OL, Quick MR, Eiland JE, Wetzler H. Residual moisture and waterborne pathogens inside flexible scopes: evidence from a multisite study of endoscope drying effectiveness. Am J Infect Control. 2018;46(6):689–96.

Sterilization

61

Abstract

Sterilization means "destruction of all forms of microbial life". A surgical instrument can be considered sterile if the probability of a single living microorganism is present is equal to or less than 10^{-6}. Use of sterile instruments and other sterile equipment is necessary to avoid infections during surgery and other aseptic processes. Sterility is dependent on a clean surface of the instruments—where all organic materials and dirt are removed, usually by a washing-disinfection process before the sterilization procedure. After this process, sterility may last for a period if handled and stored in a secure way. The following chapter is focused on practical measures to disinfect, sterilize, control, store and use surgical equipment in healthcare institutions.

Keywords

Sterilization · Heat-sensible instruments · Reusable equipment · Disinfection Sterilization · Autoclave · Infection control · Hygiene · Prevention

61.1 Purpose

- To ensure that all products undergoing a sterilization process are sterile after the process [1, 2].
- To remove pathogenic agents like bacteria, viruses, fungi, parasites and spores, from sterile instruments and other sterile equipment.
- To prevent transmission of infection from patients to other patients, staff, visitors or the environment through contaminated instruments.

B. M. Andersen, *Prevention and Control of Infections in Hospitals*,
https://doi.org/10.1007/978-3-319-99921-0_61

61.2 Comprise

- All equipment that is sterilized

61.3 Responsibility

The hospital's management ensures that written routines for sterile work and sterilization processes are available, including routine procedures against prion disease [1–5].

Management at sterile centres implement procedures for pretreating, control, packing, transport, sterilization, after-control and storage of ready-to-use sterile equipment. Resource deficiency that constitutes a risk of infection for patients and personnel must be reported to the Director immediately.

Personnel follow routines for the treatment of sterile and unsterile goods.

Preparedness in connection with deficiencies/failure (machine shutdown, flood, etc.) regarding sterilization capacity must be ensured through planned cooperation with other hospitals/sterile centres.

61.4 Practical Measures [6–12]

61.4.1 Areal

The sterile centre requires "clean room status"—in line with an operating department and is usually associated with operating departments. A sluice for entrance check and dressing is necessary. The same requirements are given for ventilation, air changes and pressure, as well as bacterial amount in the air (<100 CFU/m^3).

- The sterile centre usually has a reception area for "less clean"—equipment that is disinfected and washed other places and has to be controlled before further treatment in the centre.
- Clean room for final control and packing.
- Sterilization area—a suitable separate area—without steam and other gases leaking to other rooms.
- Clean and "dry" room for check after sterilization of the goods.
- Storage rooms for ready-to-use sterile goods; clean storage rooms (<100 CFU/m^3).
- A separate wash room for transport vehicles after use and a storage area. Transport to relevant departments should be carried out in clean, tightly closed transport vehicles that are cleaned after each use and stored clean.

61.4.2 Pretreatment of Goods Before Sterilization

All equipment coming to the sterile centre should be free of biological material. This happens during inspection, sonication of instruments (dirt and organic material release) and repeated washing in the instrument washing machine [13].

Instruments with residues of dried organic matter constitute a risk of infection (especially prions) and uncertain sterilization results.

61.4.3 Packing and Loading of the Sterilizer

The goods are packed according to defined routines, and the sterilizer is loaded correctly for which goods it is validated. Package material must be permeable to air, steam and any gas while protecting equipment against recontamination after completed sterilization process. Do not load too much goods and fill the chamber evenly each time.

61.4.4 Water Vapour Sterilization: Autoclaving

The method is safe, cheap and efficient. It is used for equipment that can withstand 120–140 °C. The autoclaving procedure treat the goods/equipment in saturated steam at elevated pressure to increase the temperature above 100 °C. In clean saturated water vapour, there is a relationship between pressure and temperature. One atmospheric pressure equals 121 °C, which kills all bacterial spores.

Physical monitoring for two systems:

1. Temperature, 134 °C; effect time (holding time), 4 min; pressure, 2 bar [14]
2. Temperature, 121 °C; effective time (holding time), 15 min; pressure, 1 bar [14]

Biological indicator (spore test) is *Geobacillus stearothermophilus* of other defined spores used for each run [14].

Chemical indicator is placed in different parts of the goods, including outside.

61.4.5 Loading

Packaging must be able to slip through air and steam. The autoclave should be loaded to let the steam circulate freely and to avoid problems with condensation and air pockets. The chamber is filled evenly each time. Too loaded autoclave or almost empty autoclave may give uncertain results.

61.4.6 Treatment Periods

The preheating period is the time from which the autoclave is started until the temperature in the chamber has reached the desired temperature.

The equilibrium period is the time from which the chamber has reached the sterilization temperature until all parts of the goods have reached the same temperature.

The sterilization period is calculated from the time the goods have reached the sterilization temperature.

At 121 °C: 15–20 min
At 134 °C: minimum 5–7 min

61.4.7 Emergency Autoclaving

Sterilization of unpackaged instruments is not recommended and should only be used in emergency situations. Aseptic coverage of the goods and short distance to the user site are a prerequisite. Instruments with cavities can only be sterilized in autoclave with pulsating pre-vacuum. Water vapour sterilization is performed at 134 °C for at least 3 min.

61.4.8 Dry Sterilization

The method uses hot air at 160–180 °C. The method is used where water vapour sterilization is not possible or practical and is suitable for metal and glassware, but not for porous materials such as compresses and textiles. The goods must withstand the high temperatures. The equipment must be completely dry before sterilization. It is packed in suitable packaging paper. The opening is sealed with sterilization tape with colour indicator that changes colour during the sterilization process. The packaging is marked with sterilization date and content.

Sterilization temperature and working time:

- 160 °C for at least 2 h.
- 170 °C for at least 1 h.
- 180 °C for at least 30 min.

The heating time until all equipment has reached the sterilization temperature comes in addition.

Maximum thermometer must be used regularly as a control, for example, every 3 months. Microbiological control with spore samples is done every 6 months. A minimum of six spores are used each time.

61.4.9 Formaldehyde: Low-Pressure Vapour Sterilization (Formalin Sterilization)

Formaldehyde sterilization is used for sterilization of equipment that cannot withstand temperatures with cycles over 65 °C or 70–80 °C. Sterilization takes place at defined sterile departments having competence for this work. The principle is to combine formaldehyde gas and bactericidal capacity from low-pressure saturated water vapour.

The formaldehyde autoclave contains three process steps:

The first step is a moisture and air extraction phase that takes place by means of a vacuum pump and thereafter filled by saturated water vapour into the autoclave chamber.

Second stage is the sterilization process, where formaldehyde and water vapour are dosed in several rounds. During the sterilization process, alternating evaporation and condensation occur within the autoclave chamber in a closed system.

In the third and final step is that formaldehyde is removed by the effect of water vapour blowing through the autoclave chamber. Afterwards equipment is dried in a vacuum, and finally filtered air is sent into the chamber.

61.4.10 Ethylene Oxide (EO) Sterilization

Ethylene oxide sterilizer is used for equipment that cannot tolerate temperatures above 55 °C. The method is performed at defined sterile departments. EO can take place at 37 °C or 55 °C, with relative humidity >60%, pressure 0.8–1.8 bar and holding time 3 h at 37 °C and 1 h at 55 °C [14].

- Biological indicator is usually *Bacillus atrophaeus* used for each run [14].
- Chemical indicator may be placed at different locations in the goods, including outside.

61.4.11 Sterilization Process

A modern EO sterilizer contains three process steps: *pre-wetting*, *sterilizing and venting* EO from the material. Sterilizers may be differently designed, some with overpressure and others with negative pressure. Results depend on several factors: the concentration of EO, temperature, relative humidity, cleaning before sterilization, packaging material, removal of gas residues from the equipment, loading the autoclave, the time sterilization process takes, etc.

Concentration of EO: The gas concentration varies from pure EO on disposable gas patrons to a mixture of 10% EO and 90% inert gas, e.g. carbon dioxide. The latter is not explosive. Autoclaves that use a gas mixture must work at over-pressure. Autoclaves where clean EO is used, works at under-pressure.

Temperature: Sterilization with EO is preceding from room temperature and upwards. When EO is used for sterilization of heat-sensitive equipment, the most common temperature is approx. 50 °C.

Relative humidity: The bactericidal activity increases with the relative humidity that should be in the range 70–100%. The wetting process should be built into the sterilization process.

Microorganisms: EO is effective both against vegetative and spore-forming bacteria and against viruses. Microorganisms in organic matter can be difficult to kill with EO as the gas has little ability to penetrate dried protein residues.

Cleaning of equipment: It is very important that equipment to be sterilized is satisfactorily cleaned.

Packaging material: The packaging must be permeable to air, moisture and EO gas. Packaging consists of one side sterilization paper and the other side plastic laminate welded together—useful in hospitals (Standard EN 868).

Removal of gas residues from the equipment: After the sterilization process has ended, the equipment may still contain large amounts of EO. The necessary aeration time depends on the temperature, chemic composition of plastic materials, equipment design, packaging and storage. For example, it takes 100 times longer to vent a semihard polyvinyl chloride than a soft one. In a hospital, it is practically impossible to operate with different air times (venting times) depending on the material in which the equipment is manufactured. Therefore, a time is chosen that cover most materials. Equipment is aired at 55 °C in the sterilizer. Then it is delivered after negative spore test.

Loading of the EO—autoclave: As with all sterilization processes, the autoclave should not be packed too tight as air, moisture and gas may otherwise be difficult to penetrate.

Sterilization period: The time sterilization takes depends on the other factors. The lower the temperature, the longer the sterilization time.

61.4.12 Plasma Sterilization

This is also a "low-temperature sterilization method" performed at 45–55 °C. The process consists of a "diffusion period" with injection of hydrogen peroxide (H_2O_2). There are produced free radicals that make the "plasma process". This is the actual sterilization process. The advantage of this sterilization method is that it does not provide any residual products after the process and hence no work environment problems.

- At a temperature of 50 °C, pressure used is 500 mtorr and effective time is 1 h.
- Biological indicator is usually *Geobacillus stearothermophilus* used for each run [14].
- Chemical indicator may be placed at different locations in the goods, including outside.

61.5 Background Information

Sterilization will destroy all microbial life except for a few infectious substances. An object is sterile when the likelihood for that a single living microbe is present is equal to or less than 10^{-6}. This is the European pharmacopoeia's requirement for sterility. Risk is 0.000001 and the security level is 99.999999%.

All equipment that comes directly or indirectly in contact with body areas that are normally sterile *should* be sterilized. All equipment penetrating the skin and mucous membranes *must* be sterile. All equipment, bronchoscope, tracheal tubes, gastroscopes, cystoscopes, endoscopes, etc.—which come into contact with respiratory tract mucosa, esophagus, urinary tract and genitalia—*should* be sterile or disinfected at high-level disinfection.

Inactivation of microbiological agents is done by burning, autoclaving, boiling in water for more than 10 min, dry heat at 140 °C for more than 90 min and moist heat at 100 °C for more than 10 min.

Nearly complete inactivation occurs by hot water/steam for more than 85 °C for 10 min, chloramine 5% in 60 min, PeraSafe 16.2% for 10–30 min and the glutaraldehyde 2–3% for 30–60 min.

The ability of the various methods to kill microorganisms is expressed by the method's inactivation factor which is the ratio of the initial number of germs to the number of surviving germs at a given time during the procedure. The inactivation factor is different for the individual microorganisms. The inactivation factor that the most resistant microorganism has is important. At a given inactivation factor, the chance of sterility for one and the same period is greater the lower the initial bacterial number is. Thorough cleaning before sterilization will reduce the microbial number and thereby ensure the sterilization procedure.

The most resistant infectious agents are called prions, protein particles that cause Creutzfeldt- Jakob's disease and bovine spongiform encephalopathy (BSE), among others. In such cases, none of our usual sterilization routines are good enough. In case of suspected prion disease, equipment used for the patient is *destroyed* by burning, after autoclaving at 134–137 °C for 1 h and other special treatment (see section on prion disease and technical disinfection).

Sterilization methods current today (Table 61.1):

- Water vapour sterilization at 121 °C for a minimum of 15 min or 134 °C for 7 min or 134 °C for 1 h on suspicion of prions
- Dry sterilization at 160 °C for 2 h or 180 °C for 30 min
- Formaldehyde/low-pressure steam sterilization at approx. 65 °C or 70–80 °C
- Ethylene oxide sterilization (EO) at 55 °C
- Plasma sterilization at 45–55 °C

Table 61.1 Methods for sterilization

Sterilization method	Benefits	Disadvantages
Steam sterilization	Can be used for everything. Non-toxic by-products easy to control and monitor Not harmful to patients, personnel and the environment Rapidly killing effect in microbes Not particularly hampered by organic matter Fast cycle Good penetration through packaging/packages Good penetration through instrument lumen	Heat-sensitive instruments can be destroyed Wet material/instruments can corrode Fire
Plasma sterilization (Hydrogen peroxide gas plasma)	Safe for the environment Non-toxic products Cycle 45–73 min. No airing required (cycle ≥24 min, ref. [1]) Heat- and moisture-sensitive instruments can be treated at <50 °C Easy to control and monitor All types of equipment and instruments Easy to establish	Cellulose (paper), textiles and liquid cannot be sterilized Often small capacity—low volume Limited use of instruments with narrow lumen and long tunnels as endoscopes (cf. producer) Special packaging—synthetic—and containers Toxic border level in the room: 1 ppm should be monitored
Ethylene oxide gas 100% (450–1200 mg/L, tp 37–63 °C, relative humidity 40–80%, time, 1–6 h) ETO	Penetrates all material and instrument lumen negative pressure chamber and good control of the gas All types of material Cycle is easy to control, monitor At increasing temperature and concentration, the sterilization time will be reduced Single dose containers—defined	Aeration afterwards to remove the gas Toxic, carcinogenic and combustible 99.9% of ETO is converted into CO_2 and water Long cycle and long aeration time Single-dose containers must be stored in fireproof cabinets
Ethylene oxide gas Mixtures	Like ETO	Like ETO

Table 61.1 (continued)

Sterilization method	Benefits	Disadvantages
Formaldehyde—low pressure Vapour sterilization vacuum, saturated water steam formaldehyde	Penetrates all material and lumen Closed system, 65–80 °C All types of material, low temperature Cycle easy to control, monitor Increasing temp and concentration reduce time Particularly useful for heat-sensitive instruments	Small volume Formaldehyde residues in equipment—control Toxic Spore tests every week Long time—cycle and airing Not so efficient at long, narrow lumen
Hydrogen peroxide steam Note—limited experience!	Safe for environment and personnel No toxic residues, aeration unnecessary Fast cycle—55 min Used for heat and moisture-sensitive objects, also metal	Restriction for instruments with cavities Limited use of instruments with narrow lumen and long tunnels as endoscopes (cf. manufacturer) **Limited experience with metal damage!** Special packaging— synthetic and containers Cellulose (paper), textiles and liquid cannot be sterilized Toxic border level in the room: 1 ppm must be monitored **Limited clinical experience** **Limited experience with microbiological effect!**

Source: Rutala WA, Weber Di. Disinfection, sterilization, and control of hospital waste. Principles and practice of infectious diseases. 2015: 3294, and edition 2005: 3331

61.5.1 Infection Risk from Contaminated Sterile Goods

An outbreak of infection among 15 orthopaedic patients who had undergone "clean surgery" was traced back to contaminated surgical instruments [15]. Most patients were infected during the operating season with normal skin flora like coagulase-negative staphylococci and *Bacillus*, and 11 out of 15 had to be reoperated. Microbiological samples from sterile goods showed the same bacterial flora on the inside of the package and on the sterile instruments themselves. Inspection of the sterile centre showed inadequate handling and control of autoclaves and bad hygienic routines. This occurred combined with the fact that surgical personnel did not observe the discoloration of outer parts of the delivered packages with sterile goods nor did good inspection of the sterile goods before opening the instrument packages [15].

References

1. Rutala WA, Weber DJ. Disinfection, sterilization, and control of hospital waste. In: Mandell, Douglas, and Bennets principles and practice of infectious diseases. 8th ed. vol. 2. Philadelphia: Elsevier Churchill Livingstone; 2015. p. 3294–309.
2. Rutala WA, Weber DJ. Disinfection and sterilization: an overview. Am J Infect Control. 2013;41:2–5.
3. Bosque PJ, Tyler KL. Prions and prion disease of the central nervous system (transmissible neurodegenerative diseases). In: Mandell GL, Douglas RG, Bennett JE, editors. Principles and practice of infectious diseases. 8th ed. London: Elsevier Churchill Livingston; 2015. p. 2142–53.
4. Government, UK. Infection prevention and control of CJD, vCJD and other human prion diseases in healthcare and community settings. Transmissible spongiform encephalopathy agents: safe working and the prevention of infection: Part 4. Revised and updated January 2014.
5. Spencer RC, Ridgway GL, vCJD Consensus Group. Sterilization issues in vCJD-towards a consensus. J Hosp Infect. 2002;51:168–74.
6. Fossum K, Baksaas I, editors. Disinfection and sterilization in health care. Oslo: State Drug Control, Department of Pharmacotherapy; 1988.
7. Hauff Ulvestad K, Hagen Sølsnæs T. Sterilforsyning i sykehus. Oslo: Universitetsforlaget; 1998.
8. Johnsen S, Hagen Sølsnæs T. Sterilization. In: Handbook in hygiene and infection control. Oslo: Ullevål Hospital; 1996. p. 191–5.
9. Andersen BM, Hagen Sølsnæs T, Hochlin K. Sterilization. In: Handbook in hygiene and infection control. Oslo: Ullevål Hospital; 1999. p. 277–83.
10. Farstad S, Hagen Sølsnæs T, Hochlin K. Sterilization. In: Handbook in hygiene and infection control for hospitals. Oslo: Ullevål University Hospital; 2003. p. 356–61.
11. Hafstad AM, Hochlin K, Tollefsen T, Andersen BM. Sterilization. In: Handbook in hygiene and infection control for hospitals. Oslo: Ullevål University Hospital; 2008. p. 496–500.
12. Andersen BM. Technical disinfection and sterilization. In: Handbook in hygiene and infection control for nursing homes, long-term institutions. Akademika. 2013. p. 467–76.
13. Kumar S, Lee WT, Szili EJ. Electrolysis-assisted sonication for removal of protein-contaminated contamination from surgical grade stainless steel. J Hosp Infect. 2012;81:41–9.
14. Basu D, Bhattacharya S, Mahajan A, Ramanan VR, Chandy M. Sterile indicators in central sterile supply department: quality assurance and cost implications. Infect Control Hosp Epidemiol. 2015;36:484–6.
15. Dancer SJ, Stewart M, Coulombe C, Gregori A, Virdi M. Surgical site infections linked to contaminated surgical instruments. J Hosp Infect. 2012;81:231–8.

Sterilization: Control and Quality 62

Abstract

Use of sterile instruments and other sterile equipment is necessary to avoid contamination and infection during surgery. Full sterility is dependent on removal of all organic materials and dirt from the instruments, a washing-disinfection process and control before, during and after the sterilization procedure. Definition of sterility is the probability of a single living microorganism present is equal to or less than 10^{-6}. Several practical indicators are used to control the sterilization process and to ensure that the instruments are sterile.

Keywords

Sterilization process · Heat-sensible instruments · Reusable equipment · Autoclave · Infection control · Hygiene · Prevention

62.1 Purpose

Ensure that all products undergoing a sterilization process are sterile after the process [1–15].

To remove pathogenic agents: bacteria, viruses, fungi, parasites, spores, from sterile instruments and other sterile equipment.

To prevent transmission of infection from patients to other patients, staff, visitors or the environment through contaminated instruments.

62.2 Comprise

All equipment that is sterilized.

All personnel working with sterile equipment.

B. M. Andersen, *Prevention and Control of Infections in Hospitals*,
https://doi.org/10.1007/978-3-319-99921-0_62

62.3 Responsibility

The hospital's management ensures that routines for sterile work and sterilization processes are available and ensure routine procedures against prion disease [1, 2].

Management at sterile centres implements procedures for pre-treating, control, packing, transport, sterilization, after-control and storage of ready-to-use sterile equipment. Resource deficiency that constitutes a risk of infection for patients and personnel must be reported to the Director immediately.

Personnel follow routines for the treatment of sterile and unsterile goods.

Preparedness in connection with deficiencies/failure (machine shutdown, flood, etc.) regarding sterilization capacity must be ensured through planned cooperation with other hospitals/sterile centres.

62.4 Practical Measures

62.4.1 Check After Each Cycle (Sterilization Process)

- *The goods must be dry.* Wet goods may be due to poor steam quality. Wet packing material does not provide protection against recontamination and growth of bacteria or fungi through the packing.
- *Physical parameters* such as temperature, sterilization time and chamber pressure must be controlled. The EN standards require that all autoclaves have a printer and diagram and that temperature, pressure and time must be printed for each time of sterilization. If a printer does not exist, a standard curve may be used to verify that the curve course is correct. The time can be checked by counting routes on the paper.
- *Chemical colour indicators* provide colour change at certain temperatures, time, humidity and eventually gas. Chemical colour indicators are available as *sterilization tape* or printed directly on the packaging material to show that the individual article has been through the sterilization process. More complex chemical indicators provide change due to temperature, time, saturated water vapour and eventually gas concentration.

62.4.2 Fixed Frequency Control

Biological indicators (BI) (spore samples) consist of certain microorganisms with known, high and stable resistance to the sterilization process [1]. Spore samples are cultures, and it takes time before the result is available. BI is suitable for testing that the sterilizer works properly. The following frequency is recommended for control using spore tests.

- *Water vapour sterilization:* At least every month. International standard every cycle [1].
- *Dry sterilization:* Every other month/every 3 months.
- *Formaldehyde sterilization:* Every other week. Preferably every cycle.
- *Ethylene oxide sterilization:* Each cycle. International standard every cycle [1]. For ethylene oxide you should wait for the result.

- *Plasma sterilization:* International standard—each cycle.

Test organisms may have varied resistance to the sterilization methods used:

- *Bacillus stearothermophilus/Geobacillus stearothermophilus* prepared for water vapour sterilization.
- *Bacillus stearothermophilus* prepared for formaldehyde sterilization.
- *Bacillus subtilis* made for ethylene oxide sterilization.
- *Bacillus subtilis* prepared for dry sterilization.
- *Geobacillus stearothermophilus* for plasma sterilization.

Thermal control is performed regularly by placing three, preferably six, adjusted thermosets, at different locations in the sterilizer to determine if there are places where the temperature does not reach the prescribed level.

Leakage test program can be found on newer sterilizers. The program should run *weekly*.

The Bowie and Dick test is used *daily* to test whether air evacuation from the chamber is satisfactory. The test consists of an accurately specified package of towels with a paper sheet with chemical indicator in a special pattern in the middle. The fabric, sterilization, temperature, packing, etc. are precisely defined. If the indicator colour has not been changed satisfactorily, this indicates air collection inside the package.

Working environment: Where gas sterilization is carried out, the work environment is to be checked annually by determining ethylene oxide and formaldehyde in the air, according to the national standard from Directorate of labour inspection (*Occupational Health and Safety*).

Formaldehyde residues in the equipment must be tested regularly by determining formaldehyde residues in standardized filter paper after sterilization. Proposed residue: maximum 100 mg/filter paper.

Maintenance and control: The EN standards require that the staff have special training in the maintenance of sterilizers. In practice, this will probably mean that such equipment should be considered as medical technical equipment. Controls: maintenance and control of printers, temperature gauges, pressure gauge and control of that spore tests are carried out according to specifications.

62.5 Background Information

There is no guarantee that the individual article is sterile after a single control (mechanically, physically, chemically or biologically). Sterility is present combined in a comprehensive quality assurance program.

Loading rate: The sterilizer must be *loaded correctly* and not overfilled.

Correct packing material is important; permeable to air, steam and any gas while protecting the equipment against recontamination.

Temperature, pressure and time must be printed for each sterilization. There are different types of printers. Some have circular sheets and a writing needle that is easily shifted by changing sheets. For documentation, these are suitable as they can be stored after one single sterilization with a control number on the sheet and on the sterilized articles. Other printers are continuous-time typewriters.

Chemical colour indicators: The simplest types produce a colour change when exposed to a certain temperature, time, humidity and eventually gas pressure. The indicator is suitable for showing whether the individual article has been through a sterilization process. Indicators can also be placed inside the packages.

If the specificity is not very high, a high sensitivity indicator will give unacceptably many false positive results for each real positive. If the sensitivity is low, true positive will not be revealed. Goods which should be rejected would be approved.

Biological indicators (BI) (spore tests). The indicator should only provide growth if the efficacy of the procedure has been significantly worse than the European Pharmacopoeia's requirements for sterility.

An advantage of using biological indicators is their ability to measure the effect of all parameters necessary to achieve sterility. The check should be performed at fixed frequency, and the international standard is for each cycle.

References

1. Rutala WA, Weber DJ. Disinfection, sterilization, and control of hospital waste. In: Mandell, Douglas, and Bennets principles and practice of infectious diseases. 8th ed. vol. 2. Philadelphia: Elsevier Churchill Livingstone; 2015. p. 3294–309.
2. Rutala WA, Weber DJ. Disinfection and sterilization: an overview. Am J Infect Control. 2013;41:2–5.
3. Bosque PJ, Tyler KL. Prions and prion disease of the central nervous system (transmissible neurodegenerative diseases). In: Mandell GL, Douglas RG, Bennett JE, editors. Principles and practice of infectious diseases. 8th ed. London: Elsevier Churchill Livingston; 2015. p. 2142–53.
4. Government, UK. Infection prevention and control of CJD, vCJD and other human prion diseases in healthcare and community settings. Transmissible spongiform encephalopathy agents: safe working and the prevention of infection: Part 4. Revised and updated January 2014.
5. Spencer RC, Ridgway GL, vCJD Consensus Group. Sterilization issues in vCJD-towards a consensus. J Hosp Infect. 2002;51:168–74.
6. Fossum K, Baksaas I, editors. Disinfection and sterilization in health care. Oslo: State Drug Control, Department of Pharmacotherapy; 1988.
7. Hauff Ulvestad K, Hagen Sølsnæs T. Sterilforsyning i sykehus. Oslo: Universitetsforlaget; 1998.
8. Johnsen S, Hagen Sølsnæs T. Sterilization. In: Handbook in hygiene and infection control. Oslo: Ullevål Hospital; 1996. p. 191–5.
9. Andersen BM, Hagen Sølsnæs T, Hochlin K. Sterilization. In: Handbook in hygiene and infection control. Oslo: Ullevål Hospital; 1999. p. 277–83.
10. Farstad S, Hagen Sølsnæs T, Hochlin K. Sterilization. In: Handbook in hygiene and infection control for hospitals. Oslo: Ullevål University Hospital; 2003. p. 356–61.
11. Hafstad AM, Hochlin K, Tollefsen T, Andersen BM. Sterilization. In: Handbook in hygiene and infection control for hospitals. Oslo: Ullevål University Hospital; 2008. p. 496–500.
12. Andersen BM. Technical disinfection and sterilization. In: Handbook in hygiene and infection control for nursing homes, long-term institutions. Akademika. 2013. p. 467–76.
13. Kumar S, Lee WT, Szili EJ. Electrolysis-assisted sonication for removal of protein-contaminated contamination from surgical grade stainless steel. J Hosp Infect. 2012;81:41–9.
14. Basu D, Bhattacharya S, Mahajan A, Ramanan VR, Chandy M. Sterile indicators in central sterile supply department: quality assurance and cost implications. Infect Control Hosp Epidemiol. 2015;36:484–6.
15. Dancer SJ, Stewart M, Coulombe C, Gregori A, Virdi M. Surgical site infections linked to contaminated surgical instruments. J Hosp Infect. 2012;81:231–8.

63 Sterile and Clean Equipment: Storage

Abstract

Use of sterile instruments and other sterile equipment is necessary to avoid infections during surgery. Full sterility is dependent on removal of organic materials and dirt from the instruments, a washing-disinfection process and control before the sterilization procedure—and afterwards to not break the sterility of the instrument before use. Definition of sterility is the probability of a single living microorganism present is equal to or less than 10^{-6}. This chapter is focused on the storage of sterile and clean equipment in healthcare institutions.

Keywords

Sterilization · Surgical instruments · Reusable equipment · Disinfection Sterilization · Infection control · Storage

63.1 Purpose

- To ensure that all products undergoing a sterilization process are sterile after the process and are stored in a hygienic satisfactory manner [1, 2].
- To remove pathogenic agents like bacteria, viruses, fungi, parasites and spores, from sterile instruments and other sterile equipment.
- To prevent transmission of infection from patients to other patients, staff, visitors or the environment through contaminated instruments.

B. M. Andersen, *Prevention and Control of Infections in Hospitals*,
https://doi.org/10.1007/978-3-319-99921-0_63

63.2 Comprise

- All equipment that is sterilized

63.3 Responsibility

The hospital's management ensures that written routines for sterile work and sterilization processes are available, including routine procedures against prion disease [1–5].

Management at sterile centres implement procedures for pretreating, control, packing, transport, sterilization, after-control and storage of ready-to-use sterile equipment. Resource deficiency that constitutes a risk of infection for patients and personnel must be reported to the Director immediately.

Personnel follow routines for the treatment of sterile and unsterile goods.

Preparedness in connection with deficiencies/failure (machine shutdown, flood, etc.) regarding sterilization capacity must be ensured through planned cooperation with other hospitals/sterile centres.

63.4 Practical Measures [1–6]

63.4.1 Storage Room for Sterile and Clean Equipment

- Sterile equipment is stored in a separate clean room, in its own closet with glass door.
- The storage room shall not be exposed to transit traffic and shall not be used for office.
- Equipment should be stored dry and at room temperature 15–25 °C.
- The ventilation should correspond to an operating department; the following limit values for clean rooms where sterile disposables/sterile disposables/multiple equipment should be stored.
  - Relative humidity: 35–70%.
  - Ventilation: 10–17 air changes per hour.
  - CFU: <100 cfu/m^3.
- Avoid strong light to prevent decomposition of material in the equipment and packaging.
- Regular check of the expiration date on the equipment package. Check any discoloration of packages.
- Always hand disinfection before handling of sterile/clean equipment.
- Avoid damage to the packaging when handling sterile/clean equipment.
- Outer packaging of transport cartons/packages is removed in a clean place *outside the* storage room, and the equipment packages are immediately placed in the storage room/closet.

- Take out only the equipment you need.
- Sterile equipment removed should be covered before shipping to the place of use.
- Sterile equipment must be traceable.
- The packaging is opened just before the equipment is put into use.
- Inspect the outside of the packaging for discoloration or moisture.
- Sterile equipment removed from the packaging should always be placed on a sterile surface under an aseptic procedure.
- One-time equipment package that has been opened should be discarded. The reusable equipment package that has been opened but not used should always be sterilized again before next use.
- Floor and bench surface in the storage room is washed daily.
- Shelves and cabinets are washed once a month—dry well before equipment is placed back.
- Main cleaning of cabinets/storage rooms at least twice a year.

63.4.2 Durability of Sterile Equipment

- The durability of sterile equipment depends on external factors such as mode of production, sterilization method, packing material, storage conditions, transportation and handling. The durability limit assumes that the product is manufactured, sterilized, transported, handled and stored in a manner that has kept the package undamaged. It is assumed that the packaging has not been opened.
- Generally speaking, two layers of textiles have shelf life 1–2 weeks, paper approximately 3 months, plastic/paper welded 1 year, metal container with filter/sterilization port 3 months. Check production date and date of exit.
- Shelf life limits for *factory-made equipment* are specified by the manufacturer. In cases where the production date is stated, may the product be expected to be durable for 5 years. Single packs are stored in the departments or shelf package, as provided.
- During handling and storage of sterile equipment/sterile disposables, must the equipment/items be protected against:
  - Damage to the packaging. Storage, handling and transportation must be carried out in such a way that the packaging is not damaged, resulting in contamination of the sterile equipment.
  - Humidity. A porous packing material that is moist can easily pass through microorganisms and other particles. Therefore, sterile articles must be stored dry.
  - Extreme temperatures/fast temperature fluctuations. Experience shows that a temperature of 18–22 °C is favourable.
  - Light. Strong light can speed up a decomposition of the material in the equipment and the packaging.
  - Insects must not have access to storage.

– Dust/particles. Each hospital must evaluate the external factors mentioned above and develop guidelines for shelf life for sterile equipment in relation to storage and handling conditions at the hospital.

63.4.3 Storage Types

Rough storage/pallet storage: Here, goods are received and stored in outer packing on pallets, in shelves preferably with adjustable shelves or directly on wheel support. Transport cartons are considered to be contaminated on the outside—often long transport by sea and land and from other continents.

Unpacking room: The outer packaging is removed, and the goods are prepared for further transport. Transport cartons must not be allowed in either clean or sterile store rooms. Outer cartons are often dirty and may contain, for example, insects. Particularly in the grooves on corrugated cardboard, dust and insects can easily accumulate. This room should have negative pressure, separate ventilation and sluice relative to sterile centres. Good access to hand hygiene.

Storage for clean and sterile equipment: Only clean and sterile items are stored, either in single pack or compartment, i.e. clean on the outside.

63.4.4 Warehouse Systems in Sterile Centres

Open shelves: The most widely used system on sterile centres is to store sterile items in open shelves. This is a reasonable solution because the shelves are easy to keep clean and require little floor space.

The downside is that the products are not protected as well as when stored in enclosed cabinets. Open shelves also provide additional requirements for environmental control. There should be a relatively good distance between the shelves so that there is plenty of space to take the items out of the shelves. The open shelves must not be placed so that the sterile articles are lying near the sink, window, door or air valves.

Closed cabinets: When picking up sterile goods from a closed cabinet, it is important to open the door carefully. A "fast" air movement will be able to extract particles and destroy the very purpose of a closed storage system. Closed cabinets are therefore suitable for articles that will be stored for a long time.

63.4.5 Warehouse Properties

When selecting building materials for floors, walls and ceiling, great emphasis must be placed on the possibility of simple and satisfactory cleaning.

Doors: Doors to rooms where sterile articles are stored in open systems should preferably have automatic sliding doors. If it is not possible, it should "turn" out of the corridor. This is to prevent dust whirling in the room. To protect the doors, it may be convenient to mount a kicking plate on the door. Due to transport vehicles entering the room, there must be no threshold.

Floor: Floors must have a smooth surface, preferably a homogeneous vinyl coating. To avoid dust collections, hollow wedges should be preferred to floorboards.

Wall and ceiling: These should be smooth, strong and painted with 20 gloss paint. Wall coverings should go butt in butt with linoleum.

Lighting: It is recommended 200 lux as backlighting, as well as spotlight at the workplace.

Windows: The windows must be tight and have a simple design. They must not be opened. There should be no curtains in the room, but the room must be shielded from solar radiation. Exterior blinds are preferable.

Washbasins: There should be no washbasin inside the room if it cannot be installed at a satisfactory distance from the sterile items. Here, dispenser with hand disinfectant can be a good alternative. There should be access to the sink at the door to the warehouse.

Cabinet: It is recommended that the cabinets are built from floor to ceiling to avoid accumulation of dust.

63.4.6 Cleaning of Storage Rooms

- Daily cleaning of floors and horizontal surfaces.
- Cleaning of cabinets and shelves as well as baskets and trays at the surgery department and sterile centre should be done once a month.
- In the hospital patient ward departments, corresponding cleaning must be performed every month. Fixed cleaning routines should be developed.
- Main cleaning should be performed twice a year at the storage rooms in the operation units and the sterile unit and once a year at the hospital departments.
- The space on the top of the cabinet (if there is any) should not be used as storage space.

63.5 Background Information [1–6]

Only sterile medical equipment and clean disposable equipment (also clean outside) should be stored in storage for sterile and clean equipment.

Sterile medical equipment, equipment used in aseptic—sterile—procedures.

- Single-use equipment/items: e.g. wound set, catheter/catheterization kit, urine bag, syringes, needles, intravascular catheterization kits, infusion set, compresses, surgical knife blade, sutures, prosthesis, sterile gloves, etc.
- Multipurpose equipment that is sterilized after each use: e.g. surgical instruments and other sterile equipment.

Clean medical equipment: equipment used for diagnostics and clean procedures.

- *Single-use equipment:* e.g. disposable gloves, disposable tongue pad, patch, Q tips, disposable stasis hose, etc. Equipment directly from manufacturer/sterile centre and clean outside.
- *Multipurpose equipment* that is cleaned/disinfected after each use: e.g. stethoscope, blood pressure device, otoscope, ophthalmoscope, multiple stasis hose, atomizer device (with single-use accessory), blood glucose meter (single-use accessory), oxygen device (disposable accessory), bedpan, urine bottle, etc.
- *Multi*purpose equipment *that is cleaned/disinfected* after each use must be in its own warehouse.
- *Bedpans, urine bottles and similar* should after cleaning and disinfection be stored in a drying cabinet—in separate storage—not in sterile storage room.

Technical large equipment/aids should be cleaned with soap and water between each use and disinfected after use by infection: crutches, wheelchair, seat cushion and so on. This should be on a separate storage for large equipment and never be placed in clean/sterile stock.

According to the separate country's law on trading; there is, for instance, in Norway "Regulations on Registration and Inspection of Medical Disposable Equipment". All products covered by the Regulations should be registered by the "Disposable Medical Device" in order to be traded.

Disease spread through air, contact and blood-borne infection.

Bacteria and other particles (>0.3 mm) are liberated from persons in varying degrees, depending on the attire and the degree of movement. In sitting position approx. 100,000 particles (mostly skin cells) are liberated per minute, while during movement up to 5,000,000 particles are liberated. The size of these particles allows them to penetrate the packing material, thus leading to contamination of the sterile equipment. Training in microbiology and hygiene is therefore necessary to create attitudes for good quality of handling of sterile equipment/products.

Work in "sterile store rooms" includes strict requirements for hygiene to prevent external contamination of the packaging material. Staff stay in the sterile storage room only as long time as they have work to perform there. Equipment or technical aids contaminated with infectious material should not be taken into storage.

References

1. Rutala WA, Weber DJ. Disinfection, sterilization, and control of hospital waste. In: Mandell, Douglas, and Bennets principles and practice of infectious diseases, vol. 2. 8th ed. Philadelphia: Elsevier Churchill Livingstone; 2015. p. 3294–309.
2. Rutala WA, Weber DJ. Disinfection and sterilization: an overview. Am J Infect Control. 2013;41:2–5.

3. Bosque PJ, Tyler KL. Prions and prion disease of the central nervous system (transmissible neurodegenerative diseases). In: Mandell, Douglas, Bennetts principles and practice of infectious diseases. 8th ed. London: Elsevier Churchill Livingston; 2015. p. 2142–53.
4. Government, UK. Infection prevention and control of CJD, vCJD and other human prion diseases in healthcare and community settings. Transmissible spongiform encephalopathy agents: Safe working and the prevention of infection: Part 4. Revised and updated, January 2014.
5. Spencer RC, Ridgway GL, vCJD Consensus Group. Sterilization issues in vCJD-towards a consensus. J Hosp Infect. 2002;51:168–74.
6. Dancer SJ, Stewart M, Coulombe C, Gregori A, Virdi M. Surgical site infections linked to contaminated surgical instruments. J Hosp Infect. 2012;81:231–8.

Medicine Storage and Preparation Room 64

Abstract

The medicine storage room is often the "heart" in the ward since nearly all patients at hospitals receive drugs of different types. Medicines are administered in many ways: tablets, fluids or drops, powders or pills, and a large amount of treatment takes place with intravascular, sterile fluids or intramuscularly. All drugs should have a minimum purity requirement, and all medicaments used in sterile areas (intravascular, intramuscular, sterile cavity, respiratory tract, etc.) must be sterile, prepared and administered. The work in medicine rooms is important concerning sterility, exactness and competence in relation to giving the right patient the right medicine. The medicine room should be a restricted area, only used by well-educated personnel, working with medicaments. An increasing incidence of various infectious agents in hospital patients can lead to contamination and spread of disease unless the staff is careful about drug delivery. The following chapter is focused on practical measures concerning storage, handling, use and control of medicaments in healthcare institutions.

Keywords

Medicine room · Medicines · Handling of medicines · Preparation of medicines Distribution of medicine · Medicine storage · Medicine cupboards · Parenteral fluids · Cleaning · Disinfection · Infection control · Hygiene · Prevention

64.1 Purpose

- Prevent infections and other complications associated with handling of medicines at the hospital wards.
- Ensure good procedures for storing and handling medication at the ward, and in particular ensure that sterile drug treatment, including extraction/additions to

B. M. Andersen, *Prevention and Control of Infections in Hospitals*,
https://doi.org/10.1007/978-3-319-99921-0_64

infusion bags by syringes, is carried out in such a way that the sterility of the product is maintained.
- Avoid single-use vials with medicaments used as multi-dose vials.

64.2 Comprise

- All who have access to the medicine room and to handling and distribution of medicines, including sterile drugs and fluids.
- This includes withdrawals from vial/ampoule, addition to infusion bags, handling of antibiotics/cytostatic agents and control of drug and dose.
- All who brings medications to the patients and ensures that the right dose is given to the right patient.

64.3 Responsibility

The hospital's management has (according to law and regulation) responsibility for ensuring that all clinical departments, outpatient clinics and other centres treating patients have defined, well-equipped and spacious medicine rooms for safe storage and space for the work with medicines. The management shall further ensure that written guidelines are available for the function, control, ventilation and use of the medicine room and for the existence of good procedures for the distribution of medicinal products.

The department management is responsible for ensuring that hygiene guidelines are updated, understood and followed for storage, control work, hygiene, distribution and access to medicines. The management is responsible for reporting errors and deviations to the hospital's management, if these can be linked to functional conditions or lack of competence among staff.

The personnel responsible for patient medication shall ensure that current procedures are followed for permanent safety checks and that good hand hygiene and personal hygiene are carried out.

64.4 Practical Measures [1]

The medical room must be located easily accessible with little walking distance for the staff. Several medicine rooms in the same department may therefore be applicable.

Controlled access work on handling and remedying medicinal products shall be carried out in a sheltered area with access only for persons certified for this work and for relevant cleaning staff.

Area should be large enough for two persons to move simultaneously in the room without contaminating the storage of medicinal products and additional equipment for drug delivery. An area of at least 16 m^2 is required for a bed ward with approximately 20 patients. There must be cabinets, large enough workbenches, suction hood, washbasin, medicine trolley, medicine trays, sterile liquids (if not stocked in a separate room), etc., and everything must be stored in a way to minimize contamination.

Floors, walls and ceilings must be of robust, washable material that can withstand disinfectants. Simple entire surfaces and cabinets with glass doors make the room more easily to keep clean.

Washbasins according to the standard should be easily accessible beside the door of the medicine room and be at least 1 m from the drug cabinet and workbenches. Avoid splashes when using the washbasin.

Hand hygiene dispenser at the door.

Workbench should be in solid and light washable material that can withstand disinfectants 2–3 m long.

LAF (laminar airflow) bench (hood) for sterile products. Antibiotics and other sterile products are prepared in the LAF bench with a suction hood. It is important that the air is not recycled to the room due to allergy/sensitization for antibacterial agents and other chemicals.

Fridge for storing medicaments (lockable) must be large enough for the ward's needs and should contain only clean medicaments that have not been in contact with patients, and cleaning should easily be carried out (one time/month). Check temperature once/week.

Cabinets and shelves: Clearly set out and easily washable. Avoid too many open shelves, especially at the floor level as dust collection is not avoidable. Prefer cabinets with glass doors. Mark shelves and cabinets.

Unauthorized items: Shoes, bags, patient medicines or samples, other patient items, food and other equipment should not be stored in the medicine room.

Cleaning, workbench and floor are cleaned daily, shelves once a week, closets and refrigerators once a month and main cleaning twice a year. Check and tidy up. Clean trolleys and trays daily and remember trolley wheels.

64.4.1 Storage of Medicines

- Medicines are stored in a separate lockable room/closet.
- Medicinal products that cannot tolerate storage at room temperature are stored at 2–8 °C in lockable refrigerator. Check the thermometer regularly, once a week.
- Medicines are sorted and placed in transparent, marked shelves in the closet/refrigerator.
- The cabinet should have glass doors for visibility.
- Drugs are discarded when the date of expiration is reached.
- The packaging is kept properly closed after each withdrawal.
- Medications taken out of original packaging *should not* be returned.
- Discarded medicinal products are stored in a closed container and are sent regularly to the pharmacy.

- The medicine/medicine refrigerator is checked, cleaned and washed every month.
- If a satisfactory aseptic working technique and work in a sheltered location, the following general guideline for use after opening of the drug- breaking the seal (when not otherwise stated by the supplier) [1–3], is:
  - Nonpreserved solutions: 24 h after opening.
  - Preserved solutions: 1 month after opening, in a refrigerator

64.4.2 Work with Medicines in Medicine Room: Hygiene Measures

64.4.2.1 Tablets, Powder, Crushing of Tablets and More

- Hand hygiene before and after.
- Clean bench, by washing over with soap and water—and disposable cloth.
- The drug is placed in clean cups with clean spoons. Do not touch directly with hands - the drug.
- When crushed in mortars, use clean equipment and wash in a washing machine at 85 °C.
- The drug tray should be clean and washed at 85 °C once a day (preferably after each medicine round).
- Drug cart with tray is cleaned daily. Remember to clean the wheels of the trolley.

64.4.2.2 Intravenous Fluids/Medications

- Hand hygiene before and after.
- Clean bench—LAF cabinets (see below).
- Rubber stoppers/additives on infusion bags *should always be disinfected* before perforating with a needle. Although the stopper is covered with a capsule, it is *not* sterile.
- It is important that hands are not kept straight over the parts of the product to be protected. This is especially important when withdrawing from ampoules.
- When opening a vial for adding medicament to a sterile bag, the date and time and name of the person who performs the procedure should be written.
- Do not work on at the washbasin when setting up intravenously! There may be splashes of gram-negative rod bacteria that are always present in the sink.

64.4.2.3 Use of LAF Benches

- Hand hygiene before and after.
- Find equipment that should be used and place on a clean bench.
- The LAF bench is no storage. The bench must be empty when not working there.
- The LAF bench should stand on continuously (exhaust). Before using the bench, disinfect all the surfaces inside the LAF bench with 70% alcohol.
- Work with calm movements.
- Work at least 15 cm inside the bench.

- Do not have more equipment than is necessary for the work procedure inside the bench.
- When opening a vial/add to a bag, the date and time and name of the person who performs the procedure should be added.
- After completion of work: Disinfect the bench with 70% alcohol. Any spillage may be wiped/washed away, preferably with soap and water before the bench is disinfected. (Spills, like albumin, cannot be washed with alcohol; soap and water must be used.)

64.4.2.4 Cleaning of LAF Benches

Daily: The bench is disinfected with alcohol 70% before and after use. Eventually spill wipes up. Wash with soap and water over the worktop once a day and when necessary.

Weekly: Once a week, wash the whole bench with soap and water. Wash all surfaces inside the bench. For vertical LAF benches (airflow from roof to bottom), lift up the grate at the bottom of the bench and clean well below this.

Note! Avoid getting water into the HEPA filter (sitting behind the lattice in the ceiling on vertical benches and in the back of the horizontal benches). When the bench is dried, disinfect all surfaces with 70% alcohol.

64.4.2.5 Control of LAF Benches

The benches should be checked regularly (once/year + smoke test every quarter) concerning leakage and air velocity. The department is responsible for checking the LAF bench and changing the filter. If there is doubt if the bench has being checked, contact the pharmaceutical department or technical department. Checks are noted on their own form available in the medicine room.

64.4.3 Handling of Medicine Doses and Distribution to the Patients

Drugs delivered to patients should always be checked by two persons.

Good hand hygiene when distributing drugs!

64.4.3.1 General Routines

- *Each patient should have his own eye drops, mixture, cream, ointment,* etc. The bottle/tube should be labelled with the patient's name and date when opened and placed in the patient's room.
- Opened cans, for instance, of laxantia for common use, should be stored in the drug trolley, and the doses should be portioned just before dispensing to the patient. Put the date on the bottle.
- "Possible drug" (medication used when needed) is taken out of the original packaging immediately before it is given.
- Provide time and calm when handling/dispensing drugs.
- *Always* check medicine card when handling drug doses.

- Medicine doses and patient name should be reviewed of two competent healthcare workers.
- Always hand hygiene before and after handling medicines.
- Avoid direct contact with medicines such as tablets, etc.
- Avoid to take medicament trolleys into patient rooms, if possible, and not into rooms with known infections.
- Use disposable equipment, like disposable drug vials and disposable gloves (changed if contact with the patient, biological material, patient-related equipment and the like).
- The patient should be advised to take his/her doses immediately/as soon as possible upon distribution.
- Use teaspoon when the patient needs help to take medications in portions and give the patient plenty to drink. The medicine is taken when the patient has swallowed it.
- Drug doses that are delivered but not taken by the patient should be discarded.

64.4.3.2 Eye Drops, Nose Drops/Spray (Aerosol), Oral Spray

- Medicine bottle is marked with the patient's name, date and when opening the bottle.
- The bottle in use must be kept hygienically safe. Keep in mind that some types of medicines must be stored in the refrigerator!
- For patients with infections (upper respiratory tract/eye), the medicine bottle should be placed on the patient's room. If possible, select single use doses, for example, eye drops, nose drops.
- Hand disinfection before handing to each patient, possibly disposable gloves as well.
- Do not let the medicine bottle come into direct contact with the skin/mucous membranes of the patient.
- Any spills on the bottle should be wiped away immediately with 70% alcohol.
- Hand hygiene afterwards.

64.4.3.3 Cream, Ointment

- The bottle/tube is marked with the patient's name and date of use.
- The bottle/tube should be in the patient room.
- The bottle/tube with expired date must be discarded.
- Hand disinfection before.
- Use gloves by application (lubricate).
- Hand hygiene.

64.4.3.4 Suppositories, Klyster

- Hand disinfection before. Use disposable gloves.
- Place the patient in the correct position and protect the surface from spillage.
- Open the pill/envelope and insert the drug into the rectum/vagina.
- Hand wash.

64.4.4 Inhalation of Drugs

64.4.4.1 Inhalation: Fluids

Equipment: Nebulizer (pari—apparatus, atomizer) with nozzle/mask, air hose, nebulizer cups and disposable gloves. Check that the apparatus has undergone proper cleaning and disinfection [4]. Avoid the patient's own equipment used at home is brought to the hospital without proper cleaning at the centre for medical equipment. Use new, cleaned and disinfected equipment. Patients with inhalation treatment should be treated at single room.

- It is important to know the operating instructions for the devices. Check that the parts of the apparatus are properly connected and check that it is functioning properly. No sharing of devices with others.
- Note the medication glass (inhalation fluid) with the patient's name, date and date of use of the glass or use single-dose vials dispensed to each patient immediately prior to inhalation.
- The nozzle and atomizer cup are washed in a dishwasher (85 °C) after each use.
- Mouthpiece/mask and atomizer vials are washed in a dishwasher and rinsed well once a day. Allow the equipment to air-dry. Parts that can withstand heat up to 100 °C may be boiled 6–10 min in water, daily. The air intake filter and the air hose to the atomizer are changed as needed and between patients.
- Hand hygiene before and use disposable gloves.
- Apply inhalation fluid directly into the vial just prior to use by the patient. Instruct and help the patient to use the device properly.
- Hand wash.

64.4.4.2 Inhalation Aerosol

Equipment: Inhalation Chamber

- Each patient must have his own device.
- Check that the parts (nozzle, flask, valve) are assembled properly. After each use, remove the parts from each other, wash them in water, add detergent and rinse thoroughly. Allow parts to air-dry. Parts that can be heated up to 100 °C: boil 6–10 min in water once a day.
- Hand hygiene and disposable gloves.
- Aerosol doses are inserted into the chamber just prior to inhalation.
- Instruct the patient for inhalation techniques and make sure that the patient is breathing properly.
- Hand wash.

64.4.4.3 Inhalation Powder

Medicinal products in powder form are stored in "Turbuhaler, Diskhaler".

- Each patient should have his own branded turbohaler/dischaler.
- The devices should be used in the patient's room.

- Get to know the operating instructions.
- Hand hygiene before any use.
- Prepare the drug dose (s).
- Instruct patient for inhalation technique.
- The nozzle is washed with soap and water every time after use, eventually in dishwasher/instrument washing machine for high-temperature equipment.
- Hand wash.

64.4.5 Blood Glucose Measurement and Other Control: Risk of Blood Infection and Other Infection

Check that all equipment is clean and that measuring instruments are disinfected between use. Do not expose equipment for blood or other contamination by placing open cotton swabs, patches, plaster and the likes together with the equipment. Single-use, disposable equipment is not used for multiple patients. Create routines that ensure purity and sterility for each patient. All equipment that comes into contact with wounds and sterile mucous membranes must be sterile. This also applies to cotton swabs and bandages that should be sterile packaged. The blood contamination problem and other infections are increasing, especially related to the sharing of reusable containers, injections and blood glucose measurements [5–13].

64.4.6 Medical Equipment to Be Reused to a New Patient

Ensure that the equipment is cleaned and decontaminated inside and outside in routine use with the patient [4]. Make good practices for this. This is especially important for patients with chronic respiratory disease, dialysis treatment, immunosuppression, infusion treatment and wound care.

Be critical of the purchase of expensive medical equipment that cannot be cleaned inside. Make sure that a new user of medical devices gets clean equipment checked and disinfected, for example, at a centre for treatment of reusable medical equipment.

64.5 Background Information

Nearly all patients at hospitals receive medicines of different types. Medicines are administered in many different ways: tablets, fluids or drops, powders or pills, and a large amount of treatment takes place with parenteral with sterile fluids or intramuscularly. All drugs should have a minimum purity requirement, and all medicaments used in sterile areas (intravascular, intramuscular, sterile cavity, respiratory tract, etc.) must be sterile, prepared and administered. The work in medicine rooms is important concerning sterility, exactness and competence in relation to give the right patient the right medicine. The medicine room should be a restricted area, only used by well-educated personnel, working with medicaments.

64.5.1 Infections: Transmitted by Medicament Treatment

One out of three hospital patients may have infections/colonisation with possible pathogenic microbes. This may be spread to other patients and to the environment, unless staff is careful about hygienic handling and delivery of, for instance, medicines. Personnel responsible for drug administration should be careful, well informed and have competence in hygiene and infection control when handling and administering drugs. It is crucial that personnel do not spread infections to patients though bad hygiene during drug handling or administration.

- Contaminated drugs with pathogenic microbes are a possible source of infection for patients and staff in direct contact.
- Pathogenic microbes can be transferred from one infected patient to another through the staff's hands and equipment used for the distribution of drug doses.
- Pathogenic microbes can be transferred from an infected patient to the staff by direct contact with, e.g. secretions, blood, sore, faeces, etc. associated with drug administration to the patient.
- Reuse of syringes, tips, lancets, intravenous agents, etc., due to time constraints, lack of knowledge, lack of information and training, savings at the hospital, etc.
- Transport, placement and contamination of medicines on patient rooms.
- Where or how the medicines are store and handled.
- Where and how the individual drug doses are handled.

64.5.2 Factors Increasing Risk of Drug Contamination

- More persons and work operations—from the ordination until the patient receives medication.
- Lack of hygiene (environment, equipment and hand hygiene)
- Time constraint and understaffing
- Delegation to personnel without knowledge and responsibility. An increasing problem
- Lack of knowledge and information. An increasing problem

References

1. Bredesen Hatlelid L, Rasch M, Hochlin K, Seljordslia B, Andersen BM. Handling of medicaments and intravenous liquids—medicine room. In: Handbook in hygiene and infection control for hospitals. Oslo; 2008. p. 510–3.

2. Andersen BM. Handling of drugs-cleaning in medicine room. In: Handbook in hygiene and infection control for long-term care. Akademika; 2013. p. 439–54.
3. Norwegian medicament—handbook for healthcare personnel; 2013.
4. Andersen BM, Hochlin K, Daling J-P. Cleaning and decontamination of reusable medical equipments, including the use of hydrogen peroxide dry-mist gas decontamination. J Microbial Biochem Technol. 2012;4:57–62.
5. Prevention of blood borne infection i healthcare. Statens helsetilsyn, IK-2552; 1997.
6. Was infected by hepatitis B at Rikshospitalet. Three patients infected by hepatitis B during treatment at the pain clinic at Rikshospitalet last year; Aftenposten 24 juli 2008.
7. CDC. Frequently asked questions (FAQs) regarding assisted blood glucose monitoring and insulin administration.
8. Klonoff DC, Perz JF. Assisted monitoring of blood glucose: special safety needs for a new paradigm in testing glucose. J Diabetes Sci Technol. 2010;4:1027–31.
9. OSHA Healthcare Advisor: hepatitis B outbreak kills six due to unsafe blood glucose monitoring. CDC; 2010.
10. McIntosh YG, Powell TA, Tipple M, et al. Multiple outbreaks of hepatitis B virus infection related to assisted monitoring of blood glucose among residents of assisted living facilities Virginia, 2009–2011. Morb Mortal Wkly Rep. 2012;61:339–43.
11. CDC. Invasive *Staphylococcus aureus* infections associated with pain injections and reuse of single-dose vials—Arizona and Delaware, 2012. Morb Mortal Wkly Rep. 2012;61:501–4.
12. WHO. Rational and safe use of injections worldwide. Clean care is safer care. The safe injection global network. www.injectionsafety.org
13. Dolan SA, Littlehorn C, Glode MP, et al. Association of *Bacillus cereus* infection with contaminated alcohol prep pads. Infect Control Hosp Epidemiol. 2012;33:666–71.

Part XII

Internal Service

65 Cleaning of Rooms in Wards

Abstract

Cleaning is increasingly relevant as an important factor to reduce spread of contaminants and infections in hospitals and other healthcare institutions. The burden of contaminants, microbes, organic materials, dirt and dust is significantly reduced by cleanliness. The air quality, working environment and comfort increase for everyone by thorough daily cleaning. In addition, the safety of patients increases when potentially hazardous microbes are being systematically and regularly removed both in bedroom departments and in operating departments. A good cleaning results in less contamination of the personnel's uniforms and thus transmission of infection to other patients. Still, cleaning is underestimated and often inadequate—(also in Norwegian hospitals)—due to savings, efficiency requirements and improper use of expertise and resources. The following chapter is focused on practical measures concerning cleaning and control in healthcare institutions.

Keywords

Cleaning of hospital room · Detergents · Cleaning methods · Frequency · Infection control · Hygiene · Prevention

65.1 Purpose

- Prevent infectious spread in the environment, between patients, personnel, visitors and equipment [1–19].
- Reduce microbes, allergenic particles, organic matter, dirt and other contaminations in the room, areas, surfaces and air.

B. M. Andersen, *Prevention and Control of Infections in Hospitals*,
https://doi.org/10.1007/978-3-319-99921-0_65

65.2 Comprise

- All floors, surfaces, furniture, sanitary facilities (sink, toilet, bathroom, etc.) and other room-associated equipment, according to the work list.

65.3 Responsibility

The hospital management is responsible (according to law and regulations) to make written routines for general sanitation and hygiene at the hospital and ensure that conditions, expertise and resources are in place for a good, systematic and quality-assured cleaning that reduces burden of infectious environment in a proper manner [20].

The department management is responsible for ensuring that correct procedures for cleaning are instituted at all times in the department and followed up in cooperation with the user, the infection control staff and the corporate health service. The department's management is also responsible for communicating to the hospital's management in case of unreasonable poor cleaning that increases the burden of infection on patients and personnel or otherwise reduces the operation, function and safety of the department.

Cleaner management, in cooperation with the department's management, is responsible for ensuring that cleaning is properly carried out in accordance with written guidelines and focused on good infection protection—at all departments. Regular quality measurements of cleaning should also be carried out.

Each cleaner is responsible for quality well-executed work in accordance with guidelines. Cleaners are also responsible for informing their managers and department managers for lack of cleaning due to lack of resources, expertise and/or personnel.

65.4 Practical Measures

A number of guidelines and routines have been established to improve the cleanliness of hospitals [3, 4, 7, 9, 11–23].

65.4.1 Dressing and Personal Protection of the Cleaner

- Cleaners use the hospital's uniform that is changed daily and when contaminated (see Chap. 6).
- Jewellery, piercing, wristwatches, etc. are not allowed.
- Hand hygiene is always important after cleaning in patient rooms.
- Follow the written procedures for use of personal protective equipment (PPE), both during normal cleaning and according to patient isolation regimes.
- Cleaners should be taught hygiene and infection prevention to protect themselves and others. It is particularly important to have knowledge of infectious diseases,

which are commonly observed in the hospital, such as MRSA, ESBL, tuberculosis, *Clostridium difficile*, norovirus and influenza (see Chaps. 14–21 on isolation routines).
- Cleaning and disinfection should be learned from scratch, as well as the use of PPE and how to handle used cleaning equipment in such situations.
- It is crucial to learn how cleaning is carried out at the different levels of cleanliness to avoid spread of infection via the actual cleaning process, for example, from the toilet to the sink.

65.4.2 Equipment for Cleaning

- Mops and cloths should satisfy the requirements for textiles used in hospitals.
- *Moisture mop*, 100% polyester, and *wet mop* in cotton/polyester [13].
- Washcloths and mops should only be used in one place or one area. Used at several sites can lead to spread of infection [24].
- Soap and detergent used should have a defined bacterial number <100 CFU [25].
- Clean equipment is used for each room.
- After cleaning in room/area, washcloths/mops are sent for wash and disinfection in textile washing machines at temperature >85 °C, following guidelines for handling used textiles.
- Other equipment like the wash stick and bucket are cleaned/disinfected in the decontaminator.
- Cleaning cart is cleaned daily.
- Keep the cleaning equipment in a suitable and separate room.

65.4.3 Methods

Studies show that wet mopping and moisture mopping are the best methods for cleaning floors and surfaces [13].

65.4.3.1 Floor

- Moisture mopping without detergent
- Wet mopping with detergent
- Glossing approx. one time/month
- Floor polish as needed

Note! Whatever method used, stains should always be removed! Dry mopping is not accepted at hospitals due to increased dust swirling from the floor.

65.4.3.2 Fixtures and Surfaces

- Dust cleaning with a moistened cloth.
- It is important that all areas that are often in contact with the patient, visitors and staff are cleaned daily such as keyboards, phone, buttons on TV, switches for

lights and calls, bedside lamps, buttons/keyboard on technical equipment, etc. Here are often large quantities of bacteria deposited [26].
- Wash furniture, chairs, tables, bedside tables, etc.
- Use of vacuum cleaner of fabric furniture, radiators, etc. should be avoided or at least in agreement with the department's management, because of spread of particles in the room. Using a dust filter—hepafilter—is necessary.

65.4.3.3 Sink, Shower, Bathroom and Other Wet Areas

In and around all wet areas (bathroom, washbasin, etc.) in the department, there are growth of gram-negative rod bacteria like *Enterobacter*, *E. coli*, *Klebsiella* and *Pseudomonas* [27]. Wash the cleanest part around the faucet and the sink first and then the faucet and around the drain. The cloth is then put into the bag for washing.

65.4.3.4 Soap

Defined bacterial count is <100 CFU, stated by the manufacturer. Soap should be used directly from the manufacturer's container and stored in such a way that it does not get contaminated. Soap can promote bacterial growth, especially of gram-negative bacteria (*Pseudomonas*, *Enterobacter*, etc.) [25].

65.4.3.5 Inspection and Cleaning Equipment After Use

- *Mops* are only used in one room at a time (one mop for the patient room, one new to the toilet, one new to the shower room, etc.). After use put mops and cloths in a bag for textiles, washed at 85 °C and dried and kept at room temperature. Washed mops can be undried if put in a clean bag, held in a clean refrigerator for up to 24 h and used for wet or moist wash.
- For *bucket* and other equipment that can withstand it, decontaminate after use.
- Wash the *nal* with clean water and soap with a clean cloth and wipe over before leaving.
- *The cleaning* cart is washed with soap and water daily.
- *Storage*. The cleaning equipment is stored in a suitable clean room that is cleaned daily.
- *Polish machines and large* floor *washing machines are* thoroughly cleaned after use and stored in a dry condition and in a clean room to prevent bacterial growth.

65.4.3.6 Special Cleaning

- Main cleaning: walls, ceiling, floor, fixtures, furniture, closets, etc., with soap and water; minimum once a year, depending on department/ward and patient groups.
- Cleaning of ventilation ducts: minimum once every 5 years or more often for valves and long air ducts and valves through the building. Contact technical department.
- Disinfection of rooms and surfaces (see below).

65.4.4 Regular Cleaning: Routine Cleaning [14–16]

Patient room, treatment room, medical treatment offices, ward office, expedition, conference rooms and corridors on the bed wards. All cleaning programs must be written and checked on a regular basis.

65.4.4.1 Patient Room

- Daily cleaned: 7 days/week (two wet mops, five moisture mops).
- *Note! Thoroughly removal of all stains with soap and water!*
- Daily washing of fixtures, all horizontal surfaces, washbasin and wall around the sink.
- Check soap dispenser, towel and dispenser for hand hygiene products.
- Weekly cleaning of lists, including floor lists and lists for patient curtains, as well as shelves and ceiling lamps.
- Valves for air intake/exhaust are washed at least once a month and more often when needed.
- Curtains are sent to wash once a month and more often when needed.
- *Floor* glossing approx. once a month and polishing when needed.

65.4.4.2 Treatment Room, Doctor's Office w/Patient, Conference Room, Ward Office, Expedition and Medicine Room

- Cleaned 5 days/week (one wet mop, four moisture mops). Simultaneous washing and dust drying of fixtures, horizontal surfaces and sink and wall around the sink. If not in use, wash accordingly. If daily use, washed daily.
- *NB! Thoroughly remove all stains with soap and water!*
- Check the soap, towel and alcohol dispenser!
- *Floor* glossing approx. once a month and polishing when needed.
- Valves for air intake/exhaust are washed outside at least once per month and if required.

65.4.4.3 Corridors on the Bed Ward, and Common Room for Patients

- Cleaned 7 days/week (two wet mops, five moisture mops).
- *NB! Thorough removal of all stains with soap and water!*
- *Floor* glossing approx. once a month and polishing when needed.
- Valves for air intake/exhaust are washed outside at least once per month and if required.
- Note that many corridors are under-ventilated and have a bad smell—often because of the coating of organic matter and microbes that decay. Therefore, good daily cleaning is particularly important here.

65.4.4.4 Ward Kitchen and Common Serving Rooms for Patients

- *Daily wet mopping—7 days a week.*
- Valves for air intake/exhaust are washed outside at least once per month and if required.
- Waste bin emptied twice a day.
- Check the soap, towel and dispenser!

65.4.4.5 Wet Rooms (Disinfection of Washrooms, Waste Disposal, etc.)

- *Daily wet mopping—7 days a week.*
- The housekeeper is responsible for daily cleaning in general on the disinfection and washrooms and other wet rooms, window frames, door handles, table and benches and shower and toilet; wash the outside of the decontaminator and of vertical surfaces around the sink.
- Check the soap, towel and alcohol dispenser!
- All of the loose fixtures and special benches for organic waste, infected equipment, etc. in the disinfection room is the nursing staff often responsible for written agreement.
- Valves for air intake/exhaust are washed outside at least once per month and if required.
- Main cleaning at least once a year and documented. More frequency must be agreed with the supervisor.

65.4.4.6 Shower/Bath Room: Attached to Patient Room

- *Daily wet mopping—7 days a week.*
- Clean the shower, remove the lint and hair from shower, and flush the shower inside with warm water.
- Clean shower chairs and all surfaces, sink, mirrors, etc.
- Check the soap, towel and alcohol dispenser!
- Valves for air intake/exhaust are washed outside at least once per month and if required.
- Main cleaning at least once a year and documented. More frequency must be agreed with the supervisor.

65.4.4.7 Shared Use of Shower/Bathroom for Several Patients

- *As above and in addition.*
- After each user, remove the used textiles, clean the shower/bathroom, wash the shower enclosure, bath and shower chair, wipe up from the floor, and the cranes and mirrors should be clear and clean. There should be good ventilation between the patients.

65.4.4.8 Toilets, Common for Patients and Visitors Entering from Corridors

- *Daily wet mopping; twice every day, 7 days a week.*
- Only "inspection" is not enough because most of the microbes and dirt are invisible! The toilet should be clean and tidy all the day—remember many helpless patients!

- Mirror, shelf, sink and toilet are washed in this order.
- The toilet is washed first from the top to the bottom and inside using the toilet brush. The toilet ring is washed with clean mop—top side first.
- The toilet brush is cleaned regularly in the decontaminator at minimum 85 °C, once a week.
- Silicone around the toilet base prevents urine from flowing under the shelf.
- Valves for air intake/exhaust in the toilet are washed at least once per month and if necessary.
- Waste bin emptied twice a day.
- Check the soap, towel and alcohol dispenser!
- Main cleaning of the rooms: two times per year.

65.4.4.9 Toilet for the Staff at the Bed Ward

- *Daily wet mopping × 7 days a week.*
- Valves for air intake/exhaust are washed outside at least once per month and if required.
- Waste bin emptied twice a day.
- Check the soap, towel and alcohol dispenser!
- Main cleaning of the rooms: two times per year.

65.4.4.10 Offices and Corridors Without Patient Access

- Wet mopping × 1/week.
- Moist mopping × 1/week.
- The corridor, door handles and railings (optionally) are cleaned 1–5 times/week depending on the activity.
- Check the soap, towel and alcohol dispenser!
- Main cleaning once a year.

65.4.4.11 Wardrobe for the Staff with Toilet and Shower

- Cleaning 5–7 days a week, depending on use (two wet mops, five moist mops).
- Check the soap, towel and alcohol dispenser!
- Main cleaning once a year.

65.4.4.12 Elevator

- Daily cleaning of floor, girder and control panel.

65.4.5 Special Cleaning

Room disinfection (disinfection and washing) when needed and in consultation with the responsible nurse. Stains and spots or organic materials are disinfected and removed by nursing staff.

Note! Whatever method, stains should always be removed!

65.4.6 Follow-Up and Control Should Not Be Time-Based

Household leaders should follow up and check cleaning at least once a week. Written check, once/month, is logged and reported to the head of the department in which the cleaning takes place. It is pointless to set minutes, etc. for each surface to be cleaned because time spent does not have anything with the quality to do [28]. The most important is that good technique and knowledge are learned and that the cleaner knows the areas that should be cleaned. Control of cleaning together with the person responsible for the cleaning is a good tool in the training process [7, 12, 13, 19, 21, 26, 29–32]. In some cases it may be appropriate to conduct certain environmental tests [33].

65.4.7 Main Cleaning Is Important

The hospital must carry out main cleaning; wash with soap and water, of all walls, ceilings, valves and air ducts every year. In some departments, main cleaning must be carried out at least twice a year: surgery department, intensive and postoperative departments and departments with patients with reduced infection resistance. In case of major outbreaks in an entire department, main cleaning should be considered after the disinfection process has been completed.

65.5 Background Information

Cleaning is an important factor in reducing the spread of infections and contaminants in hospitals and other healthcare institutions [1–10]. Effective cleaning reduces the load of biological material, dirt and dust—that patients, staff, visitors and equipment are exposed to [2, 3, 5–17]. The air quality, working environment and comfort increase for everyone by thorough daily cleaning. In addition, the safety of patients increases when potentially hazardous microbes are systematically and regularly removed both in bedroom departments and in operating departments [5, 6, 8, 11–13]. Cleaning results in less contamination of the personnel's uniforms and thus reduced transmission to patients [18]. Cleaning is underestimated and often inadequate (also in Norwegian hospitals)—due to savings and improper use of expertise and resources [8, 19].

A significant portion of the pathogenic microbes in the environment is reduced by good cleaning and thereby reduction of cross-contamination between patients via contact- and airborne microbes [11–13, 26]. However, 2 h after good cleaning of the floor, approximately the same bacterial load is present on the floor as before cleaning but now with new bacteria. A patient room that is not well cleaned can become an infection risk for the next patient [19, 34–36]. Need for cleaning varies between types of patients [37]. A good hygiene standard is cost-effective in reducing hospital infections. It is also achievable—in contrary to experience with hand hygiene and prescribing antibacterial agents [2].

Cleanliness leads to better indoor environment, healthier air (less organic material decaying) and better working conditions, is aesthetically important and gives patients and visitors a positive impression of the hospital.

65.5.1 Dust and Dirt Contain a Lot of Skin Flora

Most people release 30,000–60,000 dead skin cells from the body per minute, i.e. more than 500 million a day. This happens from patients, personnel and visitors. Dead skin cells are released continuously as small dust particles around the human body and lie as a trace after everyone in the room—and wherever you go. Dead skin cells are the main ingredient (more than 90%) in house dust and in dust in the patient's room. Approximately 10% of loose skin particles contain bacteria in the order of 5–12 per particle. The largest yield of microbes is found on the forehead, around the ears, the head itself, the upper part of the back, the axillary, the nose opening, etc., with gender variation. Also hair and beard can contain large amounts of microbes. Free skin particles will always be shed to the air from bare skin. Good cleaning of the room reduces the load of organic materials, skin cells and bacteria that come with skin shedding.

65.5.2 Area and Equipment

Floor is always coated with a certain amount of dust, skin cells, particles and microbes. A dust particle can contain 5–15 microbes. The larger the amount, the more swirls up in the air by movement in the room. By bed making, shaking out textiles, and dusting with dry cloth, large amounts of dust particles are released into the air. Generally, this is completely harmless to healthy people. However, it is a risk and source of infection for patients with chronic respiratory diseases, respiratory allergy, wounds or with a reduced immune defence/general condition.

Walls are low carriers of dust but can be contaminated with pus/secretion from patients (MRSA, influenza virus, etc.).

Shelves, *racks*, *rails in ceilings* and *all horizontal objects* carry dust and microbes, regardless of height. Movements in the room like bed making and rapid door openings may swirl bacteria-carrying particles up in the air from shelves, etc. and spread it by air currents (re-aerosol) [38].

Washbasins are always contaminated by bacteria, often with bacterial flora of the patient and the personnel who were last in the living room. Gram-negative bacteria grow well with access to water. Water directly from the tap is generally clean enough to drink if it is run for a while before use. But the opening of the crane is often grown with microbes [39, 40]. Some washbasins spray contaminated water into the air.

Toilet seats are always contaminated by the previous user's microbes. As a rule, this is normal skin microbes and/or intestinal flora. Down in the toilet itself, there is always strong contamination of the intestinal flora. In case of heavy water rinsing, aerosols can be released [41].

Air ducts/canals with air brought to and from the room often become contaminated with dust, fungi, bacteria and particles. Especially around openings of ducts for taking air out of the room, large quantities of dust and dirt are generated.

Call buttons, *light switches*, *telephones*, *radio*, *TV service channel*, *door handle* and *PC* are always contaminated with microbes from last and previous users and can be difficult to clean [42–46].

The shower/bathroom is coated on floors, walls and curtains with skin cells and intestinal flora from the last and previous users if not cleaned between each user. Bacteria and most viruses may withstand water temperatures up to 50–60 °C. Special viruses (norovirus, hepatitis E virus, etc.) and bacteria like enterococci and legionella may withstand higher temperatures.

65.5.3 Microbes

The most common microbes in dust and particles are harmless skin bacteria such as coagulase-negative staphylococci, diphtheroids, etc. and fungi.

Occasionally there are *Staphylococcus aureus*, especially in rooms where such patients are treated, and intestinal bacteria (*E. coli*, other gram-negative bacteria and enterococci). Anaerobic bacteria like *Clostridium difficile* and *Clostridium perfringens* form spores that can survive long in the environment and in the dust.

Lifetime in dust and on surfaces if not removed [47].

S. aureus	3–10 months
MRSA—methicillin-resistant *S. aureus*	Up to 10 months
Enterococci	*2–4 months*
Vancomycin-resistant enterococci	*2–4 months*
Streptococci group A	*2–4 months*
Mycobacterium tuberculosis (TBC)	*12 months*
Gram-negative rods	*Days–weeks–months*
Acinetobacter species	*10 months*
Clostridium difficile spores	*Months–years*
Hepatitis B/C/HIV	*Days–weeks–months*
Norovirus	*Days–weeks*
Influenzae	*2–3 weeks*

65.5.4 Causes and Factors Concerning "Poor Cleaning"

Some rooms/wards/departments have a bigger problem with cleaning than others, because of:

- Cracks and unevenness in floors and other surfaces that make cleaning difficult.
- Large amounts of wires on the floor/wall, etc.
- Storage of goods on the floor.

- Floor and wall covering difficult to clean/not suitable for cleaning.
- Too much equipment relative to floor space.
- Not understanding cleaning scheme.
- Changed departmental function.
- Cleaning not adapted to patient category/activity.
- Bacteria-infected wash equipment with dispersion [48, 49].
- Poorly completed washing, disinfection, aerosol formation during cleaning and poor design of the rooms, etc. [50, 51].
- Poor cleansing attracts flies and other insects that can carry potentially pathogenic microbes [52].
- Lack of cleaning personnel—infections increases [53].

References

1. Rutala WA, Weber DJ. Environmental interventions to control nosocomial infections. Infect Control Hosp Epidemiol. 1995;16:442–3.
2. Dancer SJ. Mopping up hospital infection. J Hosp Infect. 1999;43:85–100.
3. Sehulster LM, Chinn RYW, Ardunio MJ, et al. Guidelines for environmental infection control in health-care facilities. CDC MMWR. 2003;52:1–42.
4. Rutala WA, Weber DJ. Disinfection, sterilization, and control of hospital waste. In: Mandell, Douglas, and Bennets principles and practice of infectious diseases, vol. 2. 8th ed. Philadelphia: Elsevier Churchill Livingstone; 2015. p. 3294–309.
5. Boyce JM. Environmental contamination makes an important contribution to hospital infection. J Hosp Infect. 2007;65:50–4.
6. Fraise AP. Decontamination of the environment. J Hosp Infect. 2007;65:58–9.
7. Griffith CJ, Cooper RA, Gilmore J, Davies C, Lewis M. An evaluation of hospital cleaning regimes and standards. J Hosp Infect. 2000;45:19–28.
8. Hota B. Contamination, disinfection, and cross-colonization: are hospital surfaces reservoirs for nosocomial infection? Clin Infect Dis. 2004;39:1182–9.
9. Dancer SJ. The role of environmental cleaning in the control of hospital-acquired infection. J Hosp Infect. 2009;73:378–85.
10. Sie I, Thorstad M, Andersen BM. Personal- and environmental hygiene in Norwegian nursing homes. J Nurs Educ Pract. 2012;2(1):71–8.
11. Andersen BM, Solheim N, Kruger Ø, Levy F, Sogn K, Moløkken I. Cleaning of floor in patient rooms. Effect on bacteria, organic materials and particles. Tidsskr Nor Laegeforen. 1997;117:838–41.
12. Andersen BM, Røed RT, Solheim N, et al. Air quality and microbial contamination in operation rooms with and without laminar air filtration. Tidsskr Nor Laegeforen. 1998;20:3148–51.
13. Andersen BM, Rasch M, Kvist J, Tollefsen T, Lukkassen R, Sandvik L, Welo A. Floor cleaning: effect on bacteria and organic materials in hospital rooms. J Hosp Infect. 2009;71:57–65.
14. Syvrud EJ, Lukkassen R, Solheim N, Andersen BM, Hochlin K, Rasch M. Cleaning of patient rooms. In: Andersen BM, editor. Handbook in hygiene and infection control for hospitals. Oslo: Ullevål universitetssykehus; 2003. p. 408–18.
15. Lukkassen R, Rasch M, Hochlin K, Andersen BM, Seljordslia B, Tollefsen T. Cleaning at bed-departments and disinfection of rooms and surfaces. In: Handbook in hygiene and infection control for hospitals. Oslo: Ullevål University Hospital Oslo; 2008. p. 592–603.
16. Andersen BM. Cleaning of rooms, bed and equipment. In: Handbook in hygiene and infection control for nursing homes and long-term care facilities. Akademika; 2013. p. 483–92.

17. Andersen BM. Disinfection of rooms and surfaces. In: Handbook in hygiene and infection control for nursing homes and long-term care facilities. Akademika; 2013. p. 493–501.
18. Hess AS, Shardell M, Johnson JK, et al. A randomized controlled trial of enhanced cleaning to reduce contamination of healthcare worker gowns and gloves with multidrug-resistant bacteria. Infect Control Hosp Epidemiol. 2013;34:487–93.
19. Carling PC, Huang SS. Improving healthcare environmental cleaning and disinfection. Infect Control Hosp Epidemiol. 2013;34:507–13.
20. European Parliament and Council Directive 2000/54/EC of 18 September 2000 on the protection of workers from the risks related to exposure to biological agents at work.
21. Dancer SJ. How do we assess hospital cleaning? A proposal for microbiological standards for surface hygiene in hospitals. J Hosp Infect. 2004;56:10–5.
22. Griffith CJ, Obee P, Cooper RA, Burton NF, Lewis M. The effectiveness of existing and modified cleaning regimes in a Welsh hospital. J Hosp Infect. 2007;66:352–9.
23. Dettenkofer M, Spencer RC. Importance of environmental decontamination. A critical view. J Hosp Infect. 2007;65:55–7.
24. Bergen LK, Meyer M, Høg M, Rubenhagen B, Andersen LP. Spread of bacteria on surfaces when cleaning with microfiber cloths. J Hosp Infect. 2009;71:132–7.
25. Frøystad GH. Microbial contamination of cleaning tools-soap and detergents. MSIS. 1994;22:1.
26. Huslage K, Rutala WA, Gergen MF, Sickbert-Bennett EE, Weber DJ. Microbial assessment of high-, medium-, and low-touch hospital room surfaces. Infect Control Hosp Epidemiol. 2013;34:211–2.
27. Charron D, Bedard E, Lalancette C, Laferriere C, Prevost M. Impact of electronic faucets and water quality on the occurrence of *Pseudomonas aeruginosa* in water: a multi-hospital study. Infect Control Hosp Epidemiol. 2015;36(3):311–9.
28. Rupp ME, Adler A, Schellen M, et al. The time spent cleaning a hospital room does not correlate with the thoroughness of cleaning. Infect Control Hosp Epidemiol. 2013;34:100–2.
29. Larson EL, Aiello A, Gomex-Duarte C, et al. Bioluminescence ATP monitoring as a surrogate marker for microbial load on hands and surfaces in the home. Food Microbiol. 2003;20:735–9.
30. Lewis T, Griffith C, Gallo M, Weinbren M. A modified ATP benchmark for evaluating the cleaning of some hospital environmental surfaces. J Hosp Infect. 2008;69:156–63.
31. Chan M-C, Lin T-Y, Chiu Y-H, et al. Applying ATP bioluminescence to design and evaluate a successful new intensive care unit cleaning programme. J Hosp Infect. 2015;90:344–6.
32. Knape L, Hambraeus A, Lytsy B. The adenosine triphosphate method as a quality control tool to assess "cleanliness" of frequently touched hospital surfaces. J Hosp Infect. 2015;91:166.
33. Claro T, Galvin S, Cahill O, et al. What is the best method? Recovery of methicillin-resistant *Staphylococcus aureus* and extended-spectrum beta-lactamase-producing *Escherichia coli* from inanimate hospital surfaces. Infect Control Hosp Epidemiol. 2014;35:869–71.
34. Huang SS, Datta R, Platt R. Risk of acquiring antibiotic-resistant bacteria from prior room occupants. Arch Intern Med. 2006;166:1945–51.
35. Nseir S, Blazejewski C, Lubret R, et al. Risk of acquiring multidrug-resistant Gram-negative bacilli from prior room occupants in the ICU. Clin Microbiol Infect. 2011;17(8):1201–8.
36. Hamel M, Zoutman D, O'Callaghan C. Exposure to hospital roommates as a risk factor for health care-associated infection. Am J Infect Control. 2010;38:173–81.
37. Moore G, Muzlay M, Wilson PR. The type, level, and distribution of microorganisms within the ward environment: a zonal analysis of an intensive care unit and a gastrointestinal surgical ward. Infect Control Hosp Epidemiol. 2013;34:500–6.
38. Shiomori T, Miyamoto H, Makishima K, Yoshida M, Fujiyoshi T, Udaka T, et al. Evaluation of bedmaking-related airborne and surface methicillin-resistant Staphylococcus aureus contamination. J Hosp Infect. 2002;50:30–5.
39. Trautmann M, Michalsky T, Wiedeck H, Radosavljevic V, Ruhnke M. Tap water colonization with *Pseudomonas aeruginosa* in a surgical intensive care unit (ICU) and relation to *Pseudomonas* infections of ICU patients. Infect Control Hosp Epidemiol. 2001;22:49–52.

40. Bukholm G, Tannæs T, Kjelsberg ABB, Smith-Erichsen N. An outbreak of multidrug-resistant *Pseudomonas aeruginosa* associated with increased risk of patient death in an intensive care unit. Infect Control Hosp Epidemiol. 2002;23:441–6.
41. Gerba CP, Wallis C, Melnick JL. Microbial hazards of household toilets: droplet production and the fate of residual organisms. Appl Microbiol. 1975;30:229–37.
42. Neely AN, Weber JM, Daviau P, MacGregor A, Miranda C, Nell M, et al. Computer equipment used in patient care within a multihospital system: recommendations for cleaning and disinfection. Am J Infect Control. 2005;33:233–7.
43. Wilson APR, Hayman S, Folan P, Ostro PT, Birkett A, Batson S, Singer M, et al. Computer keyboards and the spread of MRSA. J Hosp Infect. 2005;61:390–1.
44. Oie S, Hosokawa I, Kamaya A. Contamination of room door handles by methicillin-sensitive/methicillin-resistant *Staphylococcus aureus*. J Hosp Infect. 2002;51:140–3.
45. Stacey A, Burden P, Croton C, Jones E. Contamination of television sets by methicillin-resistant *Staphylococcus aureus* (MRSA). J Hosp Infect. 1998;39:243–4.
46. Lemmen SW, Hafner H, Zolldann D, Stanzel S, Lutticken R. Distribution of multi-resistant gram-negative versus gram-positive bacteria in the hospital inanimate environment. J Hosp Infect. 2004;56:191–7.
47. Kramer A, Schebke I, Kampf G. How long do nosocomial pathogens persist on the surfaces? A systematic review. BMC Infect Dis. 2006;6:130–8.
48. Bartz S, Ritter AC, Tondo EC. Evaluation of bacterial multiplication in cleaning cloths containing different quantities of organic matter. J Infect Dev Ctries. 2010;4:566–71.
49. Engelhart S, Krizek L, Glasmacher A, Fischnaller E, Marklein G, Exner M. *Pseudomonas aeruginosa* outbreak in a hematology-oncology unit associated with contaminated surface cleaning equipment. J Hosp Infect. 2002;52:93–8.
50. Macve JC, Weinbren MJ. Dirty utility room design and aerosolization of organisms. J Hosp Infect. 2012;81:66–7.
51. Manian FA, Griesenauer S, Senkel D, Setzer JM, Doll JA, Perry AM, et al. Isolation of *Acinetobacter baumannii*-complex and methicillin-resistant *Staphylococcus aureus* from hospital rooms following terminal cleaning and disinfection: can we do better? Infect Control Hosp Epidemiol. 2011;32:667–72.
52. Pelli A, Kappel HB, Oliveira AG, Silva AG, Dourado PL, Bataus LAM. Characterisation of a Nocardia sp isolated from an insect (moth-fly) captured in a university hospital. J Hosp Infect. 2007;67:393–5.
53. Smith B. Britain: rise in "superbug" cases linked to decrease in hospital cleaning staff. World Socialist Web Site. wsws.org. Accessed 22 Jan 2005.

Disinfection of Rooms and Surfaces

66

Abstract

Resistant, virulent and infectious microbes lead to increasing need for disinfection of patient rooms and other areas in hospitals. Outbreaks of resistant and dangerous microbes with spread in health institutions results in that the quality of cleaning and disinfection of the hospital environment are being studied with "argus" eyes. In England, the spread of MRSA in hospitals in 2005 was considered so serious that it was taken up in the Parliament and Prime Minister Blair announced a requirement to halve the MRSA cases at English hospitals. Cleaning and disinfection then gained a significant boost.

The following chapter is focused on practical measures concerning disinfection and control of contaminated rooms in healthcare institutions.

Keywords

Disinfection of rooms and surfaces · Disinfectants · Disinfection methods Frequency · Infection control · Hygiene · Prevention

66.1 Purpose

- Prevent spread of infectious agents in the environment: between patients, personnel, visitors and equipment [1–4].

66.2 Comprise

- Infectious disease/agents; where room, equipment and environment may be contaminated with human pathogenic infectious agents.

B. M. Andersen, *Prevention and Control of Infections in Hospitals*,
https://doi.org/10.1007/978-3-319-99921-0_66

- In case of heavy burden of organic materials in the environment, in patient rooms and other areas and where limitation of possible infection is uncertain.
- After defined infectious disease/agents spread by air, contact, blood, food/water, faeces, etc., according to isolation regimens, including strict insolation. See chapter on isolation.

66.3 Responsibility

The hospital's management is responsible for the existence of written procedures for the proper disinfection of rooms and areas affected by possible contaminants and to provide enough expertise and resources to ensure that patients, personnel or visitors are not unnecessarily exposed to infectious agents [5].

The department manager ensures that disinfection procedures are implemented and understood and determine the time, level and extent of room disinfection. The leader shall also inform the hospital's management—immediately—if the necessary disinfection procedures are not followed due to lack of personnel, expertise or resources for such work. The manager should check that the cleaner follows the guidelines for the use of personal protective equipment (PPE) and disinfectants.

Personnel/cleaners follow routines for disinfection, which disinfectant to be used and areas to be disinfected. Follow procedures for taking on and removing PPE.

66.4 Practical Measures [1–4]

66.4.1 Dressing, Donning Personal Protection Equipment: PPE

The person who performs the disinfection procedure takes on PPE:

- Surgical mask and cap covering hair and ears
- Gown—waterproof with long sleeves and cuffs
- Gloves with cuffs
- Room-bound shoes or shoe covers

Follow the recommendation for PPE as outlined in the hospital's *isolation regimes* (see Chaps. 14–21).

66.4.2 Disinfectants

Follow the hospital's routines for selecting disinfectants for rooms and equipment. The most common agents are chloramine 5%, chloricide, household bleach, "perasafe" (peracetic acid) or "virkon" (pentapotassium bis). *See disinfection of instruments and equipment* (see Chap. 59).

Disinfection process and handling of washing equipment:

- In case of massive contamination, most of the spill is removed with absorbent material, packaged and treated as hazardous waste in defined, yellow waste bag.
- Suitable disinfectant—chloramine 5%—(or perasafe) is applied on contaminated surfaces (table, shelves, floor, wall and equipment such as lamp, door handle, washbasin, etc.) with cloth or sponge that is thrown away after use as infectious waste. Effect time 60 min. Exit the room during this period, but not before disinfection equipment, etc. is taken care of with regard to infection protection.
- Before taking off PPE—doffing—and before leaving the room: the equipment used, mops, cloths, etc., are packaged and treated as infectious. Mops and cloths used are handled further as infectious –brought directly to the disinfection room, put in a washing machine for mops and cloths at 85 °C and washed separately for 10 min.
- Buckets, etc. are emptied and disinfected in decontaminator in the disinfection room associated with the isolate or packaged and brought—as infected equipment—to the decontaminator in the ward's common disinfection room.
- The disinfection cart is disinfected with the same remedy and left in the room.
- PPE is removed at the exit door or in the sluice; learn how to take off PPE! Gown, cap, surgical mask and gloves are treated as infectious waste.
- Perform good hand hygiene in the end.
- Doors are marked with sign and kept closed during disinfection period (1 h).
- After the disinfection period, the infectious agent is destroyed and regular cleaning can be done.

Ventilation after disinfection of rooms: Patient room and disinfected areas are aired approximately 1 h after cleaning.

Larger areas—many room contaminated and/or much disposable equipment/medical equipment.

Larger areas—like in operation departments, intensive units and wards where many rooms/areas may be contaminated, often with a lot of disposable equipment, medical equipment, etc., gas disinfection with dry hydrogen peroxide gas is recommended, with subsequent regular washing [6–10]. Gas method should not be used in case of tuberculosis or other mycobacteria because of lack of effect [9]. Use of robot gas disinfection saves staff to be exposed to chemical fluids over time [6–8, 10].

Check the effect of gas disinfection with the use of spore tests! See chapter on disinfection of instruments and equipment.

Spot disinfection of spills, stains and other organic materials:

- Spot disinfection prevents the spread of possible contamination and organic material (urine, faeces, vomit, blood, sputum, tissue, pus, etc.) from patients to other patients, personnel, visitors and the environment.
- Spot disinfection consists of disinfecting a restricted area of blood spills and stains of organic materials on floors and other surfaces without being known or defined contagious.

The head of the department determines the extent and type of disinfection. The department's nursing staff carries out the spot disinfection immediately, in connection with the accident. It is only necessary to disinfect the area contaminated with biological material.

66.4.2.1 Indication

Limited blood spills and/or biological material on floors and other surfaces without known infectious disease:

- Spill of blood and other organic material is removed with single-use gloves and absorbent material, packaged and treated as hazardous waste.
- Suitable disinfectant—chloramine 5%—is applied on contaminated surfaces/equipment with a cloth.
- Effect time according to recommended of the disinfectant used.
- Chloramine 5% (household bleach, chloricide):
  - 30 min for dried area (removed spill)
  - 60 min for contaminated, spilled surface and if tuberculosis
- Perasafe:
  - 10 min for dried area
  - 30 min if tuberculosis
- Virkon:
  - 30 min for dried area.
  - Virkon does not have any safe effect on tuberculosis.

66.4.3 Spot Disinfection on a Clean Surface

For spot disinfection on smaller surfaces, door handles, switches, chairs, benches, etc., alcohols, 70–85%, can be used.

66.4.4 Cleaning Personnel on a 24-h Basis

There is an increasing need for disinfection of rooms and equipment in patients with different infectious diseases associated with MRSA, VRE, ESBL and other resistant gram-negative rod bacteria, *Clostridium difficile*, norovirus, rotavirus, influenza, etc. This results in additional burden and additional expenses for the hospital. It is important to have an efficient disinfection and cleaning team that remove contamination as soon as possible on a 24-h basis. This may stop more serious epidemic outbreaks and—at the same time—keep going a rational drift of the hospital.

66.4.5 Understaff of Cleaning Personnel During Periods of Sick Leave, Influenza, Etc.

By reduced staffing concerning cleaning, alternative solutions may be made with respect to prevent infections. Patient-directed cleaning and cleaning in visitor areas must therefore be prioritized.

66.5 Background Information

Outbreaks of resistant and dangerous microbes with spread in health institutions results in that the quality of cleaning and disinfection of the hospital environment are being studied with "argus" eyes. In England, the spread of MRSA in hospitals in 2005 was considered so serious that it was taken up in the Parliament and Prime Minister Blair announced a requirement to halve the MRSA cases at English hospitals. Cleaning and disinfection then gained a significant boost.

Infections and microbial agents follow patients, personnel, visitors and equipment to and from hospitals, between departments and wards and between health levels [11–14]. Many of the most resistant and/or infectious microbes have long lifetime in the environment, are robust and persist for months if they are not removed [15, 16]. Periodically, they colonize or infect patients, personnel and visitors and are carried to new areas where new equipment in new rooms is contaminated. The infection is spread through contact and air by dust and skin particles [17–23].

Before the antibiotic era, it was "good Latin" to reduce infections by good hygiene and pertinent cleaning and use of various disinfectants. Today, it is growing recognition again that cleaning, hygiene, disinfection and infection protection are the cornerstones of combating the most resistant microbes. No new antibiotics have been developed for the last 50 years—except for one antibacterial agent that bacteria now are developing resistance against [6–10, 24, 25].

A number of publications show that resistant microbes can survive in the environment after the leave of an infectious patient—for many months. The next patient may thus be exposed to environmental contamination by, for example, MRSA, VRE or multidrug-resistant gram-negative rods such as *Pseudomonas aeruginosa, Acinetobacter baumannii* and ESBL-producing *E. coli and Klebsiella* [6, 23–27]. *Clostridium difficile* spores may live forever if not removed. Also, norovirus and influenza viruses can survive for a long time in the environment [16, 27]. Microbes are spread in the environment—transmitted through contact with hands, washcloths, mops, etc. and by re-aerosols spread to other surfaces [28–32]. Roommates and the next patients staying in the same room have a clear risk of being infected [18–20, 33].

66.5.1 Disinfection of Rooms and Equipment Is a Special Work for Cleaners

There are many disinfection methods: from heat, heat vapours and chemical liquids to different gases and UVC [8–10, 34–37]. Rooms and larger equipment/surfaces are usually disinfected by chemical fluids and increasingly chemical gases are used. *See Chap. 59 for disinfection of instruments and equipment.*

Disinfectants must have a sure killer effect against microbes and not just "knocking out" so that they develop resistance to disinfectants [38–40]. Ineffective, "microbe-reducing" disinfectants/detergents in common cleaning are used in many countries. This may promote development of resistance [41–43].

Disinfection process or method is often not working [23]. The method itself can transfer microbes further into the environment if cleaning is not carried out in a hygienically thoroughly manner [21–23, 31, 32, 44]. Specially exposed are all contact points in patient rooms: all equipment used as phones, switches, PCs, bed edges, washbasins, toilet, textiles and multipurpose equipment, various auxiliary equipment such as wheelchairs and armchairs and medical examination equipment like stethoscopes and blood pressure equipment, staff's personal bags, etc. [45–51].

Cleaners must be specially trained for the work with disinfection methods and also taught in the use of chemical disinfectants and in the use of PPE [3, 4, 52, 53]. Using dedicated disinfection teams, there may be a reduction in, for instance, the spread of *C. difficile* [54].

Gas disinfection In case of larger outbreaks with more rooms and larger areas, there is an increased need of more chemical disinfectants in liquid form that may be difficult to work with. Using a robot disinfectant, gas treatment may save a lot of work and exposure to chemicals and may also save costs through decontaminating paper-wrapped disposable equipment in infected rooms [8, 10, 55]. This method is approved and used in different ways around the world [6, 8–10, 37, 55–59]. It is important that spore test are used to document the killing effect on microbes and to know that gas disinfection has no effect against mycobacteria infection [8–10, 58].

References

1. Sehulster LM, Chinn RYW, Ardunio MJ, et al. Guidelines for environmental infection control in health-care facilities. CDC MMWR. 2003;52:1–42.
2. Rutala WA, Weber DJ. Disinfection, sterilization, and control of hospital waste. In: Mandell, Douglas, and Bennets principles and practice of infectious diseases. Vol. 2. 8th ed. Philadelphia: Elsevier Churchill Livingstone; 2015. p. 3294–309.
3. Lukkassen R, Rasch M, Hochlin K, Andersen BM, Seljordslia B, Tollefsen T. Cleaning at bed-departments and disinfection of rooms and surfaces. In: Handbook in hygiene and infection control for hospitals. Oslo; 2008. p. 592–603.
4. Andersen BM. Disinfection of rooms and surfaces. In: Handbook in hygiene and infection control for nursing homes and long-term care facilities. Akademika; 2013. p. 493–501.
5. European Parliament and Council Directive 2000/54 /EC of 18 September 2000 on the protection of workers from the risks related to exposure to biological agents at work.

6. French GL, Otter JA, Shannon KP, Adams NMT, Watling D, Parks MJ. Tackling contamination of the hospital environment by methicillin-resistant *Staphylococcus aureus* (MRSA): a comparison between conventional terminal cleaning and hydrogen peroxide vapour decontamination. J Hosp Infect. 2004;57:31–7.
7. Jeanes A, Rao G, Osman M, Merrcik P. Eradication of persistent environmental MRSA. J Hosp Infect. 2005;61:85–6.
8. Andersen MR, Hochlin K, Jensen F-H, Wismar P, Fredriksen J-E. Decontamination of rooms, medical equipment and ambulances, using a dry mist of hydrogen peroxide disinfectant. J Hosp Infect. 2006;62:149–55.
9. Andersen BM, Syversen G, Thoresen H, Rasch M, Hochlin K, Seljordslia B, Snevold I, Berg E. Failure of dry mist of hydrogen peroxide 5% to kill *Mycobacterium tuberculosis*. J Hosp Infect. 2010;76:80–3.
10. Andersen BM, Hochlin K, Daling J-P. Cleaning and decontamination of reusable medical equipments, including the use of hydrogen peroxide dry-mist gas decontamination. J Microbial Biochem Technol. 2012;4:57–62.
11. Otter JA, French GL. Community-associated meticillin-resistant *Staphylococcus aureus* strains as a cause of healthcare-associated infection. J Hosp Infect. 2011;79:189–93.
12. Uhlemann AC, Knox J, Miller M, et al. The environment as an unrecognized reservoir for community-associated methicillin resistant *Staphylococcus aureus* USA300: a case-control study. PLoS One. 2011;6:e22407.
13. Kassem II. Chinks in the armor: the role of the nonclinical environment in the transmission of *Staphylococcus* bacteria. Am J Infect Control. 2011;39:539–41.
14. Lemmen SW, Hafner H, Zolldann D, Stanzel S, Lutticken R. Distribution of multi-resistant gram-negative versus gram-positive bacteria in the hospital inanimate environment. J Hosp Infect. 2004;56:191–7.
15. Kramer A, Schebke I, Kampf G. How long do nosocomial pathogens persist on the surfaces? A systematic review. BMC Infect Dis. 2006;6:130–8.
16. Yezli S, Otter JA. Minimum infective dose of the major human respiratory and enteric viruses transmitted through food and the environment. Food Environ Virol. 2011;3:1–30.
17. Shiomori T, Miyamoto H, Makishima K, Yoshida M, Fujiyoshi T, Udaka T, et al. Evaluation of bedmaking-related airborne and surface methicillin-resistant *Staphylococcus aureus* contamination. J Hosp Infect. 2002;50:30–5.
18. Hamel M, Zoutman D, O'Callaghan C. Exposure to hospital roommates as a risk factor for health care-associated infection. Am J Infect Control. 2010;38:173–81.
19. Nseir S, Blazejewski C, Lubret R, Wallet F, Courco F, Durocher A. Risk of acquiring multidrug-resistant gram-negative bacilli from prior room occupants in the intensive care unit. Clin Microbiol Infect. 2011;17:1201–8.
20. Bernard MC, Lanotte P, Lawrence C, Goudeau A, Bernard L. Air contamination around patients colonized with multidrug-resistant organisms. Infect Control Hosp Epidemiol. 2012;33:949–51.
21. D'Agata EMC, Venkataraman L, DeGirolami P, Samore M. Molecular epidemiology of ceftazidime-resistant gram-negative bacilli on inanimate surfaces and their role in cross-transmission during nonoutbreak periods. J Clin Microbiol. 1999;37:3065–7.
22. Catalano M, Quelle LS, Jeric PE, Di Martino A, Maimone SM. Survival of *Acinetobacter baumannii* on bed rails during an outbreak and during sporadic cases. J Hosp Infect. 1999;42:27–35.
23. Denton M, Wilcox MH, Parnell P, Green D, Keer V, Hawkey PM, et al. Role of environmental cleaning in controlling an outbreak of *Acinetobacter baumannii* on a neurosurgical intensive care unit. J Hosp Infect. 2004;56:106–10.
24. Rampling A, Wiseman S, Davis L, et al. Evidence that hospital hygiene is important in the control of methicillin-resistant *Staphylococcus aureus*. J Hosp Infect. 2001;49:109–16.
25. Mayhall CG. Control of vancomycin-resistant enterococci: it is important, it is possible, and it is cost-effective. Infect Control Hosp Epidemiol. 2002;23:420–3.

26. Levin AS, Gobara S, Mendes C, Cursino R, Sinto S. Environmental contamination by multidrug-resistant *Acinetobacter baumannii* in an intensive care unit. Infect Control Hosp Epidemiol. 2001;22:717–20.
27. Kuusi K, Nuorti JP, Maunula L, et al. A prolonged outbreak of Norwalk-like calicivirus (NLV) gastroenteritis in a rehabilitation centre due to environmental contamination. Epidemiol Infect. 2002;129:133–8.
28. Bergen LK, Meyer M, Høg M, Rubenhagen B, Andersen LP. Spread of bacteria on surfaces when cleaning with microfiber cloths. J Hosp Infect. 2009;71:132–7.
29. Bartz S, Ritter AC, Tondo EC. Evaluation of bacterial multiplication in cleaning cloths containing different quantities of organic matter. J Infect Dev Ctries. 2010;4:566–71.
30. Engelhart S, Krizek L, Glasmacher A, Fischnaller E, Marklein G, Exner M. *Pseudomonas aeruginosa* outbreak in a hematology-oncology unit associated with contaminated surface cleaning equipment. J Hosp Infect. 2002;52:93–8.
31. Macve JC, Weinbren MJ. Dirty utility room design and aerosolization of organisms. J Hosp Infect. 2012;81:66–7.
32. Manian FA, Griesenauer S, Senkel D, Setzer JM, Doll JA, Perry AM, et al. Isolation of *Acinetobacter baumannii*-complex and methicillin-resistant *Staphylococcus aureus* from hospital rooms following terminal cleaning and disinfection: can we do better? Infect Control Hosp Epidemiol. 2011;32:667–72.
33. Ajao AO, Johnson JK, Harris AD, et al. Risk of acquiring extended-spectrum beta-lactamase-producing *Klebsiella* species and *Escherichia coli* from prior room occupants in the intensive care unit. Infect Control Hosp Epidemiol. 2013;34:453–8.
34. Andersen BM, Bånrud H, Bøe E, Bjordal O, Drangsholt F. Comparison of UVC light and chemicals for disinfection of surfaces in hospital isolation units. Infect Control Hosp Epidemiol. 2006;27:729–35.
35. Rutala WA, Gergen MF, Tande BM, Weber DJ. Rapid hospital room decontamination using ultraviolet (UV) light with a nanostructured UV-reflective wall coating. Infect Control Hosp Epidemiol. 2013;34:527–9.
36. Anderson DJ, Gergen MF, Smathers E, et al. Decontamination of targeted pathogens from patient rooms using an automated ultraviolet-C-emitting device. Infect Control Hosp Epidemiol. 2013;34:466–71.
37. Rutala WA, Gergen MF, Weber DJ. Efficacy of improved hydrogen peroxide against important healthcare-associated pathogens. Infect Control Hosp Epidemiol. 2012;33:1159–61.
38. Speight S, Moy A, Macken S, et al. Evaluation of the sporicidal activity of different chemical disinfectants used in hospitals against *Clostridium difficile*. J Hosp Infect. 2011;79:18–22.
39. Wilcox MH, Fraise AP, Bradley CR, Walker J, Finch RG. Sporicides for *Clostridium difficile*: the devil is in the detail. J Hosp Infect. 2011;77:187–8.
40. Ali S, Moore G, Wilson AP. Spread and persistence of *Clostridium difficile* spores during and after cleaning with sporicidal disinfectants. J Hosp Infect. 2011;79:97–8.
41. Wisplinghoff H, Schmitt R, Wøhrmann A, Stefanik D, Seifert H. Resistance to disinfectants in epidemiologically defined clinical isolates of *Acinetobacter baumannii*. J Hosp Infect. 2007;66:174–81.
42. Millard J-Y. Bacterial resistance to biocides in the healthcare environment: should it be of genuine concern? J Hosp Infect. 2007;65:60–72.
43. Terpstra FG, van den Blink AE, Bos LM, et al. Resistance of surface-dried virus to common disinfection procedures. J Hosp Infect. 2007;66:332–8.
44. Hota B. Contamination, disinfection, and cross-colonization: are hospital surfaces reservoirs for nosocomial infection? Clin Infect Dis. 2004;39:1182–9.
45. Wilson APR, Hayman S, Folan P, Ostro PT, Birkett A, Batson S, Singer M, et al. Computer keyboards and the spread of MRSA. J Hosp Infect. 2005;61:390–1.
46. Oie S, Hosokawa I, Kamaya A. Contamination of room door handles by methicillin-sensitive/methicillin-resistant *Staphylococcus aureus*. J Hosp Infect. 2002;51:140–3.
47. Stacey A, Burden P, Croton C, Jones E. Contamination of television sets by methicillin-resistant *Staphylococcus aureus* (MRSA). J Hosp Infect. 1998;39:243–4.

48. Neely AN, Weber JM, Daviau P, MacGregor A, Miranda C, Nell M, et al. Computer equipment used in patient care within a multihospital system: recommendations for cleaning and disinfection. Am J Infect Control. 2005;33:233–7.
49. Schultz M, Gill J, Zubairi S, Huber R, Gordin F. Bacterial contamination of computer keyboards in a teaching hospital. Infect Control Hosp Epidemiol. 2003;24:302–3.
50. Tekerekoglu MS, Duman Y, Serindag A, et al. Do mobile phones of patients, companions and visitors carry multidrug-resistant hospital pathogens? Am J Infect Control. 2011;39:379–81.
51. Gardner P, Muller MP, Prior B, et al. Wheelchair cleaning and disinfection in Canadian health care facilities: "That's wheelie gross!". Am J Infect Control. 2014;42:1173–7.
52. Anonymous. Disinfectants for technical use in health and nursing. Norwegian Medicines Agency. Updated June 2015.
53. Havill NL, Havill HL, Mangione E, Dumigan DG, Boyce JM. Cleanliness of portable medical equipment disinfected by nursing staff. Am J Infect Control. 2011;39(7):602–4.
54. Sizlar B, Deshpande A, Fertelli D, et al. An environmental disinfection odyssey: evaluation of sequential interventions to improve disinfection of *Clostridium difficile* isolation rooms. Infect Control Hosp Epidemiol. 2013;34:459–65.
55. Otter JA, Nowakowski E, Salked JAG, et al. Saving costs through the decontamination of the packing of unused medical supplies using hydrogen peroxide vapor. Infect Control Hosp Epidemiol. 2013;34:472–8.
56. Chan HT, White P, Sheorey H, Cocks J, Waters MJ. Evaluation of the biological efficacy of hydrogen peroxide vapour decontamination in wards of an Australian hospital. J Hosp Infect. 2011;79:125–8.
57. Otter JA, Yezli S. A call for clarity when discussing hydrogen peroxide vapour and aerosol systems. J Hosp Infect. 2011;77:83–4.
58. Andersen BM. Does "airborne" hydrogen peroxide kill *Mycobacterium tuberculosis*? J Hosp Infect. 2011;77:84–5.
59. Otter JA, French GL. Survival of nosocomial bacteria and spores on surfaces and inactivation by hydrogen peroxide vapor. J Clin Microbiol. 2009;47:205–7.

67 Hospital Textiles

Abstract
The patient's textiles like bed linen are usually contaminated with skin cells and other body particles and may often contain large amounts of bacteria: 10,000 to over 100 million bacteria per 10 cm^2 textile. Samples from pyjamas and bed sheets after one night may have high yields of both normal skin bacteria and more pathogenic microbes like MRSA, enterococci and gram-negative rods. This is easily transmitted to the staff's hands and uniforms as well as to the environment and can be routed to other patients and personnel. For every day the patient uses the same bedding, the more the bacteria, skin cells and other particles are present on the laundry. The following chapter is focused on practical measures concerning healthcare textiles, laundry processes and transport and storage of textiles in healthcare institutions.

Keywords
Textiles · Bed linen · Uniforms · Laundry · Cleaning · Infectious textiles Disinfection · Transport · Storage · Infection control · Hygiene · Prevention

67.1 Purpose

- Remove microbes, body particles, skin cells and dirt from healthcare textiles, bed linen and personnel's uniforms.
- Prevent the transmission of microbes from contaminated textiles to clean textiles, patients, personnel, visitors and the environment [1–12].

B. M. Andersen, *Prevention and Control of Infections in Hospitals*,
https://doi.org/10.1007/978-3-319-99921-0_67

67.2 Comprise

All textiles used by patients and personnel and all persons who treat clean and/or contaminated textiles.

67.3 Responsibility

The hospital's management has (according to law and regulation) responsibility for written procedures for the transportation, washing and proper storage of hospital textiles and to provide safe areas for the transport, storage, washing and control of clean and unclean laundry. The management shall ensure expertise, resources and personnel for this work so that neither patients, personnel, visitors nor the environment is unnecessarily exposed to infectious agents [13].

Department management shall ensure that procedures for the treatment of clean, unclean and contaminated textiles are implemented in the daily work. Furthermore, the manager shall arrange for the storage of clean laundry in a clean room and unclean and infected laundry in defined unclean units. It must be ensured that unclean and contaminated textiles are handled and sent for wash in a proper manner to avoid exposure to microbial contamination [13].

Head of textile department and transport manager is responsible for all textile treatment regarding sorting, washing, disinfection, storage and transportation of used and clean clothes. It is important to distinguish clearly between the dirty and the clean side of the textile treatment. The manager should also inform the hospital's management—immediately—if capacity, expertise or resources cause patients, personnel, others and the environment to be exposed unnecessarily to infectious agents due to lack of professional textile treatment.

Personnel at all departments follow procedures for the treatment, storage and transportation of clean and unclean textiles.

NOTE! Remove all non-washable items, used needle tips and other sharp objects before textiles are delivered for washing! Empty your pockets and straighten the laundry!

67.4 Practical Measures

67.4.1 Patient Ward [5, 6]

67.4.1.1 Soiled Textiles in the Ward

– From beds, patients, operating clothes, personal clothing, towels, cloths and other textiles

- Protect the uniform when removing used bedding, for example, by a gown that is sent for wash after use. The uniform may easily be contaminated under such and similar procedures [14–20].

- Careful stripping and disposal of used bedding—avoid dispersion of microbes and particles from textiles to the air, hands, environment and equipment [21–27].
- Note that the mattress, quilt and pillow also may be contaminated [28].
- All loose objects must be removed from the laundry.
- Put used laundry directly in a *clean* bag or plastic bag at the user site.
- Hand hygiene.
- Do not carry unpacked, used laundry from beds, etc. out to the laundry collection point.
- Do not sort used clothes at the department.
- After the laundry bag is strapped, it will be transported as soon as possible.
- Wash the bin with wheels daily.
- Perform hand hygiene after handling laundry.

67.4.1.2 Laundry from Patients with Infection/Carrier State

- Use personal protective equipment (PPE): gloves, surgical mask and cap, gown and possibly room-bound shoes. Note that the patient's room and environment are often heavily contaminated by microbes [29, 30]. Follow the hospital's *isolation regimes*.
- Infectious laundry is textiles from patients with infection/carrier state and textiles contaminated with organic materials like faeces, pus, urine, vomit, blood, etc.
- All loose objects must be removed from the laundry.
- Directly placed in defined (yellow) bag that is strapped again, before transport to the storage room for used laundry. Wet, infectious textiles are put in a separate plastic bag that is then placed in a yellow bag for infections.
- In the isolation unit with sluice (anteroom), collecting bags can be stored until it is almost full. Close and send it to the room for used laundry—in clean bag outside.
- Wash the bag with wheels before leaving the sluice and once a day.
- Perform safe removal of PPE and hand hygiene before leaving the patient room.
- *See isolation regimes*—Chaps. 14–21.

Wash of dirty laundry at the patient ward is not recommended [5, 6].

- Not recommended at hospitals or other health institutions due to infection risk

Wash of patient clothing at the department is not recommended [5, 6].

- Not recommended at hospitals or other health institutions due to infection risk

67.4.1.3 Storage of Used, Dirty Laundry

- Avoid storage of laundry bags at the department—send it for wash as soon as possible.
- During up-filling, the sack is stored on disinfection room/garbage disposal, together with waste bags.

- The storage room should have negative pressure and be cleaned daily.
- There should be good routines for collecting used laundry at the hospital.
- Departments with sluices like operating and intensive units shall have storage rooms for unclean laundry and waste in the transition zone between the department and other units and shall be subject to negative pressure in relation to the department.

67.4.1.4 Transport of Unclean Laundry

- The bags must be solid enough to withstand transport. Plastic bags must be solid, minimum P-5. Nylon and textile bags should be of dense weaved fabric.
- Close tightly before transport, and retighten with metal plastic string about 10 cm from the upper edge or otherwise.
- Avoid the use of person lifts, if possible.
- Trolleys/carts used for laundry transport should not be used for clean transport without proper cleaning. All trolleys are cleaned in special washing machines at 85 °C for 10 min.
- Personnel transporting laundry should afterwards change work clothes and wash their hands well before clean transport.

67.4.1.5 Textile Chute for Unclean Fabrics

- Associated storage room for unclean laundry.
- Textile chute and underlying collection rooms shall have negative pressure.
- The chute should not be designed to cause overpressure in the tube under the bag (piston effect).
- The shutters and door to the collection room shall be airtight and should not be opened at more than one place at the same time (negative pressure).
- The chutes should be metal lined and should be cleaned once a year.
- Storage room under the chute must be provided with locks and washbasins and must be cleaned once a day.
- Location of collection room against outer wall with loading ramp outside.

67.4.1.6 External Transport

- *Clean and unclean transport should not be mixed!*
- Before clean transport, car/trailer cargo area must be thoroughly cleaned with soap and water.
- Trolleys must be cleaned properly in the laundry, damp heat of at least 85 °C and wiped dry before packed with clean textiles for transport to user.
- Return transport of used textiles in trolleys and other packaging must take place in an "unclean" car.
- External transportation assumes that all unclean laundry is well and properly packed. If this is taken cared of, cleaning the car's load compartment is sufficient.

67.4.2 The Laundry [3–6]

The laundry is responsible for all textiles: from arrival as a laundry and until they are deposited clean and in use in the bed wards. The laundry company, in cooperation with the hospital's management, is responsible for procurement, quality, textile types, ease of use and capacity. There should never be a lack of textiles for patients or personnel. If there are too little/too bad textiles, it could reduce the hospital's activity. Infection protection of patients and personnel is more important than the hospital's goal of savings [13].

The laundry staff should be protected against microbes, high levels of particles, large amounts of organic materials, fungi and chemical agents [13]. It is important to have good training in hygiene and infection control and control of the amount of particles and microbial levels in the laundry, both on the clean and unclean side. The laundry must be checked routinely for ventilation, clean air, daily cleaning and main cleaning once a year,—and particle and chemical load.

67.4.2.1 Do Not Store Textiles Outside!

- Do not put textiles unprotected outside due to the general risk and access to birds and animals!
- Textiles that stand outside will be damaged by prolonged wetting where decay and wet rot easily occur, which will propagate to the laundry and back to the patients! There have been several outbreaks due to water-damaged fabrics with bacterial spores that survive the washing process.

67.4.2.2 Unclean Side: Input and Sorting of Used Laundry

- The inlet section—reception of used laundry—is separate from the laundry itself.
- Here there can be a massive concentration of contaminants.
- An effective vacuum with negative pressure prevents contaminants from this area to penetrate to the clean part of the laundry.

67.4.3 Ordinary Unclean Laundry from the Wards

- Sorting unit for textiles is physically separated from the rest of the laundry with separate room and negative pressure.
- The personnel working on unclean laundry side should not work on a clean side the same day due to the danger of cross-contamination.
- All the staff should have wardrobes and canteen.
- Laundry facilities must have a sluice function. In the sluice there should be cap, shoes, gown, gloves, surgical mask or respiratory protection (tuberculosis and particle load), as well as hand wash and shower.

- If the sluice function is not possible, clean donning should be carried out on the clean side and uncleaned doffing on the unclean side.
- On the unclean side, there must be a separate toilet and sink.
- When sorting, wear protective clothing, gown, gloves, cap, shoes and surgical mask/respirator.
- Wet-wash the floor daily.

67.4.3.1 Infected Textiles: From Patients with Infection/Carrier State

- Treated in separate rooms with separate ventilation and vacuum.
- Infected textiles are treated separately and carefully by staff wearing their PPE.
- Washed in separate machine; do not sort before washing.
- After washing, the laundry can be sorted for regular washing.
- Eventually wash twice at 85 °C.

67.4.3.2 Sharp Objects and Other Wastes Found in Textiles

- Make registration and feedback to wards, if possible!
- Report accidental injury, and contact the manager.
- Note and evaluate actual vaccinations.

67.4.3.3 Clean Side: Clean Treatment of Clean Laundry

- Overpressure relative to the unclean side: look for doors and windows so the pressure balance is functioning.
- Minimal handling reduces the number of microbes on clean clothes!
- Staff with clinical signs of infections should not handle clean clothes!
- Staff should wear clean uniforms every day.
- Good personal hygiene.
- Good hand hygiene and shower (after work on the dirty side).
- The finished and clean laundry is packed clean on clean trolleys for each department.

67.4.3.4 Washing Process: Textiles

- All textiles (patients and personnel) are washed at >85 °C for 10 min.
- All textiles (patients and personnel) are dried in the tumble dryer at >85 °C for 10 min.

67.4.3.5 Surgical Textiles

- Washed separately.
- Control and packing unit for sterile laundry is separated from clean laundry unit due to particle release.
- After checking and packaging, textiles go for autoclaving.
- Allow everything to be done at the textile supply.

67.4.3.6 Cleaning

- Daily washing of floor and dust drying of work surfaces and table.
- Weekly dust drying of pipe hangers, roof beams and shelves.
- Routine for cleaning machines and internal trolleys.

67.4.3.7 Control

- Control of bacteria in the air (CFU/m^3) on the clean side once a year.
- Check particle amount in the air on the clean and unclean sides to check exhaust/air quality every year.
- Control of positive pressure and negative pressure (clean and unclean sides, once a month).
- Control of cleanliness in the working area (ATP and similar) 1–2 times a year or more often.
- Take samples from 100 cm^2 clean clothes on the clean trolley; 10 random samples/year.

67.4.3.8 Transport of Clean Clothes

- Trolley is cleaned before use and closed.
- Transported from the clean side of the laundry by car or trailer with clean and closed cargo area.
- Purity should be checked 1–2 times a year.

67.4.3.9 Patient Ward: Treatment of Clean Laundry

- Store dry and dust free in separate storage room for clean textiles. Only clean textiles should be stored here.
- Always wash/disinfect hands before entering textile storage room.
- No transit traffic through stores.
- The floor of the textile room is not a storage area.
- Daily cleaning of floors.
- Do not store clean textiles in patient rooms! There is risk of infection to the next patient!
- Textiles from the patient's room must not be returned to clean textile storage. There is risk of infection!

67.4.3.10 Personnel's Uniform

- The work suit must be cleaned every day.
- Wash at 85 °C for 10 min and dry at 85 °C for 10 min, and should tolerate this.
- Winter clothes for ambulance personnel, etc. must withstand washing at 60 °C for at least 20 min.
- Work clothes should not be taken home and washed there. It is not allowed due to infection risk.
- Working clothes are adapted to the working situation.

67.5 Background Information

67.5.1 Risk of Infection

Healthcare textiles are often contaminated with blood, tissues and infectious agents and must therefore be packed, transported and washed hygienically satisfactorily so that no one else is exposed to infection or organic matter [1–10].

Microbes survive on fabrics for hours to days and weeks, depending on which agent it is [1, 2, 10, 14, 16, 22]. It is therefore important to change clothes if contaminated with blood, pus or tissue fluids. Depending on endemic or epidemic situations and the patient categories taken cared of, there may be large amounts of microbes on staff uniforms—such as resistant gram-negative rods, MRSA, VRE, *Clostridium difficile*, norovirus, rotavirus, influenza virus, etc. [14–22, 29, 31]. Problems are often that patients with infection are detected late after admission and may therefore contaminate the environment and other patients before the infection is detected [32].

The patient's textiles are usually contaminated with dead skin cells and other body particles and often contain large amounts of bacteria: 10,000 to over 100 million bacteria per 10 cm^2 textile [1]. Samples taken from 18 patient's pyjamas and bed sheets who spent one night in a hospital showed in a sampled area of 10 cm^2 different potentially pathogenic microbes [33]. There was a flora varying from normal flora such as coagulase-negative staphylococci, corynebacteria and *Bacillus* spp. to enterococci (9/18 patients), MRSA (5/18), *E coli*, *Proteus mirabilis* and *Pseudomonas aeruginosa* [33]. The amount of bacteria was in many cases up to 100,000/10 cm^2 [33]. This is reflected in the staff's hands and uniforms as well as in the environment by the patient's care and examination and can be routed from there to other patients and personnel [1, 10, 34]. The more days the patient uses the same bedding, the more the bacterial load and particle load on the laundry increase [1, 10, 33].

The staff in nursing situation in contact with the patient's bedside, bed sheet, duvet, pillows, etc., have a great chance of acquiring a patient's microbes on the front of their own uniform unless patient-bound gowns are used [10, 14–20]. Therefore, frequent shifts and washing of textiles are very important in health institutions. The number of microbes increases on the uniform for each day it is used, and for this reason, the staff have to change outfits every day and more frequently if contaminated [5, 6]. A high degree of safety is achieved by treating all organic material as potentially infectious.

Note! Personnel working with transport and sorting of dirty textiles are particularly exposed to contamination and organic materials if not handled in a hygienically sound manner!

Note! Avoid grading of "contagious"!

67.5.2 The Washing Process

The washing process should remove dirt and contaminants through prewash, main wash and rinse.

- *Patient/personnel textiles* are heat disinfected through a 10-min wash process at 85 °C and corresponding drying process. Then the textiles are free for ordinary bacteria, viruses and fungi, but not sterile. Spore-forming bacteria such as *Bacillus* and fungal spores can survive the washing process and accompany the textiles further to storage. Such agents have become more relevant as a cause of outbreaks in other countries and may be a challenge for patients with severe immune defences, including premature babies.
- *Other fabrics* like curtains, tablecloths, etc. can be washed at lower temperatures (60 °C).
- *Bedside curtain/cloth on display panel* is sent for washing after each patient; there are often large amounts of patient microbes on these textiles [35].
- *Operation* textiles are specially treated and sterilized.
- *Sterile textiles* are packaged in as special textiles and autoclaved.

67.5.3 All Treatment of Unclean, Dirty Laundry: Separated from the Treatment of Clean Textiles

Unclean laundry is a source of infection in all healthcare institutions. Special bedding and patient textiles are often contaminated with tissue fluids, infectious agents and blood. It is important that unclean laundry such as bed linen, towels, washcloths, patient clothing and personnel work clothes are handled in a hygienically sound manner. Remember hand hygiene since contaminated hands can spread microbes between patients, textiles and other equipment and personal clothing [1, 10, 18, 26, 34].

Most microbes can be airborne by swirling from surfaces and bedding by care and nursing, opening and closing of doors, cleaning, etc. [21–27]. Microbes are easily spread to patient clothes and the staff's uniform. Therefore, gowns are recommended for care and washing of patients. Clothes that are contaminated must be replaced. Personnel involved in transportation and sorting of unclean laundry are particularly exposed to contaminants if the textiles are not secured through hygienic treatment.

References

1. Sehulster LM, Chinn RYW, Ardunio MJ, et al. Guidelines for environmental infection control in health-care facilities. CDC MMWR. 2003;52:1–42.
2. Centers for Disease Control and Prevention. Laundry: washing infected materials. CDC; 2011.
3. Hygienic requirements and procedures for treatment of textiles used in healthcare. IK 1941. Norwegian Board of Health; 1994.
4. Anonymous. Textile supply, Ullevål hospital, has sat the standard for quality system (NS-ISO 9002 standard) in laundry, textile storage, sewing room.
5. Dufseth IS, Andersen BM. Textiles, cleaning, control, transport and storage. In: Handbook in hygiene and infection control Håndbok i hygiene og smittevern for sykehus. Ullevål universitetssykehus; 2003. p. 419–25, og 2008, 604–9.

6. Andersen BM. Cleaning and control of textiles. In: Handbook in hygiene and infection control for nursing homes and long-term care facilities. Akademika; 2013. p. 493–501, 503–9.
7. Doncaster and South Humber Healthcare NHS trust infection control laundry policy NHS; 2009.
8. Bloomfield SF, Exner M, Signorelli C, Nath KJ, Scott EA. The infection risks associated with clothing and household linens in home and everyday life settings, and the role of laundry. International Scientific Forum on Home Hygiene [Internet]; April 2011. p. 1–47. http://www.ifh.homehygiene.org.
9. Barrie D. How hospital linen and laundry services are provided. J Hosp Infect. 1994;27:219–35.
10. Mitchell A, Spencer M, Edminston C Jr. Role of healthcare apparel and other healthcare textiles in the transmission of pathogens: a review of the literature. J Hosp Infect. 2015;90:285–92.
11. Fijan S, Gunnarsen JTH, Weinreich J, Sostar-Turk S. Determining the hygiene of laundering industrial textiles in Slovenia, Norway and Denmark. Tekstil. 2008;57:73–83.
12. Sie I, Thorstad M, Andersen BM. Personal- and environmental hygiene in Norwegian nursing homes. J Nurs Educ Pract. 2012;1:71–81.
13. European Parliament and Council Directive 2000/54 / EC of 18 September 2000 on the protection of workers from the risks related to exposure to biological agents at work.
14. Neely AN, Maley MP. Survival of enterococci and staphylococci on hospital fabrics and plastic. J Clin Microbiol. 2000;38:724–6.
15. Hambraeus A. Transfer of *Staphylococcus aureus* via nurses' uniforms. J Hyg. 1973;71:799–814.
16. Zachary KC, Bayne PS, Morrison VJ, Ford DS, Silver LC, Hooper DC. Contamination of gowns, gloves, and stethoscopes with vancomycin-resistant enterococci. Infect Control Hosp Epidemiol. 2001;22:560–4.
17. Treakle AM, Thom KA, Furuno JP, et al. Bacterial contamination on health care workers' white coats. Am J Infect Control. 2009;37:101–5.
18. Munoz-Price LS, Arheart KL, Mills JP, et al. Associations between bacterial contamination of health care workers' hands and contamination of white coats and scrubs. Am J Infect Control. 2012;40:245–8.
19. Wiener-Well Y, Galuty M, Rudensky B, Schlesinger Y, Attias D, Yinnon AM. Nursing and physician attire as possible source of nosocomial infections. Am J Infect Control. 2011;39:555–9.
20. van der Reijden WA, Heijers JM, Vandenbroucke-Grauls CM, de Soet JJ. Survival of bacteria on uniforms in relation to risk management in dental clinics. J Hosp Infect. 2009;73:283–5.
21. Shiomori T, Miyamoto H, Makishima K, Yoshida M, Fujiyoshi T, Udaka T, et al. Evaluation of bedmaking-related airborne and surface methicillin-resistant *Staphylococcus aureus* contamination. J Hosp Infect. 2002;50:30–5.
22. Macias, et al. Controlling the novel (H1N1)—do not touch your face! J Hosp Infect. 2009;73:280–91.
23. Macve JC, Weinbren MJ. Dirty utility room design and aerosolization of organisms. J Hosp Infect. 2012;81:66–7.
24. Best IE, Fawley WN, Parnell P, et al. The potential for airborne dispersal of *Clostridium difficile* from symptomatic patients. Clin Infect Dis. 2010;50:1450–7.
25. Gehanno JF, Louvel A, Nouvellon M, Caillard JF, Pestel-Caron M. Aerial dispersal of methicillin-resistant *Staphylococcus aureus* in hospital rooms by infected or colonised patients. J Hosp Infect. 2009;71:256–62.
26. Albrich WC, Harbarth S. Health-care workers: source, vector, or victim of MRSA? Lancet Infect Dis. 2008;8:289–301.
27. Bernard MC, Lanotte P, Lawrence C, Goudeau A, Bernard L. Air contamination around patients colonized with multidrug-resistant organisms. Infect Control Hosp Epidemiol. 2012;33:949–51.
28. Ndawula EM, Brown L. Mattresses as reservoirs of epidemic methicillin-resistant *Staphylococcus aureus*. Lancet. 1991;337:488.
29. Wendt C, Dietze B, Dietz E, Ruden H. Survival of *Acinetobacter baumannii* on dry surfaces. J Clin Microbiol. 1997;35:1394–7.

30. Blythe D, Keenlyside D, Dawson SJ, Galloway A. Environmental contamination due to methicillin-resistant *Staphylococcus aureus* (MRSA). J Hosp Infect. 1998;38:67–70.
31. Hirai Y. Survival of bacteria under dry conditions; from a viewpoint of nosocomial infection. J Hosp Infect. 1991;19:191–200.
32. Chang S, Sethi AK, Stiefel U, Cadnum JL, Donskey CJ. Occurrence of skin and environmental contamination with methicillin- resistant Staphylococcus aureus before results of polymerase chain reaction at hospital admission become available. Infect Control Hosp Epidemiol. 2010;31:607–12.
33. Malnick S, Bardenstein R, Huszar M, Gabbay J, Borkow G. Pyjamas and sheets as a potential source of nosocomial pathogens. J Hosp Infect. 2008;70:89–91.
34. Ludlam HA, Swayne RL, Kearns AM, et al. Evidence from a UK teaching hospital that MRSA is primarily transmitted by the hands of healthcare workers. J Hosp Infect. 2010;74:296–9.
35. Ohl M, Schweizer M, Graham M, et al. Hospital private curtains are frequently and rapidly contaminated with potentially pathogenic bacteria. Am J Infect Control. 2012;40:904–6.

68 Patient Beds

Abstract

Beds are important resources for drifting an effective hospital and should be provided with expertise, resources and personnel. Neither patients, personnel, visitors nor the environment should be exposed to infections from contaminated beds or bed equipment. The following chapter is focused on practical measures concerning patient beds, bed equipment and bed linen and washing, transport and storage in healthcare institutions.

Keywords

Patient beds · Bed linen · Pillows · Mattresses · Quilts · Cleaning · Disinfection · Transport · Storage · Infection control · Hygiene · Prevention

68.1 Purpose

- Prevent transmission of infections between patients or between patient and personnel [1–10].
- Remove microbes, body particles, skin cells and dirt from patient beds, mattresses, pillows and quilts.

68.2 Comprise

- Everyone who work with patient beds and everyone who is washing, transporting and storing beds

B. M. Andersen, *Prevention and Control of Infections in Hospitals*,
https://doi.org/10.1007/978-3-319-99921-0_68

68.3 Responsibility

The hospital's management has (according to law and regulation) responsibility for written procedures for the treatment and control of the hospital beds and bedding equipment: that there are good procedures for transport, washing and proper storage of beds when not in use. In addition, satisfactory facilities for bed washing and washing of quilts, pillows and mattresses and maintenance of this shall be provided. There must be clean areas for the storage of clean laundry and for bed linen.

The department management ensures that written procedures for the treatment of clean, unclean and contaminated patient beds are implemented in the daily work. Furthermore, the manager shall ensure that clean and used beds are separated and treated in a proper manner.

Head of the textile department and head of transport service are responsible, respectively, for textile processing and transport as regards textiles and bedding.

Cleaning units are responsible for local or central cleaning of beds.

All personnel who treat patient beds are responsible for ensuring that clean bed is not contaminated by others than the patient and that the unclean bed does not pollute the environment or other patients.

68.4 Practical Measures [5–8]

No isolation regime, no suspected contagion.

There are at least two solutions: with and without access to professional washing systems for beds. Either way, bed linen should be treated with care so that no infection is spread to personnel, patients and the environment.

68.4.1 Used Bed: Cleaning on the Patient Room

- Linen is carefully taken off so that bacteria and dust are not swirled up in the air.
- The bed is washed with soap and water.
- The mattress is wiped off with soapy water and cloth.
- Pillow and duvet that are not visibly contaminated are sent to wash approx. Once per month. Wash at 85°°C for 10 min, optionally, in bed washing machine.
- Pillow and duvet that are visibly contaminated are packaged and sent to wash.
- After washing the bed, wash hands before putting on a new bed linen.
- Uniform should be clean when bed-making.
- Clean linen is taken from clean textile store.
- The bed is made ready in a clean room, separate from the laundry room.
- The bed is stored covered by clean cover/plastic—in a clean room.

68.4.2 Used Bed: Cleaning in a Bed Wash Central

- In the patient's room, remove the bed linen carefully so that the bacteria and dust do not swirl up in the air.
- Used bed is carefully transported to the bed central.
- If there is a bed washing machine, use this.
- Pillow and duvet that are not visibly contaminated are sent to wash approx. Once per month (85 °C, 10 min).
- Pillow and duvet that are visibly contaminated are packaged and sent to wash. It is done by the person who strips the bed.
- The bed is washed with soapy water at approx. 60 °C and then dried.
- Mattress is washed the same way and is wiped.
- Flushing should be avoided to protect the personnel and environment against aerosols.
- There must be a careful distinction between clean and unclean sides. Clean beds must not be exposed to splashes from washing of unclean beds.
- The bedmaker's hands and clothes must be clean. The bed is covered with clean cover/plastic and stored on clean rooms that are cleaned daily.
- The transport of clean bed takes place as the transport of other clean goods with hand hygiene and clean outerwear.

68.4.3 Infections and Isolation Regimes

- See isolation regimes for contact-, blood- and airborne infections or strict isolation. The type of infection protection is decided by the management at the section/department.
- The patient's bed and mattress are disinfected in the patient's room.
- Duvet and pillow are packaged as contaminated and sent as contaminated laundry.

68.5 Background Information

Microbes from a patient can survive for hours or days in bed linen and on the bed itself. Also, duvet, pillow and mattress can be infected as found for methicillin-resistant *S. aureus* (MRSA), *Acinetobacter* and other bacteria [2, 9–12]. Cleaners at Good Hope Hospital in the UK were in 2007 told to not wash sheets and bed linen between patients but to turn them over to save 500,000 £ [12]. There was a significant increase of MRSA cases and doubling of *Clostridium difficile* cases: "Is that all the safety of a patient's life is worth? 0.275 pence?" [12]. Therefore, it is important to clean the bed, bed linen and mattress between each patient.

See also Chap. 67.

References

1. Sehulster LM, Chinn RYW, Ardunio MJ, et al. Guidelines for environmental infection control in health-care facilities. CDC MMWR. 2003;52:1–42.
2. Centers for Disease Control and Prevention. Laundry: washing infected materials. CDC; 2011.
3. Hygienic requirements and procedures for treatment of textiles used in healthcare. IK 1941, Norwegian Board of Health; 1994.
4. Anonymous. Textile supply, Ullevål hospital, has sat the standard for quality system (NS-ISO 9002 standard) in laundry, textile storage, sewing room.
5. Dufseth IS, Andersen BM. Textiles, cleaning, control, transport and storage. In: Handbook in hygiene and infection control for hospitals. Ullevål universitetssykehus; 2003. p. 419–25, og 2008, 604–9.
6. Andersen BM. Cleaning and control of textiles. In: Handbook in hygiene and infection control for nursing homes and long-term care facilities. Akademika; 2013. p. 493–501, 503–9.
7. Syvrud EJ, Lukkassen R, Andersen BM, Solheim N. Patient beds. Textile treatment, wash, transport and storage. In: Handbook in hygiene and infection control for hospitals. Ullevål universitetssykehus; 2003. p. 426–8.
8. Lukkassen EJ, Rasch M, Brekke H, Andersen BM. Patient beds. Textile treatment, wash, transport and storage. In: Handbook in hygiene and infection control for hospitals. Ullevål universitetssykehus; 2008. p. 610–2.
9. Mitchell A, Spencer M, Edminston C Jr. Role of healthcare apparel and other healthcare textiles in the transmission of pathogens: a review of the literature. J Hosp Infect. 2015;90:285–92.
10. European Parliament and Council Directive 2000/54/EC of 18 September 2000 on the protection of workers from the risks related to exposure to biological agents at work.
11. Ndawula EM, Brown L. Mattresses as reservoirs of epidemic methicillin-resistant *Staphylococcus aureus*. Lancet. 1991;337:488.
12. "Don't wash sheets-turn them over. Astonishing order at a hard-up hospital." Daily Mail; Saturday 14 April 2007.

69 Hospital Waste

Abstract

Waste is produced in large amounts in hospitals: organic and not organic materials, infectious materials, disposable used equipment, outside packing, etc. It is important that waste is handled, packaged, stored and transported to the destruction place without exposing anybody to infectious materials. Patients, personnel, visitors, people who handle waste and the environment should not be exposed to infections from not well-treated, packed or stored waste. The following chapter is focused on practical measures concerning treatment of waste in hospitals: storage, cleaning and control.

Keywords

Waste · Organic waste · Infectious waste · Waste transport · Waste collection Waste package · Infection control · Hygiene

69.1 Purpose

Prevent contamination from biological waste to patients, personnel, visitors, the environment and others who treat waste from hospitals [1–7].

69.2 Comprise

- All human biological waste (tissue, organs, blood), including sticking/cutting objects used on patients or in experiments
- All microbiological agents and other contaminants from diagnostic or experimental work
- Anyone who treats, packs, stores and transports waste containing human biological agents

B. M. Andersen, *Prevention and Control of Infections in Hospitals*,
https://doi.org/10.1007/978-3-319-99921-0_69

69.3 Responsibility

The hospital's management has (according to law and regulation) responsibility for written procedures for the treatment and control of hospital waste - both infectious and non-infectious. This is the case from the waste is generated, through packaging, storage and transport - until left to municipal or central disposal [6].

The department management is responsible for ensuring that proper procedures for sorting, packaging and storage of waste are carried out.

The defined department treating waste is responsible for the proper sorting and transportation of pre-packaged waste, proper storage and delivery to destruction adapted to the waste and providing feedback to each department by deviation. It must also be verified that the infection protection is being taken care of for each individual who works with waste and that it is carefully distinguished between clean and unclean transport.

Personnel dealing with waste should have the knowledge, expertise and time to implement appropriate personal protective measures, including hand hygiene and personal hygiene, with a change of uniform when needed.

69.4 Practical Measures

69.4.1 Department or Ward: Producer of Waste [3–5]

69.4.1.1 Packing of Waste

Practise good hand hygiene and wear gloves when packing. Avoid spill of waste on the uniform. In case of infectious waste, personal protection equipment—PPE—is used.

All waste is packed and closed securely in the user's place, in thick plastic packaging that withstands the weight of the contents and is completely sealed. The packaging should be clean *outside* when carried to the store room. The outside packaging must always be marked. This first phase is the most important part of the waste treatment.

69.4.1.2 Waste Store Room

This room must be suitable for storage of waste. It should have "wet room quality" and preferably with negative pressure to other rooms. If small amounts of waste or frequent collection, the department's disinfection room can be used.

- Washbasins should be easily accessible, preferably in the waste room.
- Daily cleaning of floor and rubbish racks and main cleaning once a year and when needed.
- Large enough room (usually 10–12 m^2) adapted to function, with wet room quality of walls and floors and outlet grating in the floor.

Table 69.1 Problem waste; solutions must be adapted to the hospital's own routines and collectors of waste

Problem waste	Package often used
Wastes from infection patients	Yellow sack/container—robust
Highly soggy bandages	Yellow sack/container—robust
Blood soiled waste	Yellow sack/container—robust
Liquid, liquid-filled waste	Plastic can—solid
Biological materials, organs, placenta, amputation, test materials	Plastic can—solid
Sticking/cutting waste	Box/can with lid
Waste that cannot be compressed	Box/can or risk container[a]
Infusion set with the whole set—complete	Box/can or risk container
Medicinal products	Box/can or risk container
Pleur-vac and other closed vacuum/draining systems	Box or risk container

[a]Yellow thick plastic bag in cardboard box labelled hazardous waste. Remember, label the outer packages. Hand hygiene is very important after handling waste

69.4.1.3 Waste Sorting [3–5]

- Packaged contaminated waste is placed in thick yellow plastic bag.
- Packed other waste is placed in another thick black plastic bag (or another colour).
- Liquid, liquid-filled waste or larger biological parts of biological material are stored in solid plastic boxes with lid.
- Sticking/cutting waste is placed in solid boxes with lid. Before the jar is full, put the lid well in place, and place it in a yellow plastic bag in a labelled risk box. It is important that sticking/cutting waste is placed directly in a tight container at the user site.
- All waste *that should not be compressed* is placed in a yellow plastic bag in boxes labelled hazardous waste or in a thick plastic bag/plastic cap with lid.
- All outer packaging is marked (Table 69.1).

69.4.2 Transport of Waste

69.4.2.1 Check the Packaging

- Wear gloves and gown when handling waste bags.
- Waste bags are closed properly. Secondarily, package is marked outside.
- Make sure that the packaging is not contaminated outside and that there is no hole. Feedback to the department if packaging/sorting fails.
- Handle the bag so that there is no damage to it during transport.
- During transport, waste bags must be free from contamination on the outside and without risk to the personnel.
- In case of special risk of infection, the department shall report on how the waste is to be handled.

- Avoid the use of person lifts, if possible.
- The waste may be collected in larger movable containers, according to the hospital's routines. The containers are closed with a tight lid after use.
- Infectious wastes (yellow bags/cans/boxes) are placed in a separate container for infectious materials. Close with a tight lid and lock.
- Containers are flushed once a week or more frequently if necessary after defined routines.
- Avoid aerosols/water spray on clothing/face during this procedure.
- Wash hands immediately after transport of waste, also after wearing gloves.
- Change uniform when the waste treatment and transport are completed, especially important if clean work is to be carried out afterwards (e.g. transport of clean equipment, patients, etc.).

69.4.2.2 Cleaning and Control

- All trolleys/carts used for waste transport must be thoroughly cleaned before any clean transport (trolley wash at 85°°C for 10 min). Otherwise daily cleaning with soapy water. Wear gloves, surgical mask/cap and gown when washing trolleys and carts used for transportation of waste.
- Personnel transporting waste should afterwards change work clothes and wash hands well before clean transport.
- Infectious accident: follow routines and contact healthcare worker in charge for further treatment.
- Problems with infectious waste: contact responsible department or infection control personnel.

69.4.2.3 Note!

Waste containers should not be standing with lock open outside the buildings!

Containers with infectious waste should always be locked and never be compressed—to avoid leakage of infectious materials!

69.5 Background Information

69.5.1 Infection Risk

1. *General risk of infection.* All human biological waste is defined as potentially infectious and must be treated as such in a general protective manner, e.g. blood, urine, other secretions/excretions and tissues. This waste may contain unknown contaminants.
2. *Known/suspected infectious substance.* In some cases, the infectious agent is known, for example, *Salmonella*, *Shigella*, *Staphylococcus aureus*, *Mycobacterium tuberculosis* and other resistant bacteria and viruses like hepatitis viruses A, B, C, D and E, HIV, influenza virus, norovirus, etc. The contaminated waste comes *directly* from the patient (pus, bandages, blood samples, blood, urine, faeces, vomit, expectorate, tissue, organs, etc.) or *indirectly* through contaminated disposables, textiles and other items placed in infectious waste. It

can also be waste from diagnostic or experimental work with microorganisms and other contaminants.

Both groups, 1 and 2, must be secured with good packaging at the user's place (patient room, operating room, etc.) before the waste is packed in a sack/carton/defined packaging for further transport. Packaging for infectious materials/organic material should be defined in consultation with the hospital's health/environment/safety and infection control personnel, responsible for waste in the municipality.

69.5.1.1 Sorting

Due to the large amount of waste per day, it is important that the waste is already sorted at the user site. Secondary packaging should always be labelled. Infectious waste varies from one department to another. Total hazardous waste accounts for 5–10% of total waste. In many hospitals, this percentage is very high (30–75%).

69.5.1.2 Compression

Waste from the hospital is often voluminous and, for that reason, is often compressed before transport. However, this should not happen with contaminated waste or other hazardous waste. Total waste at somatic hospitals in a city like Oslo (500,000 inhabitants) is estimated to be at 2–5 kg/bed/day, corresponding to 16–42 L/bed/day of non-compressed waste.

69.5.2 Destruction of Human Biological Waste

69.5.2.1 Sewage System: Without Treatment

Large quantities of human biological waste, both with and without various contaminants, go directly untreated out in the common sewer system. The dilution effect and microbiological and chemical degradation eventually destroy the contaminants which, in addition, may have a limited life outside the body. The microbes that adapt to sea and brackish water are usually not very infectious to humans; however, this is dependent on climate and type of microbes.

69.5.2.2 Incinerators

In combustion of human biological material, all contaminants are destroyed. However, a serious disadvantage is the pollution of exhaust gases and smoke during the combustion process and relatively expensive transportation costs. Most packaged waste is incinerated—especially organic materials and infectious waste.

69.5.2.3 Other Heat Inactivation of Waste

Large collecting autoclaves can heat-inactivate 25,000 L or more waste per day. This can be run on regular waste disposal site. Such autoclaves can reduce significantly the amount of waste for combustion. There are a number of *disinfection machines* for heat treatment of waste.

See also Chap. 59 on disinfection.

References

1. Sehulster LM, Chinn RYW, Ardunio MJ, et al. Guidelines for environmental infection control in health-care facilities. CDC MMWR. 2003;52:1–42.
2. Rutala WA, Weber DJ. Disinfection, sterilization, and control of hospital waste. In: Mandell, Douglas, and Bennets principles and practice of infectious diseases. Vol. 2. 8th ed. Philadelphia: Elsevier Churchill Livingstone; 2015. p. 3294–309.
3. Ullevål hospital procedure: handling biological waste; 1998.
4. Brekke H, Hochlin K, Rasch M, Andersen BM. Biological waste. In: Handbook in hygiene and infection control for hospitals. Oslo; 2008. p. 613–7.
5. Andersen BM. Handling of human biological waste. In: Handbook in hygiene and infection control for nursing homes. Akademika; 2013. p. 511–5.
6. European Parliament and Council Directive 2000/54/EC of 18 September 2000 on the protection of workers from the risks related to exposure to biological agents at work.
7. WHO. Healthcare waste and its safe management. 1.12.2006.

Food and Beverages

70

Abstract

Hospital patients are highly dependent on a good food control, clean kitchen and clean food.

Practical measures concerning food and other nutrients; cooking processes, serving, transport, storage and control are central in healthcare institutions. The following chapter is focused on kitchen hygiene; practical measures to handle, prepare, cook and serve food and beverages in hospitals in a safe way; and how to treat and wash dishes and cutlers to avoid transfer of infections between patients, personal and environment.

Keywords

Food · Nutrients · Beverages · Cooking · Preparation · Serving · Dish washing Transport · Storage · Food supply · Control · Water · Hygiene

70.1 Purpose

To prevent transmission of infectious agents via food, other nutrients and beverages to patients and staff [1–5].

70.2 Comprise

- All serving that takes place at the ward, clinic and outpatient clinics, patient hotels and at cafeterias
- Everyone who is offered food and beverages at the hospital: patients, personnel and visitors

B. M. Andersen, *Prevention and Control of Infections in Hospitals*,
https://doi.org/10.1007/978-3-319-99921-0_70

70.3 Responsibility

The hospital's management ensures that official, national written requirements for food hygiene, nutrients and handling/serving of food are available and followed [1–6]. In Norway, the Norwegian Food Safety Authority regularly check the hospital regarding the preparation and supply of food, as well as hygiene around the kitchen, ward kitchen and food serving [1–6].

The central kitchen's management and preparation of food follows national guidelines and orders and ensures that patients, personnel, relatives or visitors are not exposed to food contamination [6].

The department management facilitates the serving of food in a hygienically safe manner to the patients. The national guidelines and instructions should be followed by the ward kitchen, which has no admission for visitors or patients.

Everyone who handles food, dishes, etc. must follow the hospital's routines. Personnel responsible for the production and presentation of foodstuffs must not have infections or be carriers of infectious agents [7].

70.4 Practical Measures [8–10]

70.4.1 Personal Hygiene

- Wash hands before and after handling food/serving.
- Use clean uniform, do not use jewellery or piercing, and long hair should be covered/set up.
- Perform hand hygiene before and after helping a patient to eat.
- Wash hands after handling unclean dishes.
- Personnel with gastrointestinal infection should be on sick leave until healthy/no-carrier state (see gastrointestinal infections).
- In case of infections on the hands (herpes simplex, staphylococci, streptococci, etc.), go on sickness leave.
- Small wounds/scrapers must be covered with waterproof plastic (optionally with gloves on the outside).
- Avoid unhygienic habits (contact with the nose, mouth and hair or sneeze over food).
- Do not cough in the bend of the arm or other places on the uniform; use a paper towel and wash your hands afterwards.
- Potted plants and other plants should be removed from the kitchen.

70.4.2 The Patient

- The patient is offered to wash or disinfect hands *before the* meal.
- Ask the patient not to use the phone during the meal as it is often heavily contaminated with microbes (wipe over with a cloth and disinfect afterwards).

- The food is placed on a clean table or bedside table. Make sure the surface of the board is clean. Wash with soap and water if necessary.
- Food is best taken in clean, proper surroundings.
- Offer hand hygiene *after the* meal.
- Do not allow the patient to touch food/drink or equipment/service that others should eat/use.
- Open, self-service buffets where patients and visitors can touch directly the food are *not acceptable!* Everything (slices of bread, cheese, jam, etc.) must be packed separately.

70.4.3 The Food, Nutrient and Beverage [1–5]

- Do not let hot food stand at room temperature over time. Bacteria can grow and form toxins. If the food is not eaten immediately, it should be cooled quickly and warmed up immediately before it is eaten. Keep the food covered. Particularly "bulk food" in large portions is subjected to growth of microbes and toxin production over time when there is a slow cooling (*Clostridium perfringens*, *Bacillus cereus*, *Staphylococcus aureus*).
- Lightly decaying foods must be quickly placed in a refrigerator (never more than 2 h at room temperature).
- Warm food should be kept above 60 °C and the time limit for eating is maximum 2 h.
- The food trolleys should be clean outside and inside when loaded from the central kitchen.
- Food trolleys/cabinets/and dispensers should be checked regularly to ensure that they maintain proper temperatures and are clean.
- The food trolley should be brought to the ward kitchen. It is not allowed to ladle out the food from the food trolley on the corridor.
- All cold foods are stored in the refrigerator at −1 to +4 °C or freezing at −18 °C or colder. Thawing of frozen foods should take place in a refrigerator.
- Food to be served must not be mixed with food that has been served.
- Make sure the food is served in a hygienic and aesthetically satisfactory manner (clean bedside/board, clean surface).
- Do not touch directly on food or on the used parts of the dishes!
- If food is made at the ward kitchen, good hygiene must be carried out. Check the expiration date of the foods. There should be adequate bench space and washing facilities.
- *Do not serve the patients food like* unpasteurized cheeses, milk or other foods made from unpasteurized milk or other foods that may—due to food source, production, storage or limited shelf life—contain *Listeria* or other pathogenic microbes!
- See the health institution's official food procedures, where there should always be a list of foods that are *not suitable* for serving patients.
- There must be a log and report on cleaning and temperature control of the refrigerator.

70.4.4 Portion for Microwave/Heating

Portion packs for heating/microwave are treated as easily decaying products and placed in refrigerator at maximum +4 °C until use. When heated, the temperature should exceed 72 °C. The portions are sealed and must be broken first during serving.

70.4.4.1 Food Waste

- Food waste must be handled in a hygienically safe manner.
- In the case of a board serving, food waste must be returned to the central kitchen or processed according to custom routines.
- Infectious waste should be taken care of at the department.
- It must be ensured that the waste does not contaminate other foodstuffs and that it does not bother in other ways (smell, attraction of pests, etc.).
- Local solutions are followed.

70.4.4.2 Infected Patients: How to Treat Food Waste and Dishes—See Isolation Routines

- *Contact-borne agent/blood-borne agent*: Tray/board with food waste after use is treated as infected. Equipment from patient, contaminated with blood/tissue fluids, etc., is heat disinfected (dish, cup, cutlery, tray, etc.) in the decontaminator (decontamination room) before being treated as normal used dishes.
- *Airborne agent/strict isolation:* All equipment is thermal (heat) disinfected in the isolation unit before treatment as regular washing.
- *Heat decontamination*: takes place at a minimum of 85 °C for 10 min (eventual autoclaving when strict isolation).
- *Regular decontaminator* can be used, where another machine is not available. It is assumed that the goods are properly placed (e.g. in the basket) and do not disappear into the machine.

70.4.4.3 Washing of the Dishes, Service Sets, Equipment, Trolleys/Carts/Trays, Etc.

- Dishes and cutlery are washed at the central kitchen in a dishwasher (rinse at 40 °C, wash at 60 °C and steam treat at 85 °C); at least 85 °C for 5 min with final rinsing and at least 85 °C if measured between cutlery/plates. Local solutions.
- Trolleys and steel boxes can to be returned to the central kitchen for cleaning. Local solutions.
- Clean and unclean tableware must be treated completely separate, i.e. storage of clean equipment must be well spaced—at least 2 m from the washing area and put in a closed cabinet.
- Avoid open rinsing and prewashing of dishes, etc. which cause aerosol formation. In such cases, washing should be carried out in a separate room—separate from storage of clean equipment.
- Wash hands after touching unclean equipment and before touching clean equipment.

- If the dishes are washed at the ward kitchen (post-kitchen), wash them in a dishwasher with the same temperature requirements as above. The hot water from the tap does not meet the requirement for temperature. This also applies to the kitchen equipment for the staff.
- Remember washing cans, thermo-cans and serving tables on the corridors! This is very important since it is a contact point between patients and visitors with risk of transmitting infections. During outbreaks, serving on corridors in hospitals should be prohibited.

70.4.4.4 Kitchen Hygiene

- Daily cleaning is important: benches, stove and floor.
- Weekly cleaning of drawers, cabinets and refrigerators.
- Use clean cloths and clean towels, and send them for laundry at each shift or more often when needed.
- There should be a separate hand washbasin in the kitchen and preferably a utility sink.
- Coatings on benches and floors should be complete so that cleaning can be effective.
- If used dishes are brought back the kitchen, separate the clean and unclean side carefully.
- Check cleaning of exhaust valves and possibly fan and filter in the exhaust fan every month.
- Cutting machines that cannot be heat-treated are thoroughly cleaned after each use and every day. Afterwards, disinfect with 70% alcohol.
- The microwave must be clean—it loses the effect when dirty. Remember the lid placed over the food tray is put in the dishwasher after each use.
- See separate routines for cleaning of ice machines.
- The dishwasher is cleaned inside each week and temperature control weekly.

Employee food (packed lunches, cakes and the like).

These should be stored in a separate refrigerator and should not be mixed with patient food.

70.4.4.5 Family or Visitor's Food

Visitors who bring food to the patient should not enter the ward kitchen, and the food should not be mixed with the hospital's patient food.

Food traded outside the hospital, for example, directly from a ward or department:

Do not take this to the ward kitchen and do not mix in with the hospital's patient food.

70.4.4.6 Canteens for Patients

- It should always be kept clean and tidy, also at the cafeteria's kitchen.
- It should not be self-service or buffet style.

- Work in the canteen is dependent on good personal hygiene, clean uniform and cap that effectively cover the hair.
- All types of food served must be wrapped in/covered separately to avoid transfer of microbes between patients.

70.4.4.7 Food and Beverages on the Corridor, Living Room, Etc.

- Food services (meals) on the corridor for patients are not hygienically acceptable.
- Juice, hot drinks, water, etc. may be served in periods but should be omitted.
- Cans, etc. are cleaned daily and all equipment is replaced daily.
- Avoid that patients/visitors are touching food that others should eat—separate wrapping of cake, biscuits, etc.
- During outbreaks of gastroenteritis, norovirus or other contagious agents at the department, the corridors are emptied and food/beverages are served directly from the kitchen.

70.4.4.8 Internal Control: Food

Follow the hospital's IC food procedures.

70.5 Background Information

Hospital patients are highly dependent on a good food control, clean kitchen and clean food. Globally very large exchange of food and beverages, and a serious lack of food control, constitutes a high infectious risk, especially for patients and personnel in healthcare.

70.5.1 Food Control, For Example, Norway

Even well-developed and rich countries, like Norway (ca 5 mill inhabitants), have been haunted by many and extensive food- and waterborne epidemics, also in hospitals. Typhoid fever, bacterial dysentery and cholera from food and water were common until the twentieth century and epidemics of streptococci, diphtheria and tuberculosis via unpasteurized milk, ice cream and other foods; milk-borne epidemics were common in the middle of the last century. Contagious jaundice virus (hepatitis A) and poliovirus in food and water were at risk until the 1960s. In Norway, the *Health Act* came in 1860 with local food control, followed by the *Slaughterhouse and Meat Control Act* (1924), the *Food Control Act* (1933) and the *Coordinated Nutrition Control Act* (1978). Good hygiene eliminated most infectious diseases related to nutrition, anchored in health management with *health and integrity* in focus [11].

The *Norwegian Food Safety Authority* ("Statens næringsmiddeltilsyn-SNT") (1988) was the first control line of public and private enterprises. Accredited laboratories controlled microbiology, resistance patterns, chemical agents, additives, pests and other indicators of foodstuffs, including water and supervised food producers, serving places and grocery stores. All imported food and beverages were checked. *SNT* was later on (2004) replaced by national food supervision ("Mattilsynet"), responsible for control of food, seafood, animal health and agricultural surveillance. The anchor to the health administration disappeared, and the industry and manufacturers got into the public food control [11, 12]. *Self-declaration and random sampling* were introduced instead of a routine control of all imported food [11]. Lack of control contributed to a variety of food scandals. Antibiotic-resistant bacteria increased in fish, animal and poultry herds and also in animal and fish feed and entered the food production [12–14]. A new type of contagious jaundice (hepatitis E) is spread among pigs and transferred to humans. Blood donors are still not tested for hepatitis E [12].

Today, the Norwegian Food Safety Authority reports annually 1400–1800 food-borne bacterial intestinal infections, infected in Norway, and this is the top of the iceberg. The Authority conducts infection detection at outbreaks and places the preventive responsibility on the manufacturer: "The individual food business that produces or markets food is responsible for ensuring that food is safe and that this is indeed the case. The Norwegian Food Safety Authority is responsible for supervising that food business is in compliance with its obligations" [11].

However, it is impossible to control food producers in other countries. Requirements for training in hygienic and proper animal husbandry have been removed or reduced, also in Norway. This leads to an increased incidence of serious infections among animals such as listeriosis from bad silo feed and other feed. About 50% of animal feed is imported and assessed by the Norwegian Veterinary Institute as "both biological and chemical risk" [12].

70.5.2 Bacteria: Food-Borne [12–28]

Dangerous *E. coli* bacteria (EHEC; entero-haemorrhagic *Escherichia coli*) infected 18 children with 1 death in Norway in 2006 [12, 15]. The source was slicing sausage from Norwegian animal herds. Food control would probably have prevented the outbreak. On May 2014 there was an outbreak of EHEC in England in connection with visits on animal farms, "lamb petting zoo", and the same is observed in the United States and in Denmark. Infected sprout seed from Egypt, grown in Germany, infected 4000 patients; hence, 900 with haemolytic uremic syndrome (HUS) and 60 died in 2011. The bacterium was in addition antibiotic resistant (ESBL). Import control would have prevented the outbreak [15].

Drug-resistant *E. coli* (ESBL) is detected in Norwegian-produced chickens, as a result of uncontrolled imports.

Salmonella outbreaks from food increase in Norway as in other developed countries. From 2004 to 2013, the National Institutes of Health registered at least 13 outbreaks with more than 420 infected persons. Outbreaks were traced back to imported foodstuffs such as Italian rucola salad, frozen minced meat from Poland, Italian salami sausage, catering company serving food from abroad, Spanish bacon, alfalfa sprouts with contaminated seeds from abroad and minced meat from Sweden, which came from Danish meat companies [14, 16].

Salmonella was also detected in imported animal feed in 2012, such as soya, meat-bone flour, animal fat and flour and also in fish feedstocks (16 of 827 samples) [13]. *Salmonella* was detected in 2 of 690 investigated chicken flocks [13]. One of 198 samples from fish-contained salmonella was imported from Vietnam [13].

Salmonella diarizonae is found in almost half of samples from sheep [13]. Norway is special globally by the wide spread of this bacterium. *S. diarizonae is* usually detected in reptiles (snakes, lizards and turtles as pets) and in fish, but in Norway, they have come across to sheep. It's not normal either in sheep or humans. In sheep it produces diarrhoea and lamb foetal dead, and in humans it has been registered as increasing cause of severe infection in blood, urine, respiratory tract, etc., in patients with impaired resistance against infections. *S. diarizonae* can be a challenge for young children and patients with immunodeficiency [12, 17].

S. diarizonae is now found in up to 45% of samples from sheep and described as an endemic, under-reported zoonosis in Norway [12, 17]. It is the second most frequent cause of abortion in sheep and can induce diarrhoea in all animals. The spread in the crews must be limited by, among other things, routine control of animals and of imported feeds.

Shigella bacteria imported via fresh sugar peas from Africa started outbreaks of diarrhoea both in Denmark and Norway during spring 2009 and were also registered in other outbreaks [14, 18, 19]. *Shigella* in food products is not registered in Norway.

MRSA in food production comes with uncontrolled import of livestock/animal and foodstuffs and poses a risk of food-transmitted disease in Norway [14]. Pig production in the Netherlands and Denmark is most often infected with MRSA [20–22]. In 2012, animal-associated MRSA (LA-MRSA) was the second most common cause of human disease in Denmark, and in 2013 it completely dominated. In Danish pig farms, 16% were infected with MRSA, 44% infected at the slaughter and 77% of all animals brought to the slaughterhouses [20–22]. It is estimated that at least 30–40% of Danish pork for sale is MRSA-infected, which Norwegian importers now take into account. The infection is also detected in chicken meat and in milk tanks in Denmark, the Netherlands and England [12, 22]. In Denmark, children are warned of "visiting farms" due to infection [20]. Denmark's food minister launched a five-point plan in the summer of 2014 to reduce MRSA among animals [21]. Norway is moving towards the same development, but all pig farms are negative today concerning MRSA.

Listeriosis [12, 23–28]. The food scandal in Denmark in 2014, where 38 people were infected with listeria bacteria from Danish roll sausage (Deli meat), resulted in 15 deaths [23]. The food control was poor. Caramelized apples led to listeria disease in 32 people in 2014, of which 6 died in 11 states in the United States [24]. In the autumn of 2007, there was an outbreak at a hospital in Oslo (Rikshospitalet) in Norway with a total of 11 patients infected from Norwegian-produced soft cheese. There are still many outbreaks of listeriosis, and particularly vulnerable to this type of infection are patients with impaired resistance to infections, pregnant women and persons with pathological conditions in the intestine (cancer, diverticles, etc.) [25–28].

70.5.3 Virus

The hepatitis E virus (HEV) that infects animals (pig and chicken—zoonosis) is robust with great ability to survive in the environment and can withstand temperatures up to 70 °C for 20 min and 60 °C for 1 h [29]. The virus is closely linked to animal food production and poor animal hygiene.

The hepatitis E virus was rare in Europe. However, from 2009 on, HEV has been widely distributed in pig production in Denmark, Sweden, the Netherlands, Italy (50%) and Spain (40%) [12, 29]. A total of 85% of British pigs are infected while at the same time infecting the population. It is believed that one in ten British sausages and pork meat is infected with the heat-resistant virus [30]. It is therefore now recommended heating for 20 min at 70 °C or higher temperature to destruct the virus [30]. Let the sausage/meat lay for a while after the warming—before eating [30]. The virus that spreads in pigs is also in Norway [12]. HEV is most serious (liver affected) for pregnant women—especially during third trimester—and for people with affected liver or severe immune defences [31].

Widespread HEV infection among pigs, combined with poor kitchen hygiene, increases infection in the population. The Netherlands calculates a HEV-positive blood transfer every day since they do not test blood donors. In Norway HEV infection is present in pig farms; the extent is unknown nor is it tested in blood donors.

Norovirus is associated with contact and airborne transmission and causes outbreaks from contaminated water and food [32–37]. It is resistant to high temperatures and to chemicals, survives up to a year in the environment, has very low infective dose (one to ten virus particles) and gives almost no immunity. A high proportion of the population globally is infected every year.

70.5.4 Parasites

Toxoplasmosis infects half of Norwegian sheep farms and can cause serious infection to animals and humans [38]. The parasite survives drying, salting, smoking and partly freezing and is in a red risk area for humans and domestic animals [38].

70.5.5 Reasons for Spreading Resistant and Dangerous Microbes via Food

- *Lack of hygienic import control and national control.* Animals, feeds, food and other foodstuffs. For the last 10 years, no food has been routinely controlled. When the hygiene control is out, there is often a lower level of hygiene in the production of food [12].
- *Poor hygiene in agriculture and slaughterhouses.* Large-scale drift and robotization lead to major contamination in animal—living areas with production of large amounts of dust-bearing bacteria and with special requirements for good hygiene [12]. The same happens in slaughterhouses and can be followed further

up in the food chain. Infection via milk, milk products and meat products with, for example, salmonella, MRSA, *Listeria* and resistant bacteria is also a fact in Norway. Large animal herds, increased animal density, poor hygiene and trading with livestock and pigs/calves are increasing risks for spread of infection. Antibiotics for animals and fish and growth promoters (pleuromutilin, copper, zinc, etc.) also select for antibiotic resistance in the herd. One third of Norwegian chickens carry antibiotic-resistant bacteria [12].

- *Infectious spread from cattle*. MRSA can be detected in the air up to 150 m from infected cattle and can be spread from colonized animals on pasture with dirt—via air to people passing through the pastures, as recently shown in Pennsylvania. Such contamination creates major problems for the entire animal production with cleaning and disinfection, ventilation systems and the building as a whole. Farmers and families are particularly vulnerable to infection, which in turn can affect the work situation and health.

70.5.6 Measures to Reduce the Rate of Food-Borne Infections

- Establish a solid and effective food control, control of all production units—both domestic and imported. Animals and poultry with MRSA or other serious infections (resistant bacteria, hepatitis E) may not be imported to the country. Visits at farms abroad must lead to a number of preventive measures. Infected flocks must not be able to spread the infection (infection control measures), and infected animals must not be delivered to the open market [12].
- Good hygiene—washing and disinfection and personal protective equipment (PPE) must be used properly. Butchers, veterinarians and production units must be followed up with regular hygiene and infection controls. Good and local animal welfare in spacy and hygienic areas will lead to less infection.
- Kitchen hygiene, including kitchen hygiene at health institutions, must be placed on a higher level than today. The bacteria present on the surface of the meat die by cooking and frying, while the virus usually sits inside the meat and will withstand more heat. Pre-cooked foods should not be contaminated by using the same equipment on raw and cooked foods. Raw and cooked/fried foods should not be mixed. The salad should be washed separately [16].Good kitchen hygiene includes good hand hygiene, dishwashing with high enough temperature and good cleaning.
- *Better food control* would lift the food control back on a more correct track for *health and integrity* over profit and bad and unhygienic animal care [11, 12].

70.5.7 Nosocomial Infections via Food and Beverages

70.5.7.1 Hospital Microbes

After a day in hospital, the microbial flora in the intestinal tract and in the oral cavity is somewhat displaced by "hospital flora". It comes with food, water, equipment, other patients, personnel and the environment around the patient. In most cases this is not important for the patient's hospital stay. However, if the hospital environment is loaded with resistant or virulent (pathogenic) microbes, "hospital microbes" may pose a risk, especially for surgical and intensive patients and in immunosuppressed patients.

Resistant bacteria like gram-negative rods (ESBL), VRE and MRSA can easily be spread into the environment via contaminated food and water. In order to prevent the spread of hospital microbes, it is particularly important with a high level of hygiene concerning serving food and beverages at hospitals.

Intestinal Pathogenic Microbes in Hospitals

- Intestinal pathogenic bacteria, like *Salmonella*, *Shigella*, *Campylobacter*, *Yersinia* and pathogenic strains of *E. coli*, rarely occur as a hospital infection, but may spread in hospitals during lack of infection control [39–41]. The greatest risk may occur outside hospitals, during holidays and travel activity. A total of 75 persons—mostly patients—at a hospital in Southern Norway were infected with *Salmonella infantis,* an outbreak that started from the central *kitchen* [15]. The workers at the kitchen had recently been for holidays in the South of Europe, got some stomach problems there, but were healthy carriers when returning to job. *S infantis* was found in food and in the kitchen environment [15].
- *Listeria monocytogenes* is an actual hospital bacterium for special patient groups. *Listeria* is normal flora in animals, associated with contaminated foods such as unpasteurized dairy products and other refrigeration products, cold cuts and fish toppings, grows in the refrigerator and is living in water amoebas, thereby surviving chlorine treatment of water.
- Intestinal pathogenic viruses such as noro-, sapo- and other caliciviruses, as well as rotavirus, are frequently transmitted via contaminated water and food and can be spread by healthy carriers working with food and beverages.
- Hepatitis A can be an epidemic problem, especially if a healthy virus carrier is working in central kitchens.
- Hepatitis E may probably be a new and underestimated virus brought into hospitals via infected food and beverages.
- "Food poisoning" occurs in response to toxins in the food (re-heated food). Good healthcare and kitchen practices today make such episodes rare.
- *Clostridium difficile* often causes antibiotic-associated diarrhoea (colitis) in patients treated with antibacterial agents. The bacterium is a resistant, spore-forming microbe that easily infects other patients. It is the most frequent cause of acute diarrhoea in hospitals. Spores of bacteria may be transferred via salads, other food, beverages, etc.

70.5.8 Spread of Infections

Lack of hygiene control concerning food and beverages may increase the risk of carrier status or infection of resistant and special microbes. This problem is very relevant for hospital patients. Infection is most often transmitted from a healthy carriers or a person in the recovery phase.

Visitors', relatives' and/or patient's participation in cooking and serving and using "patient refrigerator", ice machines and other kitchen equipment is a risk of infection that is to be avoided. Resistant bacteria may be brought to hospitals via contaminated meat, fish and other foodstuffs—delivered to the central kitchen and post-kitchen at the hospital [42, 43].

Infection from contaminated equipment, dishes and cutlery may occur in case of failure of routines or technical faults on the dishwasher. Temperatures >85 °C kill most bacteria, viruses, parasites and fungi, while some microbes survive 75 °C [1–5].

Infection via drinking water may cause major epidemic outbreaks. Visibly clear drinking water may contain up to 10,000 bacteria per mL.

Ice machines that never are cleaned, with ice baler that rarely is cleaned and with free access from all users, patients and visitors, constitute a high risk of contamination and growth of bacteria, especially *Pseudomonas aeruginosa* [44–48]. Also parasites and fungi survive here (*Pneumocystis carinii*, *Giardia lamblia*, *Cryptosporidium*). The area around the opening of the machine is easily contaminated. Ice machines, impossible to clean inside, should not be used. The entire interior of ice machines must tolerate disinfection, for example, with chloramine 5% once a week. Ice machines should not be used in case of infectious outbreaks in the department.

1. When purchasing a new type of ice machine, contact the technical department, the kitchen management and infection control personnel. Ice machines may be registered at the technical department. It is recommended to use ice machines with closed systems where no one is in contact with the ice.
2. The machine must be directly connected to a water outlet, no recirculation or backflow in the system. The machine is placed in a clean place in the kitchen.
3. The machine must be easily accessible for cleaning all parts that are in contact with ice water.
4. Daily cleaning in the dishwasher of equipment (cans ol) used to pick up ice. Ensure that this is not contaminated during use. Wash hands before ice is collected. Patients/relatives should not handle the ice machine.
5. Weekly cleaning with soapy water. Rinse with clean water and finally with chloramine; 40 mL of chloramine 5% are added to 5 L of water. Rinse with clean water.
6. Every quarter, a more comprehensive cleaning and inspection of the system should be carried out; refer to the instruction manual for each ice machine registered.
7. Maintenance and inspection should be routinely performed by the technical department and recorded.
8. Patients with severely impaired infection defence should not use ice from the ice machines even if the machine is well controlled and cleaned. They should always use frozen sterile water.

See Chap. 71 on water.

References

1. Norwegian Nutrition Act of 19 May 1933.
2. Regulations for hygiene and food. Hygiene regulations for production and supply, etc. of Foodstuffs. 8 July 1983. Norway. p. 1253.
3. Regulations on internal control systems to comply with the Nutrition Act (IK-Food 1994). Norway.
4. Operating conditions in food business. NMT Info D1 17.11.1995. Norway.
5. Nutrition hygiene regulations No. 1239-2005, 12 Nov 1997. Norway.
6. European Parliament and Council Directive 2000/54/EC of 18 September 2000 on the protection of workers from the risks related to exposure to biological agents at work.
7. Norwegian Public Health Authority. Regulations on pre-examination of healthcare workers—antibiotic-resistant bacteria IK-36/1996.
8. Arnesen V, Rasch M, Solheim N, Hochlin K, Andersen BM. Food and dishwashing. In: Handbook in hygiene and infection control for hospitals. Ullevål University Hospital Oslo; 2003. p. 443–50.
9. Arnesen V, Rasch M, Hochlin K, Tollefsen T, Seljordslia B, Andersen BM, Nielsen E. Food and dishwashing. In: Handbook in hygiene and infection control for hospitals. Ullevål University Hospital Oslo; 2008. p. 625–32.
10. Andersen BM. Kitchen hygiene and serving food. In: Handbook in hygiene and infection protection for nursing homes. Long-term-care-institutions. Akademika publisher; 2013. p. 517–25.
11. Elvebakken KT, Rykkja LH. Norwegian food control conflicts for control purposes and values. Norsk Statsvit Tidsskr. 2006;22:119–40.
12. Andersen BM. Food contamination is a neglected problem. Aftenposten Viten. 2014;28:10.
13. Hofshagen M, Tafjord Heier B, Lange H, Hauge K. Salmonellose. Zoonosis report 2012. About diseases that can infect between humans and animals. Norway's situation. Veterinary Institute July, 2013.
14. Lange H, Tafjord Heier B, Nygård K, Vold L, Wester AL, Kapperud G. Nutrition-borne infections and outbreaks in 2011. Bethesda: National Public Health Institution; 2012.
15. Andersen BM. Gastrointestinal pathogenic bacteria. In: Handbook in hygiene and infection protection. Part 1. Microbiology and infection control. Fagbokforlaget. p. 95–108.
16. Takkinen J, Nakari UM, Johansson T, Niskanen T, Siitonen A, Kuusi M. A nationwide outbreak of multiresistant *Salmonella typhimurium* var Copenhagen DT 104B infection in Finland due to contaminated lettuce from Spain, May 2005. Eurosurveillance. 2005;10:194–6.
17. Abbott SL, Ni FCY, Janda JM. Increase in extraintestinal infections caused by *Salmonella enterica* subspecies II-IV. Emerg Infect Dis. 2012;18:637–9.
18. Pillay DG, Karas JA, Pillay A, Sturm AW. Nosocomial transmission of *Shigella dysenteriae* type 1. J Hosp Infect. 1997;37:199–205.
19. Schimmer B, Meldal H, Perederij NG, et al. Cross-border investigation of a *Shigella sonnei* outbreak in a group of Norwegian tourists after a trip to Russia. Eurosurveillance. 2007;12:159–62.
20. Kolmos HJ. Pat a pig—and get resistant bacteria with home. Ugeskr Laeger. 2011;173:527.
21. Food Minister Dan Jørgensen. New plan should limit pig MRSA to the barns. Ministry of Food, Agriculture and Fisheries. Denmark. 3 June 2014.
22. Andersen BM. MRSA. Handbook in hygiene and infection control. Part 1. Microbiology and infectious diseases. Fagbokforlaget; 2014. p. 39–59.
23. Promed mail September 9, 2014. Listeriosis—Denmark: copenhagen, fatal, deli meat suspected, more cases.
24. Promed mail December 31, 2014. Listeriosis—USA: fatal-caramel-coated and pre-packaged apples, update, alert.

25. Dawson SJ, Evans MRW, Willby D, Bardwell J, Chamberlain N, Lewis DA. *Listeria* outbreak associated with sandwich consumption from a hospital retail shop, *United Kingdom*. Eurosurveillance. 2006;11:89–91.
26. Koch J, Stark K. Significant increase of listeriosis in Germany—epidemiological patterns 2001-2005. Eurosurveillance. 2006;11:85–8.
27. Grahek-Ogden D, Lassen J. Listeriose in Norway 2005. MSIS Rep. 2006;34:16.
28. Gerner-Smidt P, Ethelberg S, Schiellerup P, et al. Invasive listeriosis in Denmark 1994-2003; a review of 299 cases with special emphasis on risk factors for mortality. Clin Microbiol Infect. 2005;11:618–24.
29. Andersen BM. Hepatitis E. Handbook in hygiene and infection control. Part 1. Microbiology and infectious diseases. Fagbokforlaget; 2014. p. 187–90.
30. Promed mail November 11, 2014. Hepatitis E UK: undercooked pork sausage.
31. Pfefferle S, Frickmann H, Gabriel M, et al. Fatal course of an autochthonous hepatitis E virus infection in a patient with leukaemia in Germany. Infection. 2012;40:451–4.
32. Andersen BM. Outbreak of acute gastroenteritis inside and outside. Ullevål Hospital, December 1994–February 1995. MSIS Epiuke 8 1995.
33. Andersen BM, Størvold G, Vainio K. Norovirus gastroenteritis at Ullevål University Hospital. Tidsskr Nor Laegeforen. 2003;123:1239.
34. Vestergaard LS, Olsen K, Stensvold R, Bøttiger B, Adelhart M, Lisby M, et al. Outbreak of severe gastroenteritis with multiple aetiologies caused by contaminated drinking water in Denmark, January 2007. Eurosurveillance. 2007;12:72–4.
35. Verhoef L, Depoortere E, Boxman I, et al. Emergence of new norovirus variants on spring cruise ships and prediction of winter epidemics. Emerg Infect Dis. 2008;14:238–43.
36. Lee N, Chan MCW, Wong B, et al. Faecal viral concentration and diarrhoea in norovirus gastroenteritis. Emerg Infect Dis. 2007;13:1399–401.
37. Kroneman A, Vennema H, Harris J, Reuter G, von Bonsdorff C, Hedlund K, Vainio K, Jackson V, Pothier P, Koch J, Schreier E, Bottiger B, Koopmans M, Foodborne Viruses in Europe Network. Increase in norovirus activity reported in Europe. Eurosurveillance. 2006;11(12):E061214.1.
38. Høgåsen HR, Valheim M, Hektoen L, Framstad K, Nesbakken T. Risk and vulnerability analysis of Norwegian sheep production: consequences for animal health and public health. Report 10. Veterinary Institute. 2011.
39. Bjørnestad H, Herikstad H, Hasseltvedt V, Kuusi, Aavitsland P. Outbreak of campylobacteriosis among health care personnel after sports activities in Stavanger. MSIS. 1998;26:26.
40. Melby KK, Svendby JG, Eggebø T, Holmen LA, Andersen BM, Lind L, Sjøgren E, Kaijser B. Outbreak of *Campylobacter* infection in a subarctic community. Eur J Clin Microbiol Infect Dis. 2000;19:542–4.
41. Seto EYW, Soller YES, Colford JM. Strategies to reduce person-to-person transmission during widespread *Escherichia coli* O157: H7 outbreak. Emerg Infect Dis. 2007;13:860–6.
42. Mannix M, Whyte D, McNamara E, et al. Large outbreak of *E coli* O157 in 2005, Ireland. Eurosurveillance. 2007;12:54–6.
43. Marshall BM, Levy SB. Food animals and antimicrobials: impacts on human health. Clin Microbiol Rev. 2011;24:718–33.
44. Wilson IG, Hogg GM, Barr JG. Microbiological quality of ice in hospital and community. J Hosp Infect. 1997;36:171–80.
45. Burnett IA, Weeks GR, Harris DM. A hospital study of ice-making machines; their bacteriology, design, use and maintenance. J Hosp Infect. 1994;28:305–13.
46. Andersen BM, Bøe E, Arnesen V. Ice machines, cleaning and control. In: Handbook in hygiene and infection control for hospitals. Ullevål University Hospital Oslo; 2003. p. 451–52.
47. Andersen BM, Rasch M, Arnesen V. Ice machines, cleaning and control. In: Handbook in hygiene and infection control for hospitals. Ullevål University Hospital Oslo; 2008. p. 633–34.
48. Kanwar A, Cadnum JL, Xiu D, Jencson AL, Donskey CJ. Hiding in plain sight: contaminated ice-machines are a potential source for dissemination of gram-negative bacteria and *Candida* species in healthcare facilities. Infect Control Hosp Epidemiol. 2018;39:253–8.

Water and Water Systems in Hospitals 71

Abstract
Drinking water is generally clean enough for use by healthy people in most countries. However, breakage of sewage pipes into drinking water may happen, or the actual drinking water source may be heavily contaminated by accidents. Floods and natural disasters cause global problems with regard to drinking water; with outbreaks of cholera, other bacteria and hepatitis A and E; and with norovirus and other viral types, protozoans and a variety of other microbiological agents. Legionella has often been linked to outbreaks in healthcare institutions. The following chapter is focused on practical measures concerning water and water systems in hospitals: source, use and control.

Keywords
Water · Water systems · Drinking water · Ice machines · Bacteria · Fungi Parasites · Hygiene · Infection control

71.1 Purpose

There may still be rather large, waterborne outbreaks on in industrialized countries like Norway, in spite of being a country exceptionally rich on clean water [1–3]. However, water and sewage systems may often be old, damaged by building activities and not well maintained.

- Therefore, it is very important with preventive measures to prevent transfer of microorganisms from water systems at the hospital to patients, personnel, visitors or the environment.

B. M. Andersen, *Prevention and Control of Infections in Hospitals*,
https://doi.org/10.1007/978-3-319-99921-0_71

71.2 Comprise

- *All water systems for clean water*—from water source through hospital intake (piping systems, central hot water units) and for washing (all types), showers, bathrooms, toilets, pools or machines (instrument washers, decontaminators, dishwashers, laundry dishes, autoclaves, machines that are cooled by water, machines for drinking water, ice machines, coffee machines, etc.).
- *All wastewater systems*—from the sink, shower, bathroom, toilet, etc. through collector's pipes back into the sewer system. Especially older hospitals are exposed to flooding of sewage from old, broken sewage pipes or incorrect treatment of wastewater.
- *All patients*, *personnel*, visitors, equipment and environment at the hospital.

71.3 Responsibility

The hospital's management provides written guidelines for water treatment and use and control of water and sewage in the hospital and that patients, personnel and visitors are not exposed to contaminated water [4].

Technical department follows procedures for water treatment and control and reports to the director—immediately—in case of serious risk of infection. Notices from local water authority about contaminated drinking water shall be communicated immediately to the director, infection control unit, chief of the central and ward kitchens and after local agreement.

Property/building department shall ensure water and drainage.

71.4 Practical Measures [1, 5–9] (Tables 71.1 and 71.2)

71.4.1 Aerosol-Producing Devices

"Plumbing systems at hospitals and other healthcare institutions constitute a significant risk of spread of infection. It is therefore important that preventive measures are determined and implemented on the basis of thorough risk assessments" [8].

Table 71.1 Cooling tower: control

Cooling towers	Drain off and cleaning Control of growth and biofilm	Full-year operation: ×2 Part-time operation: ×1
	Disinfection	Risk assessment determines how often the system is disinfected (legionella growth/other growth)
	Monitor and measure inhibitor level	Monthly
	Colony count tests Legionella test	Monthly (weekly with dip slide) + 1 week after cleaning At outbreaks—and preferably once a year

Table 71.2 Water distribution network: control

Internal water distribution network	Shock heating Control of growth and biofilm	Full-year operation: ×2
	Disinfection with chlorine (replacement or addition to shock heat)	Risk assessment
	Water temperature minimum in – Water heater: 65 °C – Regular tap points: 55 °C after 1 min	Monthly
	Colony count test Legionella test	Monthly At outbreaks—and preferably once a year
Shower heads and hose	Clean	Quarterly
Drains rarely in use	Rinse trough with hot water	Weekly

Source: Guidance for the prevention and control of legionella infection. Public Health Institute 2003, updated 2010 and 2013 [7–9]

Legionary disease was discovered in 1976. The disease causes many outbreaks around the world, linked to the cooling tower and to hospitals [1, 5], see Table 71.3. *Legionella* is an environmental bacteria that "survives everything and can withstand everything"—even high temperatures [1, 5–16].

In Norway, few cases have been registered each year, but without preventive measures against legionella growth in the plumbing systems, infection risk is considered to be significant [7–9]. The basis for risk assessments is described [8].

71.4.2 Risks: Especially for Legionella Infection [1, 6]

- Cooling towers and scrubbers or similar are predominating; see Table 71.3 [1, 5–9, 12–28].
- Travel and foreign stays [16, 17, 22].
- Irrigation systems in agriculture, for vegetables, shops and moisture systems for patients [29, 30].
- Electronic sinks, splashes and aerosols around sink and stationary water systems [31–34].
- Failing control of water systems in hospitals [25, 26].
- Window cleaner systems with growth in flushing containers [18].
- Soil, dust and plant products [1, 6].

71.4.3 Internal Water Distribution Network: Citations from Norwegian Water Report 115 [7–9]

- The temperature in the circulation pipes for hot water should be kept constant above 60 °C, and the hot water at all tap points should reach at least 60 °C within 1 min of opening.

Table 71.3 *Legionella* species

Some outbreaks of legionella infections associated with water systems or unknown						
Place		Year	Number	Died	Infection source	Comment
America	USA, Philadelphia, VA	1976	221	34	Cooling tower, hotel	"Veterans" *Legionnaires' disease*
	USA, Oklahoma	2004	66		Hotel	Pontiac fever—tourists
	USA, Pennsylvania, VA	2012	21	5	Water distribution	Control failure, hospital Identical to 1976! CDC
	USA, Ohio	2013	35	5	Cooling towers	Nursing homes
	USA, Wisconsin	2013	31		Source unknown	
	USA, Alabama	2014	9	2	Water distribution	Control failure, hospital
	USA, New York City	2015	128	12	Cooling towers	Lack of control, CDC
	Canada, Toronto	2005	127	21	Cooling towers	Institution for elderly
	Canada, Quebec	2012	176	11	Cooling towers	
Europe	United Kingdom, Stafford	1985	175	28	Cooling towers	Hospital
	England, Hereford	2003	26	2	Cooling towers	Cider production
	United Kingdom, Edinburgh	2005	100		Cooling towers?	Wind direction
	United Kingdom, Edinburgh	2012	100	3	Cooling towers?	
	England	2014	1		Birth under water	Home birth
	Spain, Murcia	2001	800	3	Cooling towers	Hospital cooling tower
	Spain, Zaragoza	2004	28	2	Cooling towers	Hospital cooling tower
	Spain, Catalonia	2012	8		Cooling towers	Tourists
	Spain, Catalonia	2013	14		Unknown	
	France, Pas-de-Calais	2004	86	17	Cooling towers	Noroxo factory
	Norway, Stavanger	2001	28	7	Cooling towers	Many passed by
	Norway, Nesodden	2003	10		Whirlpool	"Pontiac fever"
	Norway, Fredrikstad	2005	103	11	Air scrubber, cleaning	Borregaard factory
	Norway, Radiumhospitalet	2013	5	1	Water distribution	Control failure, hospital
Australia	Australia, Melbourne	2000	125	4	Cooling towers	Aquarium
	Australia, Victoria	2013	5	1	Cooling towers	
Sum			2428	169		
Died				7%		

Source: Promed—mail, [1, 5, 6]
Cooling tower is often associated with outbreaks

- The temperature of the cold water system should not exceed 20 °C.
- Regular or continuous treatment of the hot water system must be carried out.
- Blind pipes should be removed, and if this is not possible, drain valve should be mounted so that regular flushing can be performed. There should also be routines for regular flushing of other slightly used tap points.
- Flushing the shower with water that holds 70 °C, some repeated times each year will prevent legionella growth.
- To prevent growth of legionella bacteria, shower hoses and shower heads should be regularly flushed with water holding at least 70 °C for 5 min.
- A program must be developed for checking the technical facilities, like including temperature recording.
- A program for sampling and analyses of germ numbers and *Legionella* spp. must be prepared [8].

71.4.4 Preventative Measures [1, 5, 6]

- Heat >75 °C (heat resistant). Central hot water heaters should be set at least 75–85 °C to inhibit growth of the microbe.
- Avoid uncontrolled use of the cooling tower. Check that venting from the cooling tower is not drawn into the nearest air intake. Avoid local air cooler/heating systems that can promote the growth of microbes in condensation water and spread it into the room on collected dust particles. Follow routines that prevent such spread (such as cleaning routines).
- Chlorine has good disinfecting effect on bacteria in water. Chloramine 5% disinfectant (less effect if a lot of protein is present). The bacteria are also rapidly killed by 70% alcohol.
- Hot water (>75 °C) for flushing pipes approximately in 30 min is effective.
- Control of water systems, cooling towers, water distribution networks, hot water, humidification systems [30], cleaning systems, showers, baths for birth [27, 28], irrigation systems, etc. All stagnant water, growth inside pipes, biofilms, etc. provide a basis for legionella.
- Colony count test (most often number of coliform bacteria) from defined taps (growth at 36 °C)—preferably monthly to quarterly. The number of bacteria (most often gram-negative rods) should not exceed 100/mL clean drinking water [1, 5, 6].
- At high germ numbers, flush with warm water for 15–30 min. Then check the test.

71.5 Background Information

Drinking water is generally clean enough for use by healthy people in most countries. However, breakage of sewage pipes into drinking water may happen, or the actual drinking water source may be heavily contaminated by other accidents. Floods and natural disasters cause global problems with drinking water, causing outbreaks of cholera, other bacteria and hepatitis A and E and norovirus and other viral types, protozoans and a variety of other microbiological agents. Legionella has often been linked to outbreaks in health institutions.

There are still large, waterborne outbreaks in industrialized countries like Norway, in spite of being exceptionally rich on clean water [1–3]. However, water and sewage systems may often be old, damaged by building activities and not well maintained. During Christmas 1978, several hundreds were sick of *Shigella sonnei* in two communities in Norway (Brandbu and Røyken) due to contaminated drinking water [1]. In 2000, hundreds of people were infected with *Campylobacter jejuni* via contaminated drinking water in Skjervøy in northern part of Norway [2]. In Bergen 2004, approximately 5000 were infected with *Giardia lamblia* from contaminated drinking water source, hence many with long-lasting effects [3].

71.5.1 Other Waterborne Microbes That May Be Pathogenic

Most gram-negative rod bacteria grow and propagate unharmed in water, such as *Pseudomonas aeruginosa*, *Enterobacter cloacae*, *Klebsiella* sp., *Citrobacter*, *Serratia*, *Acinetobacter*, *Burkholderia*, *Stenotrophomonas*, etc [31–43]. In New Delhi, multidrug-resistant gram-negative bacteria are detected in drinking water *cisterns*—even *Vibrio cholera* with NDM-1 super-resistant gene [34, 43].

In southern parts of Europe, the incidence of mycobacteria in water increases and is associated with infections during surgery and infections among patients with highly impaired infections [44]. Outbreaks may also occur due to improper location, design or use of washbasins, too close to patients, electronic water mixture on too low temperatures and use as sinks for sewage [31–34, 41].

Large collectors under the sink, plumbing traps or "gypsum knee", where the container is containing sewage that becomes a growth of many types of gram-negative bacteria, are a risk [34, 37, 45].

- A nosocomial outbreak of multiresistant *Enterobacter cloacae* among patients after heart surgery and among leukaemia patients at Tromsø Regional Hospital, Norway, was linked to contaminated plumbing trap of a sink made for collecting used plaster (gypsum) in the operation department (1989) [34, 37, 46].
- Multidrug-resistant *Pseudomonas aeruginosa* in the tap water at the intensive care unit at Akershus University Hospital, Norway, led to several outbreaks and deaths among patients (2002) [38].
- Aerosols generated from a washbasin placed too close to patient's beds caused contamination, colonization and infection with multidrug-resistant *Pseudomonas aeruginosa* [41]. Aerosols with bacteria contaminated the environment at a large distance around the sink (2009) [41].
- A washbasin in an intensive care unit was the reservoir and source for an outbreak of multidrug-resistant *Acinetobacter baumannii*—which also contaminated the entire drainage system (2010) [42].

- For an 18-month period, there were 84 secondary cases of multidrug-resistant *Acinetobacter baumannii* at an intensive department in France (2013) [33]. The outbreak started with two index patients from abroad transferred to the department with *A. baumannii*, which was further spread through the staff's hands, by air, poor hygiene and splash of contaminated water in the sink [33].

Biofilm and heavy growth in water systems, as well as a lot of humus, protect bacteria and keep the growth at the same rate. Persons with severely impaired immunity defence should not drink tap water, and open wounds or urine catheters should not be rinsed in running water!

In hospitals, in addition to regular legionella control, a routine control of water is important for detection of germ numbers (numbers of gram-negative rod bacteria). Water systems with a higher yield of coliform bacteria than 100/mL water should be treated by flushing with hot water.

In case of outbreak of legionella, start tracing of the infection with the cooling tower and "dead ends"—if there exists! [46, 47].

References

1. Andersen BM. *Legionella pneumophila*. In: Bacteria and diseases. Epidemiology, infections and infection protection. Oslo: Gyldendal Academic; 2005. p. 318–29.
2. Melby KK, Svendby JG, Eggebø T, Holmen LA, Andersen BM, Lind L, Sjøgren E, Kaijser B. Outbreak of *Campylobacter* infection in a subarctic community. Eur J Clin Microbiol Infect Dis. 2000;19:542–4.
3. Nygård K, Schimmer B, Søbstad Ø, et al. A large community outbreak of waterborne giardiasis-delayed detection in a non-endemic urban area. BMC Public Health. 2006;6:141.
4. Ministry of Labor and Administration. Regulations on protection against exposure to biological factors (bacteria, viruses, fungi and more) in the workplace. FOR OSLO: 1997-12-19 nr.1322.
5. Andersen BM. Legionella. In: Handbook in hygiene and infection control for hospitals. Oslo: Ullevål University Hospital; 2008. p. 40–2.
6. Andersen BM. Legionella. In: Handbook in hygiene and infection control for hospitals. Microbiology and infection protection. Norway: Fagbokforlaget; 2014. p. 116–20.
7. Guideline for the prevention and control of legionella infection. Oslo: National Public Health Institute; 2007.
8. Pettersen JE. Prevention of linfection—a guide. 2nd ed. Oslo: National Public Health Institute; 2010.
9. Pettersen JE. Prevention of legionella infection—a guide. 3rd ed. Oslo: National Public Health Institute; 2012.
10. Sehulster LM, Chinn RYW, Ardunio MJ, et al. Guidelines for environmental infection control in health-care facilities. CDC MMWR. 2003;52:1–42.
11. Rutala WA, Weber DJ. Disinfection, sterilization, and control of hospital waste. In: Mandell, Douglas, and Bennets principles and practice of infectious diseases, vol. 2. 8th ed. Philadelphia: Elsevier Churchill Livingstone; 2015. p. 3294–309.
12. CDC. [Increasing incidence of] Legionellosis in the United States, 2000-2009. MMWR. 2011;60:1083–6.
13. CDC. Surveillance for waterborne disease outbreaks and other health events associated with recreational water-United States, 2007-2008. MMWR Surveill Summ. 2011;60:1–32.

14. CDC. Surveillance for waterborne disease outbreaks associated with drinking water-United States, 2007-2008. MMWR Surveill Summ. 2011;60:38–68.
15. CDC. Legionellosis resource site. Updated 5 Feb 2013.
16. Joseph C, Lee J, Van Wijngaarden J, Drasar V, Pastoris MC. European guidelines for control and prevention of legionnaires disease. European Commission; 2003.
17. Burnsed LJ, Hicks LA, Smithee LM, et al. A large, travel-associated outbreak of legionellosis among hotel guests: utility of the urine antigen assay in confirming Pontiac fever. Clin Infect Dis. 2007;44:222–8.
18. Promed mail September 14, 2010. Legionellosis, fatal- UK: Wales.
19. Promed Mail July 12, 2012. Legionellosis - UK: Scotland, more cases, fatal.
20. Promed Mail May 24, 2012. Legionellose-New Zealand -fatal.
21. Promed Mail September 7, 2012. Legionellosis Canada: Quebec, Fatal *L Pneumophilia*.
22. Promed mail September 10, 2012. Legionellosis-Spain: Catalonia, tourists.
23. McCormick D, Thorn S, Milne D, et al. Public health response to an outbreak of Legionnaires' disease in Edinburgh, United Kingdom, June 2012. Euro Surveill. 2012;17:20216.
24. Promed Mail January 24, 2013. Legionellosis Australia: Victoria. Fatal, cooling tower suspected.
25. Promed Mail February 23, 2013. Legionellosis- USA: Pennsylvania, nosocomial, CDC investigation.
26. Dommerud T. The hospital admits failure after legionella deaths. Aftenposten 26 May 2013.
27. Teare L, Millership S. *Legionella pneumophila* serogroup 1 in a birthing pole. J Hosp Infect. 2012;82:58–60.
28. Promed Mail July 1, 2014. Legionellosis UK: England neonatal underwater birthing.
29. Moore G, Walker J. Presence and Control of *Legionella Pneumophilia* and *Pseudomonas Aeruginosa* biofilms in hospital water systems. In: Percival SL, Williams DW, Randle J, Coioper T, editors. Biofilms in infection prevention and control. Boston: Academic; 2014. p. 311–37.
30. Moran-Gilad J, Lazarovitch T, Mentasti M, et al. Humidifier-associated pediatric Legionnaires' disease, Israel, February 2012. Euro Surveill. 2012;17(41):20293.
31. Assadian O, El-Madani N, Seper E, et al. Sensor-operated faucets: a possible source of nosocomial infection? Infect Control Hosp Epidemiol. 2002;23:44–6.
32. Charron D, Bedard E, Lalancette C, Laferriere C, Prevost M. Impact of electronic faucets and water quality on the occurrence of *Pseudomonas aeruginosa* in water: a multi-hospital study. Infect Control Hosp Epidemiol. 2015;36:311–9.
33. Landell C, Legrand P, Lesprit P, et al. Protracted outbreak of multidrug-resistant *Acinetobacter baumannii* after intercontinental transfer of colonized patients. Infect Control Hosp Epidemiol. 2013;34:119–24.
34. Andersen BM, Sørlie D, Hotvedt D, Almdahl SM, Olafsen K, George R, Gilfillian A. Multiply beta-lactam resistant *Enterobacter cloacae* infections linked to the environmental flora in a unit of cardiothoracic and vascular surgery. Scand J Infect Dis. 1989;21:181–91.
35. Andersen BM, Teige B, Hochlin K, Elsebutangen N, Fagerbakk L, Seljordslia B, Syversen G. Failure of ionized water produced by activeion ionator to kill harmful bacteria. Microbiol Biochem Technol. 2012;4:3.
36. Hollyoak V, Allison D, Summers J. *Pseudomonas aeruginosa* wound infection associated with a nursing home's whirlpool bath. Comm Dis Rep CDC Rev. 1995;23:100–2.
37. Olafsen K, Hotvedt R, Andersen BM, Almdahl SM, Sørlie D. Nosocomial infection with resistant *Enterobacter cloacae*. Tidsskr Nor Legeforen. 1989;109:332–6.
38. Bukholm G, Tannæs T, Kjelsberg ABB, et al. An outbreak of multidrug-resistant *Pseudomonas aeruginosa* associated with increased risk of patient death in an intensive care unit. Infect Control Hosp Epidemiol. 2002;23:441–6.
39. De Boeck HD, Miwaqnda B, Lunguya-Metlia O, et al. ESBL-positive *Enterobacteria* isolates in drinking water. Emerg Infect Dis. 2012;18:1019–20.
40. Nordmann P, Naas T, Poirel L. Global spread of carbapenemase-producing *Enterobacteriaceae*. Emerg Infect Dis. 2011;17:1791–8.

41. Hota S, Hirji Z, Stockton K, et al. Outbreak of multidrug-resistant *Pseudomonas aeruginosa* colonization and infection secondary to imperfect intensive care unit room design. Infect Control Hosp Epidemiol. 2009;30:25–33.
42. La Forgia C, Franke J, Hacek DM, et al. Management of a multidrug-resistant *Acinetobacter baumannii* outbreak in an intensive care unit using novel environmental disinfection: a 38 month report. Am J Infect Control. 2010;38:259–63.
43. Promed Mail July 28, 2012: NMD-1 carrying *Vibrio cholerae*- India.
44. Andersen BM. Other mycobacteria. Microbiology and infectious disease. In: Handbook in hygiene and infection control. Part 1. Norway: Fagbokforlaget; 2014. p. 140–1.
45. Gbaguidi-Haore H, Varin A, Cholley P, Thouverez M, Hocquet D, Bertrand X. A bundle of measures to control an outbreak of *Pseudomonas aeruginosa* associated with P-Trap contamination. Infect Control Hosp Epidemiol. 2018;39:164–9.
46. Andersen BM, Dahl IMS, George RC, Gilfillian A. Septicaemia caused by an *Enterobacter cloacae* strain varying in resistance against cephalosporins. Infection. 1989;17:156–9.
47. CDC. Keeping cool under pressure: NYC Legionnaires' disease outbreak, summer 2015. CDC; 6 Oct 2015.

72 Technical and Medical Technical Equipment

Abstract
Hospitals have large amounts of medical technical and other larger and smaller technical equipment that need routines for cleaning, maintenance and repair. The technical devices may be used in patient rooms, operation departments, laboratories, examination rooms, intensive units, etc. and may be shared by many users and moved between departments and rooms. Microbes usually follow these devices if no hygienic measures are used. Large systems for water and drainage, ventilation, air pressure conditions and heating should be cleaned, maintained, repaired and treated so that patients, personnel, visitors or the environment is not exposed to infection.

Keywords
Technical equipment · Medical technical equipment · Hospital · Water sewage system · Ventilation · Air filtration · Air pressure systems · Room heating Hygiene · Infection control

72.1 Purpose

Protect technical and medical technical personnel, other personnel, patients and visitors against infection from medical and other equipment and against contamination in connection with building and ventilation measures [1, 2].

72.2 Comprise

- All equipment, medical devices and technical installations in direct/indirect contact with human biological material and/or microbes.

B. M. Andersen, *Prevention and Control of Infections in Hospitals*,
https://doi.org/10.1007/978-3-319-99921-0_72

- *Medical technical equipment* is defined as any instrument, device, aid, material or any object used to diagnose, monitor, treat or alter the patient's anatomy or physiological process. Laboratory equipment where the answers are used for diagnostics of patients is defined as medical devices.
- *Other technical equipment* that comes into contact with the blood or other tissues should be *handled in a similar manner*. This also applies to decontaminator, instrument washing machine, dishwashers, other disinfection machines, autoclave, sewage systems, ventilation systems, outlet and extraction systems, etc.
- Be aware of the possibility of spreading contaminants via pipes, slides over ceilings and ventilation and through elevator, lift shaft and technical routes, by accidental pressure changes and diffusion.
- Respiratory equipment—see separate Chaps. 29–31.

72.3 Responsibility

The hospital's management provides written procedures for the purchase, maintenance, repair and use of technical equipment and medical equipment and for clear and defined hygiene and protection requirements for the equipment [2].

The department's management contacts the infection control unit and medical devices unit *before purchase* for evaluation of hygiene and infection prevention in terms of cleaning and use.

All users requiring maintenance, repair or checking of above-mentioned equipment, either at their own department or sent to the technical department or any other entity, shall ensure that the equipment is properly cleaned and disinfected if necessary—or treated at another secure way.

Departments that have practical responsibility for the maintenance, inspection and repair of technical equipment follow procedures for personal protection and hygiene during supervision, repair, inspection and maintenance of medical devices/equipment and when working with connections of decontaminator and similar equipment to water and drainage.

72.4 Practical Measures [3, 4]

Disinfect equipment as much as possible.

All medical devices must be disinfected before being sent for repair. Those who "own" the equipment and order the work must ensure that the equipment is disinfected or chemically disinfected before it is sent for repair, maintenance and evaluation.

72.4.1 Infected Equipment

If disinfection of the equipment is impossible, this is reported in writing on the equipment. Carefully clean the equipment on the outside and pack it in yellow plastic bag before sending. On the label, set "Infected".

72.4.2 Hand Hygiene

When receiving equipment for repair, hand hygiene is important before and after technical work. Wear gloves where the equipment seems unclean, even if it is cleaned from the sending unit.

72.4.3 Work Attire During Normal Work with Cleaned Machines/Equipment

- Use the hospital's work outfit. Private clothing should not be used due to the risk of infection.
- Work clothes are changed daily.
- Visor/exhaust hood if splash and dust.
- Wear gloves when needed and always when equipment is contaminated. Perform hand hygiene after removing gloves.
- Remove the workwear before leaving the room, during dinner break, etc.
- Do not eat or drink in rooms where technical equipment is repaired.
- Always practice good hand hygiene after leaving the machine/equipment.

72.4.4 Work Attire When Working with Possibly Infected Device

In case of possible infection, work in a separate room or distance from others. Avoid blowing/suction. Consider whether the equipment should be gas disinfected before cleaning and repair.

- Use the hospital's uniform. Private clothes must not be used.
- Learn to take on and off personal protective equipment—PPE!
- Wear surgical mask or respiratory protection, P3 mask, if there is airborne infection or a lot of dust.
- Use cap that covers the hair and ears.
- Use eye protection.
- Wear gloves with long cuff.
- Use gown with long cuffs, waterproof if splashes.
- Exhaust hood if splash and dust.
- Perform hand hygiene after removing gloves.
- Remove the gown and other PPE before leaving the room—treated as infected waste.

72.4.5 Ventilation and Exhaust in Patient Rooms and Service Rooms

If high risk for spread of infection, for instance, when removing hepafilters from exhaust hoods in infectious isolates or laboratories, the infectious agent should be deactivated in advance. Formaldehyde damp evaporating is often used in the disinfection of exhaustion hoods. Note allergy to formalin!

Also hydrogen peroxide dry gas ("mist") can be used [1, 5–8]. There are also good systems of hydrogen peroxide gas with higher humidity, but this can corrode instruments more than dry gas, if moisture is not removed immediately [9–12]. Proper guidelines including control of effect should be available for such procedures if used. Contact infection control personnel if questions. *See Chap. 59 on disinfection.*

72.4.6 Work with Aggregates and Channels

When working in aggregate rooms and with channels serving isolates and other risk areas, a negative pressure in the room must be established. It will often be necessary to use a mobile exhaust fan with exhaust to the outside. Protective equipment and written procedures must be followed. Use respiratory protection—P3 mask, hood and gloves, gown/boots/shield/tight glasses. Contact infection control personnel in advance and learn procedures for using infection protection equipment, on and off. *See Chaps. 14–21 on isolation.*

72.4.7 Cleaning of Rooms for Technical Work

- Daily cleaning of benches and floors.
- It is important to have good cleaning in rooms where technical equipment is being worked with because of the infection risk.
- The same cleaning principle in the store room for repaired equipment.
- Main cleaning once a year.
- *See Chap. 65 on cleaning.*

72.4.8 Disinfection of Medical Devices Before Returning

After repair and cleaning of internal technical parts, gas disinfection of the equipment is carried out again. Dry hydrogen peroxide gas 5% has been found to have a good disinfectant effect without destroying metals or other fine-scale equipment [5, 7]. Spore test ensures that the disinfection process has been active. Performed by treatment aids centres or equivalent. NB medical devices used in patients with tuberculosis are discarded [5, 7].

See Chap. 59 on disinfection.

72.4.9 Return of Repaired Equipment

Upon return of repaired equipment, the recipient must ensure proper cleaning and—if necessary—disinfection/sterilization of the equipment before reuse of the unit.

72.5 Background Information

Medical equipment/patient equipment often come in direct or indirect contact with organic materials and contaminants. This results in infection risk. Therefore, the equipment must be cleaned and disinfected in a hygienically acceptable manner after use. The operating instructions of the device must contain cleaning procedures adapted to the equipment and the hospital's routines.

Chemical disinfection (chlorine compounds, glutaraldehyde, perasafe, etc.) is used where instruments and equipment cannot be treated with thermal disinfection or sterilization. Chemical disinfectants in combination with heat are used for flexible endoscopes that have been in contact with mucous membranes, etc. Devices like blood gas analyser should have routines for inactivating (killing), infectious blood agents.

In many cases, the disinfection process cannot be carried out for the internal mechanical structures of equipment, for instance, apparatus using air cooling systems or systems associated with water and drainage or ventilation ducts. In such cases, the device/equipment must be treated as contaminated or, if possible, be treated with gas disinfection, while the device is on—air/gas is pulled through the internal machine parts [5, 7].

It may be appropriate to decontaminate equipment with formaldehyde gas or other gaseous forms such as hydrogen peroxide, chlorine gas, etc. before working, such as laboratory extractors and exhaust ducts from infectious isolates. Gas exposure for patients or personnel must be avoided. *See Chap. 59 on disinfection.*

References

1. Rutala WA, Weber DJ. Disinfection, sterilization, and control of hospital waste. In: Mandell, Douglas, and Bennets principles and practice of infectious diseases. Vol. 2. 8th ed. Philadelphia: Elsevier Churchill Livingstone; 2015. p. 3294–309.
2. Ministry of Labour and Administration. Regulations on protection against exposure to biological factors (bacteria, viruses, fungi and more) in the workplace. FOR OSLO: 1997-12-19 nr.1322.
3. Berge JA, Laugerud F, Hochlin K, Andersen BM, Solheim N, Rasch M. Technical and medical-technical activity. Cleaning, maintenance and repair. In: Handbook in hygiene and infection control for hospitals. Oslo: Ullevål University Hospital; 2003. p. 453–7.
4. Berge JA, Hochlin K, Rasch M, Laugerud F, Andersen BM. Technical and medical technical activity. Cleaning, maintenance and repair. In: Handbook in hygiene and infection control for hospitals. Oslo: Ullevål University Hospital; 2008. p. 635–8.
5. Andersen BM, Rasch M, Hochlin K, Jensen FH, Wismar P, Fredriksen JE. Decontamination of rooms, medical equipment and ambulances, using a dry fog or hydrogen peroxide disinfectant. J Hosp Infect. 2006;62:149–55.
6. Andersen BM, Syversen G, Thoresen H, Rasch M, Hochlin K, Seljordslia B, Snevold I, Berg E. Failure of dry fog or hydrogen peroxide 5% to kill *Mycobacterium tuberculosis*. J Hosp Infect. 2010;76:80–3.
7. Andersen BM, Hochlin K, Daling JP. Cleaning and decontamination of reusable medical devices, including the use of hydrogen peroxide dry-fog gas decontamination. J Microbiol Biochem Technol. 2012;4:57–62.

8. Landelle C, Legrand P, Lesprit P, et al. Protracted outbreak of multidrug resistant *Acinetobacter baumannii* after intercontinental transfer of colonized patients. Infect Control Hosp Epidemiol. 2013;34:119–24.
9. French GL, Otter JA, Shannon KP, Adams NMT, Watling D, Parks MJ. Tackling contamination of the hospital environment by methicillin-resistant *Staphylococcus aureus* (MRSA): a comparison between conventional terminal cleaning and hydrogen peroxide vapor decontamination. J Hosp Infect. 2004;57:31–7.
10. Jeanes A, Rao G, Osman M, Merrcik P. Eradication of persistent environmental MRSA. J Hosp Infect. 2005;61:85–6.
11. Otter JA, Nowakowski E, Salked JAG, et al. Saving costs through the decontamination of the unpackaged medical supplies using hydrogen peroxide vapor. Infect Control Hosp Epidemiol. 2013;34:472–8.
12. Chan HT, White P, Sheorey H, Cocks J, Waters MJ. Evaluation of the biological efficacy of hydrogen peroxide vapour decontamination in wards of an Australian hospital. J Hosp Infect. 2011;79:125–8.

Laboratories

73

Abstract

Patient test samples are taken and examined at outpatient clinics, in bed posts and at policlinic consultations and treatment units. They are collected and transported to central laboratories or examined by smaller laboratory units, adapted to the patient group. Samples are sent in pipes or transported by defined methods to the laboratory. A large number of samples are also sent to other hospitals, laboratories or diverse private laboratories.

The following chapter is focused on laboratory safety for patients and personnel to avoid spread of infections between patients, personnel and environment.

Keywords

Laboratory tests · Safety · Blood-borne infections · Sampling · Storage · Transport Control · Hygiene

73.1 Purpose

Protect staff, patients, other persons and the environment against infection [1–10].

73.2 Comprise

- All who work with patient testing, sampling, transport and investigation.
- All who work with further examinations of organic test samples from patients.
- Anyone who otherwise handles organic and/or biological material.

B. M. Andersen, *Prevention and Control of Infections in Hospitals*,
https://doi.org/10.1007/978-3-319-99921-0_73

73.3 Responsibility

The hospital's management provides written procedures and resources for proper handling of sample materials and other organic material, and that personnel, patients and visitors are not exposed to infection [1, 2].

The department's management provides for hygienic guidelines and training of personnel and to report to the Director in case of laboratory activities that may expose personnel and patients to infection.

Personnel follow guidelines for personal and general infection protection and report accidents or injuries that expose patients or personnel to infection.

73.4 Practical Measures [11, 12]

Patient samples often pass multiple links, from when they are taken to when they are analysed and destroyed. The entire sampling-packaging-transport-analysis-waste system must be ensured so that patients, personnel, others and the environment are not infected [1, 2, 5, 6].

73.4.1 Sampling from the Patients in the Wards

- The patient should be informed and placed at ease, and there should be peace and quiet during the procedure.
- Personal good hygiene, clean work clothes—not jewellery or personal clothing, and carry out good hand hygiene before and after testing/sampling from patients.
- Wear gloves and gown/surgical mask/shield/cap in case of a risk of splash and spill.
- Perform spot disinfection if spill of organic materials; wear gloves when disinfecting.
- Avoid storing of sampling equipment in patient rooms and do not place the "sampling basket" in the patient's bed.
- Wash or clean stasis hose, etc. with alcohol between each use.
- Fixed routines for cleaning of sample trolley/sample basket—once per week.
- Do not place the sampling equipment in the textile store or room for sterile equipment!
- In case of infection, the hospital's isolation regimes and procedures are followed.
- If any questions, contact the responsible head of the ward *before* going to the patient.

73.4.2 Laboratory Work: Personal Infection Protection

- Follow the laboratory procedures and regulations.
- Always wear gloves on contact with biological material.

- It is not allowed to eat, drink or smoke in the laboratory! Mouth piping is forbidden!
- Hand hygiene after use of gloves/contact with biological agent.
- Hand hygiene before leaving the laboratory and before food break.
- Change clothes if contaminated with biological material, new outfits every day.
- Do not eat in the same clothes as you work in, eventually use an "eating/pause gown" over laboratory clothes.
- Do not pour biological material from pipes or glasses; use pipette.
- Avoid spills and splashes! Think about what you do and work calmly!
- If spills, splashes and aerosols of biological material are expected/risk:
  - Work in a separate exhaust hood with gloves and gown
  - Or if exhaust hood is not present, work with gloves, surgical mask/cap, eye protection and single-use gown in a separate room with negative pressure.
- Carefully follow the instructions for routine cleaning of equipment.
- Avoid equipment where blood must be wiped away manually between each sample!
- If such equipment is still in use, protect hands with gloves, practise good hygiene and use eventually surgical mask/cap/eye protection (risk of aerosols).
- Provide instructions placed on safety benches, doors of rooms with higher risk of infection, centrifuges, etc.
- All equipment must be disinfected regularly. Make routines for this.
- All equipment must be disinfected before repairs. If this cannot be done, it must follow the guidelines for handling/personal protection during repair.

73.4.3 Workplace Functions in Laboratory

The laboratory should be spacious with proper placement of doors, exhaustion hoods and other major equipment in relation to ventilation requirements and working procedures.

- *Reception for samples* with registration and distribution of samples must be adapted to a level of hygiene that also takes care of unknown infection.
- *Division of samples* into separate tubes/glasses, by opening primary samples, should take place under the exhaustion hood/shield with gloves, gown and optional surgical mask/cap.

Note: Special treatment of rare types of risk samples, special microbes (Biosafety Laboratory 3–4).

Regular laboratory with good control over procedures must meet the following requirements:

- Hand wash and hand disinfection on all sections.
- Note! There should be *hot water* in the wash basin! At tapping, the temperature should reach 75 °C to avoid biofilm formation and growth of legionella and gram-negative environmental microbes.

- Good distance, at least 2 m between each workplace to avoid cross-infection (aerosol).
- Benches shall be easily washable and withstand disinfectants like 5% chloramine.
- Centrifuges should be in separate technical rooms, separate from regular laboratory work to prevent accidents (aerosol). Alternatively, place in exhaustion hood with negative pressure and at a good distance from workplace.
- Washing centrifuges should be treated in the same way.
- All fixtures must be washable and withstand disinfectants such as chloramine, including chairs. Textile-covered chairs are not suitable for laboratories.
- *Wastewater* from laboratory analysers should be treated as infected waste.

Risk laboratories/rooms where the risk of infection is greater than elsewhere (aerosol-forming procedures, known infection, work with specific pathogenic viruses or bacteria, autopsy, etc.).

- Limited access, interlocking doors that open the right way and with clear warning sign on the door.
- Negative air pressure with pressure gauge (25–70 pascal) and controlled airflow against separate extract via hepafilter/UVC/electrostatic filter.
- A separate decontamination system and autoclave for the destruction of contaminated waste and water/liquids, if necessary.
- Sluice function with the possibility of high-level personal protective equipment and a decontamination unit after work in the laboratory.
- Dedicated personnel, trained in and understanding the importance of high-risk mitigation and infection protection.

Service room with disinfection room, autoclave room, waste room, laundry room, clean storage, storage for samples, media, and other equipment; toilet, shower and washbasins, office, rest room, etc. must be carefully planned for each laboratory.

Note! Carefully separate between unclean and clean areas in the laboratories using sluice systems or corridors.

Technical rooms are planned for technical equipment such as robots and centrifuges.

Waste room Human biological material and/or contaminants/microbes must be handled as potentially infectious. It can be disinfected or autoclaved at the laboratory before it is disposed of as ordinary waste. Particularly contaminated waste (e.g. from microbiological laboratory) must be destroyed before it leaves the section/department.

- Handwash in the waste room.
- The waste room must be under negative pressure and there should be floor drain for cleaning.
- Infectious waste should not be compressed if it has not been disinfected beforehand.

73.4.4 Cleaning in Laboratories

- Benches are washed daily with soap and water. Organic material is removed first with spot disinfection.
- Chloramine 5% has a good effect against viruses, fungi, bacteria and spores.
- Floors are washed daily in laboratories that are in daily use, as well as toilets. Waste of organic material is removed immediately by the person who is soiling on the floor; spot disinfection.
- Equipment, etc. should not stand on the floor, preventing cleaning.
- Sampling carts and similar equipment are cleaned daily.
- See chapter on room cleaning.

73.4.5 Spot Disinfection

It is usually only necessary to disinfect the area contaminated with biological material.

1. Spilled blood and other organic materials are removed using gloves and absorbent material. It is packaged and treated as hazardous waste.
2. Suitable disinfectant—like chloramine 5%—is applied on contaminated surfaces/equipment with cloth or sponge.
   Acting time:
   - 30 min (dried surface)
   - 60 min (dirty surface)

73.4.6 Transport of Biological/Organic Samples

Transport pipes should not be used in case of high risk of infection. There must be a negative air pressure in the system. Routines for cleaning of transport containers should be implemented; cleaned in a decontaminator once a week or more frequently if contaminated/spill. All paper material should be replaced. The transportation system should be gas disinfected once a year or more often if contaminated.

Manual transport should be performed with packaged sample material in containers that are cleaned in a decontaminator once a week. Samples should stand upright—opening up—during transport.

See Chap. 74 on transport of samples.

73.4.7 Accidents with Samples: Blood or Tissue

Accidents occur most often in connection with centrifugation, tube/glass opening, test tube crushing and sampling and procedures that may cause spills/stab wound/cut.

- Immediate action: see *accidents with blood—or tissue*
- Registration, corporate health service
- Accident registration for the laboratory for measures:
  - New equipment due to less risk
  - New work procedures to reduce risk

73.4.8 Prophylactic Measures for Specialty Laboratories

Local routines and guidelines should be made for each laboratory specialty (microbiology, pathology, clinical chemistry, blood bank, immunology, medical genetic).

73.5 Background Information

All biological material is considered to be potentially infectious and should be treated as such [1, 2, 5, 6].

Laboratory infections are well known.

- A survey of 4079 people infected at work at microbiological laboratories showed that 168 died of infection [13]. Dominant agents were *Brucella* sp., Q fever, hepatitis, typhoid fever, tularaemia and tuberculosis [13].
- In an English survey of 24,000 laboratory workers, 45 were infected with *Shigella* sp., 38 with hepatitis, 21 with tuberculosis and 1 with brucellosis [14].
- In 2012, a laboratory outbreak with a fatal course of meningococcal meningitis was reported in San Francisco [15]. This type of infection is rare today. Globally, in the period 1985–2001, 16 laboratories reported infections with *Neisseria meningitidis*, half of which were fatal.
- HIV and hepatitis C are newer microbes that represent a clear risk for laboratory personnel, as well as resistant mycobacteria. The SARS virus has been documented to have infected laboratory personnel, as well as *Sabia virus* and other high-pathogenic viruses despite alleged use of protective equipment. Current agents are also prions—infectious, resistant protein molecules.
- By 2015, 309 laboratory infections were published in 47 reports worldwide—reviewed by a group in Belgium [16]. Infections with *Salmonella* dominated; 42%, followed by *Brucella;* 40%, *Neisseria meningitidis* 4%, vaccinia virus 4%, *Francisella tularensis* 2%, Ebola and Marburg virus 2%, *E. coli* (O157: H7) 1%, *Mycobacterium* sp. 1%, *S. aureus* 1%, *Bacillus anthracis and Bacillus cereus* 1%, *Burkholderia pseudomallei and B. mallei* 1%, *Clostridium difficile* 1%, West Nile virus 1%, *Chlamydia psittaci* <1%, cowpox <1%, dengue virus <1%, leptospirosis <1%, SARS <1% and *Shigella sonnei* <1% [16].
  - The infection routes recorded in this material were 46% inhalation, 28% parenteral inoculation—cut injuries—20% oral infection and only 6% contact infection [16].

  - The main reason for infection was lack of compliance 73% (did not follow routines) and indifference/lack of knowledge 2%.
  - Bio-accidents were the cause of 24% of cases, hence technical error 8% and human error 93% [16].
- Laboratory infections are usually highly under-reported as they often cause mild symptoms [16].
- The study also showed that the staff perceived that accidents were associated with lack of experience, insufficient training, excessive workload, lack of knowledge about work risk, distraction in work and lack of respect for personal protection [16].

73.5.1 Risk of Infection

The accident hazards in laboratories are many, especially because *aerosols* are easy to generate in laboratory work [16–19]. Drop of bottles, agar plates with microbes, etc. have been investigated and generally show significant formation of aerosols [19]. It is well known that in the case of blood spills, most of it will be invisible aerosols or splashes [18]. This is important because bacteria, viruses and fungi can penetrate the mucous membranes of the upper respiratory tract and conjunctivae.

Risk work depends on the material and what to investigate. By "known" infection status, the personnel are most often carefully following preventive guidelines. If "unknown" infection status, it is easier to break the routines for personal preventive measures if no good general precautions are taken.

Risk situations are procedures that are especially known to cause infection to personnel.

- Sampling
- Opening of tubes/containers
- Distribution of samples
- Analyses of blood samples
- Work with blood cultures
- Resistance determination of microbes
- Aerosol-forming procedures (centrifugation, splash on distribution of samples, resistance studies, splash and stabbing at sampling, etc.) [16–19].

73.5.2 Spread of Infection

- Contact: direct, indirect, and contact with drops that fall onto the surface/equipment/textiles.
- Airborne: "dust", droplets (particles <10 μm), droplet nuclei and microscopic drops of blood, microbes and tissues. This is probably the most frequent and dangerous infection in the laboratory [16–19].
- Inoculation/puncture/stab: transmission of blood/tissue from one person to another; direct or indirect vie contaminated equipment, etc.

73.5.3 Safety/Security Cabinet

In case of known or suspected risk of infection, and in the case of possible aerosol-forming procedures, the laboratory work should be carried out in safety cabinet class I–III. Glass cabinet is often better and easier to keep clean than plastic. The location of the cabinet in the room is important, not too close to the door or to exterior wall.

Class I with hepafilter is a clean cabinet and provides good personal protection if the air extractor works satisfactorily. Hepafilter protects the exhaust duct from contaminants.

Class II with hepafilter and recirculated air in the cabinet provides good personal protection and also protection for the material in the cabinet (cell cultures, etc.).

Class III with hepafilter for intake and exhaustion of air and work through gloves connected to cabinet provides maximum protection. Used only at risk laboratories at particularly hazardous agents to public infections (Ebola, Lassa, Marburgvirus mm.). The cabinet is heavy to work in and requires training/competence.

73.5.4 Infection from High-Risk Laboratories

There have been a number of—probably more than 200 "leaks"—infectious agents from high-risk laboratories both in the United States and in Europe. In the United States, a congressional hearing was done in 2014 after a laboratory accident with anthrax, smallpox and a fatal bird flu virus. During the period 2008–2012, there were more than 1000 laboratory accidents in the United States—involving bacteria, viruses and toxins that could pose a bioterror threat to the population. In 2012, CDC documented 727 unfortunate laboratory events and 11 laboratory infections, including theft of microbiological agents.

In summer 2014, it was at Tulane Primate Research Center in Louisiana that laboratory studies were made for vaccine production on the highly virulent bacterium *Burkholderia pseudomallei*—first and foremost present in Australia and Asia [20, 21]. During the autumn 2014, it was discovered that four monkeys located outside the complex and far from the laboratory and not involved in the project were infected with this bacterium. At the same time, a man who was to investigate the cause of the spread of infection in the laboratory was infected [20].

In July 2014, CDC closed high-risk laboratories after accidents with bird flu virus and anthrax spores that were not inactivated before shipment to other laboratories [22]. There were more than 100 people exposed to infection, but no one became ill.

73.5.5 Transport and Shipment Risk

There is a very large shipment of human biological material and microbes in most countries in the world. Accidents can happen here as well. A Canada post office car crashed during transport between laboratories with samples containing among others anthrax, *E. coli*, *Salmonella*, tubercle bacteria and influenza virus [23].

References

1. Norwegian Directorate of Labour Inspection. Regulations on protection against exposure to biological factors (bacteria, viruses, fungi and more) in the workplace, 19 Dec 1997.
2. European Parliament and Council Directive 2000/54/EC of 18 September 2000 on the protection of workers from the risks related to exposure to biological agents at work.
3. Stratton C. Tuberculosis, infection control, and the microbiology laboratory. Infect Control Hosp Epidemiol. 1993;14:481–7.
4. Anonymous. Update: universal precautions for prevention of transmission of HIV, hepatitis B virus and other bloodborne pathogens in health care settings. MMWR. 1988;37:377–88.
5. Rutala WA, Weber DJ. Disinfection, sterilization, and control of hospital waste. In: Mandell, Douglas, and Bennetts principles and practice of infectious diseases, vol. 2. 8th ed. Philadelphia: Elsevier Churchill Livingstone; 2015. p. 3294–309.
6. Edmond MB, Wenzel RP. Infection prevention in the healthcare setting. In: Mandell, Douglas, and Bennets principles and practice of infectious diseases, vol. 2. 8th ed. Philadelphia: Elsevier Churchill Livingstone; 2015. p. 3286–93.
7. Digranes A, Haukenes G, Hovig B, Iveland H. Prevention of infections in laboratories for medical microbiology. Norway: Society of Medical Microbiology; 1989.
8. Bolyard EA, Tablan OC, Williams WW, Pearson ML, Shapiro CN, Deitchman SD, et al. Guideline for infection control in healthcare personnel, 1998. Infect Control Hosp Epidemiol. 1998;19:407–63.
9. Mahoney FJ, Stewart K, Hanxian H, Coleman A, Alter MJ. Progress towards the elimination of hepatitis B virus transmission among health care workers in the United States. Arch Intern Med. 1997;157:2601–5.
10. Lymer UB, Schutz A, Isaksson B. A descriptive study of blood exposure incidents among healthcare workers in a university hospital in Sweden. J Hosp Infect. 1997;35:223–35.
11. Andersen BM, Syversen G. Laboratories. In: Handbook in hygiene and infection control for hospitals. Oslo: Ullevål University Hospital; 2003. p. 458–65.
12. Andersen BM, Syversen G. Laboratories. In: Handbook in hygiene and infection control for hospitals. Oslo: Ullevål University Hospital; 2008. p. 639–45.
13. Pike RM. Laboratory-associated infections: summary and analysis of 3921 cases. Health Lab Sci. 1976;13:105–14.
14. Harrington JM, Shannon HS. Incidence of tuberculosis, hepatitis, brucellosis, and shigellosis in British medical laboratory workers. Br Med J. 1976;1:759–62.
15. Standen A. Lab accident at San Francisco VA leaves man dead of bacterial meningitis. KQED News, 2 May 2012.
16. Willemarck N, Van Vaerenbergh B, Descamps E, et al. Laboratory-acquired infections in Belgium (2007–2012). ISPWIV, February 2015.
17. Aintablian N, Walpita P, Sawyer MH. Detection of *Bordetella pertussis* and respiratory syncytial virus in air samples from hospital rooms. Infect Control Hosp Epidemiol. 1998;19:918–23.
18. Cole EC, Cook CE. Characterization of infectious aerosols in health care facilities: an aid to effective engineering controls and prevention strategies. Am J Infect Control. 1998;26:453–64.
19. Bennett A, Parks S. Microbial aerosol generation during laboratory accidents and subsequent risk assessment. J Appl Microbiol. 2006;100:658–63.
20. Willgress L. Safety fears after potentially deadly bacteria are accidentally released from high-security Louisiana research lab. Mail-Online, 2 March 2015.
21. Peacock SJ, Schweitzer HP, Dance DA, et al. Management of accidental laboratory exposure to *Burkholderia pseudomallei* and *B mallei*. Emerg Infect Dis. 2008;14:e2.
22. CDC lab incident: anthrax. CDC, Updated 19 July 2014.
23. Doyle P. FedEx truck carrying microbes crashes in Winnipeg. CBC News 3-7-5.

74 Transport in Hospitals

Abstract
In hospitals, there is a busy transport activity between departments of equipment, technical instruments, textiles, food and beverages, patient samples, waste, etc. This activity may spread infectious diseases between wards and departments if not taken care of by good hygienic methods. The following chapter is focused on transport of clean equipment, food and other clean items, contaminated equipment and other goods, and patient samples.

Keywords
Transport in hospitals · Clean and unclean equipment · Goods · Food and beverages · Patient samples

74.1 Purpose

Protect staff, patients, other persons and the environment against infection.

74.2 Comprise

All who work with transport in hospitals of clean or unclean equipment and goods, food and beverages, patient samples, other organic materials and waste.

74.3 Responsibility

The hospital's management provides written procedures and resources for proper handling and transport of clean or unclean equipment and other goods, food and beverages, patient samples and other organic materials and waste, and that personnel, patients and visitors are not exposed to infection.

B. M. Andersen, *Prevention and Control of Infections in Hospitals*,
https://doi.org/10.1007/978-3-319-99921-0_74

The department responsible for all internal transport at the hospital provides hygienic guidelines and training and control of personnel and reports to the Director in case of activities that may expose personnel or patients to infection.

Personnel follow guidelines for general infection protection, and report accidents or injuries that may expose patients or personnel to infection.

74.4 Practical Measures [1, 2]

74.4.1 Clean Equipment, Food and Other Clean Goods

- Perform hand hygiene and wear clean clothes.
- Check that the transport equipment is clean before transport.
- Check that clean goods are well covered with clean packaging.
- Do not transport clean and unclean goods together.
- Place clean goods as directed by the recipient but never in unclean rooms as a waste room or disinfection room.

74.4.2 Used, Unclean Equipment

- Used medical equipment, aids, etc.
- Used equipment to be transported must be cleaned/disinfected outside of the department before transport.
- Protection (gloves, etc.) during transport is not necessary if the equipment is cleaned.
- Wash hands well after finishing the transport.

74.4.3 Patient Samples

From the department/ward to different laboratories:

- The patient sample (tube, box, etc.) shall be clean *outside* and marked during transport.
- The sample must be transported in containers that can be cleaned with common disinfectants.
- Use disposable gloves when placing the sample in containers.
- Remove the glove and close the container.
- Carefully transport the sample to the receiver.
- Routines for cleaning and disinfection of transport containers are followed at the laboratory.

References

1. Syvrud EJ, Hochlin K, Andersen BM, Rasch M. Transport of clean and unclean equipment, textiles, samples and waste. In: Handbook in hygiene and infection control for hospitals. Oslo: Ullevål University Hospital; 2003. p. 442.
2. Brekke H, Hochlin K, Andersen BM, Rasch M. Transport of clean and unclean equipment, textiles, specimens and waste. In: Handbook for hygiene and infection control for hospitals. Oslo: Ullevål University Hospital; 2008. p. 624.

Ambulances, Emergency Medical Service (EMS) and Other Transports of Patients 75

Abstract

Ambulance personnel are often the first healthcare personnel who meet and take care of the patient in different situations outside the hospital. Patients may have unknown or known infections or carrier states like MRSA, other resistant microbes, blood-borne viruses or respiratory infections. Most often the infection status is not known. During epidemics of influenza or noroviruses, for example, the transport in ambulances may be challenging, concerning infection control. Very seldom, there may be questions about special dangerous infectious agents. Acute patient treatment during transport to hospitals, often require use of sterile or disinfected equipment. Good hygienic routines during work in ambulances are very important to prevent transmission of infections between patients and personnel. During the last 10–15 years, a number of guidelines have been provided for emergency medicines and other transports of patients with infection—both on land and in the air. The following chapter is focused on emergency and transport safety for patients and personnel to avoid transmittance of infections between patients, personnel and environment.

Keywords

Emergency medical service · EMS · Ambulances · Safety · Patient transport Infection control · Hygiene

75.1 Purpose

To avoid transmission of infections between patients and personnel during emergency medical service, transport/treatment and care [1–15].

B. M. Andersen, *Prevention and Control of Infections in Hospitals*,
https://doi.org/10.1007/978-3-319-99921-0_75

75.2 Comprise

All personnel involved in emergency medicine/transport system related to the hospital and patients treated in ambulances and other transport systems.

75.3 Responsibility

The hospital's management provides written procedures for hygiene and safety during transportation and emergency medical treatment [15]. Competent personnel and necessary resources for infection protection must be available.

The management of ambulances/emergency medicine/transport follows procedures for infection control, competence and quality, so that personnel, patients or the environment are not exposed unnecessary to infection [15]. The Director of the hospital is immediately informed if patients, personnel or others may be at risk of infection during this activity.

The management of clinical departments/outpatient clinics/nursing homes/healthcare centres, etc. shall provide information to ambulance personnel concerning patients with/suspected infections and infection control procedures and special measures to protect patients with increased susceptibility to infections.

Everyone involved in the emergency medicine/patient transport system follows guidelines and is educated in hygiene and infection control.

75.4 Practical Measures [11, 12, 14]

("Transport" here is meant emergency medical treatment/ambulances-car-flight-boat/patient transport.)

75.4.1 Ambulance Station, Other Locations and Service

- The ambulance station must have a laundry and decontamination area. Chemical disinfectants in liquid and in gas form should be used, if necessary [16–18].
- There should be separate, clean stores for textiles, sterile equipment, clean equipment and decontamination—and washing facilities for instruments—and access to packing and sterilization of instruments.
- Larger medical-technical equipment (ECG, heart starter, ventilator, etc.) that may extract dust and microbes from the ambulance's coupe is routinely sent to the medical-technical treatment centre for cleaning and disinfection of internal parts.

- Ward office must be clean. All floors and other surfaces in common areas, restrooms and toilet must be washed daily.
- Washing of work clothes and textiles should be carried out professionally as a routine at the hospital's textile department or at the approved laundry. Work clothes are changed after each shift or more frequently if contaminated, and there must be enough work clothes to ensure that this is carried out safely. *See textiles.*

75.4.2 General Infection Control Measures

- Hand hygiene before and after transporting/treating a patient.
- Working clothes should be clean, possibly clean gown outside of other work clothes.
- Transport of patients shall not present a risk to the person who treats the patient in the ambulance.
- All health units/levels should report infection risk when the ambulance is ordered.
- External ambulance transports are ordered via emergency centrals/transport/ambulance, etc., or otherwise in the local system.
- Avoid large storage of clean equipment and textiles in the ambulances, etc., which collect dust and microbes from patients and personnel in the ambulance.
- *Patient with (suspected) respiratory tract infection*: put a surgical mask on the patient and mask/cap on yourself.
- *Biological materials*: always wear single-use gloves when in contact with biological material, including injections, IV treatment and the like.
- *Respiratory system/intubation/suction*: use surgical mask/eye protection/cap/gloves, and change the gown/dress/uniform afterwards.
- *Trauma/acute wound treatment/stop bleeding,* etc.: use surgical mask/eye protection/cap/gloves and change the gown/dress/uniform afterwards.
- *Much spill of biological material during transport*: cover the patient (not head) with clean cloth/blanket, etc., as far as this does not inhibit observation and therapy!

75.4.3 Risk of Infection During Emergency Treatment

- Follow routines for using personal protection equipment and for safe donning and doffing.
- *Risk of infection*: the person who arranges the transport must be informed of any person who is exposed to and suspected for or has symptoms of infection. Follow the hospital's guidelines for transport, according to isolation regimes. See Chap. 47 on early measures to prevent spread of infections.

- Transport of patients with *increased susceptibility to infections* (placement of bed/stretcher, contact with other patients, etc.); follow current guidelines and notify to the ambulance unit. See Chap. 20 on protective isolation.
- Ambulance personnel/emergency medical personnel with severe respiratory tract infection, gastroenteritis or wounds on their hands, or other possible infectious diseases that can easily be transmitted, should not be in close contact with patients and clean goods. See Chap. 8 on personal hygiene and infection control.

75.4.4 Internal Transport Within the Hospital

Transporting the patient in bed and wheelchair, following and supporting a patient for examination or treatment, etc.:

- Hand hygiene before transport begins.
- The uniform must be clean. The work clothes often come into contact with the patient when lifting and other help.
- In case of infection, infection control measures should be informed by the responsible nurse at the patient's department/ward (see below).
- In case of protective isolation, the infection protection regime must be informed from the patient's department/ward.

75.4.5 External Transport Between Hospital Buildings

Transport of the patient in a stretcher, wheelchair or car; follow and support a patient for examinations, transfer to another department, treatment, etc.:

- Thoroughly clean the transport car—at least one time per week—and disinfect after transport of the patient with infection. Clean the wheelchair and stretcher before and after each transport.
- Do not use the patient transport car for transportation of unclean goods. If this is still necessary, wash the car thoroughly with soap and water before patient transport.
- When transporting an infected patient, the requester must provide the infection prevention regime to be used. The car is disinfected and washed inside after the transport of the patient with infection/potential infection according to the infection regime given by the department (see below).
- In case of protective isolation, the infection protection regime must be stated from the patient's department.

75.4.6 Ambulance, External Transport: Outside Hospital

Transport to and from the hospital in an ambulance stretcher, wheelchair or regular seat:

- The car is thoroughly cleaned with soap and water once a week.
- The car is disinfected and cleaned thoroughly after each transport in case of suspected infection.
- Depending on the amount of organic material spilled, such as blood, vomiting, etc., spot disinfection or complete disinfection and cleaning are performed (see below).
- When transporting an infected patient, the requester must provide the infection regime to be used. The car is disinfected inside after transport according to the infection regime specified by the department (see below).
- The infection regime may vary according to patient handling and activity.
- In case of protective isolation, the infection protection regime must be stated from the patient's department.

75.4.7 Ordinary Cleaning Routines of the Ambulance

75.4.7.1 Between Each Patient Transported on Stretcher

- The bed sheets, pillowcases and duvet covers are changed, and the stretcher cover/mattress is washed with soap and water.
- Carpet without cover is sent to wash after each use. Store in a clean room/bag before reuse.
- Pillows/duvets that are soiled by blood and tissue secretion and excretion are sent to the laundry. Keep it clean in the storage afterwards.
- The chair that the patient or staff has used is washed with soap and water (damp cloth) between each use.
- All medical equipment, laryngoscopes, etc., which have been used are sent for disinfection and/or sterilization. Clean equipment is placed in a clean suitcase/unit.
- Disinfect stethoscopes, blood pressure equipment and other items that have been used for the patient.
- Used equipment is placed in a separate unit—do not return in the medicine box together with clean equipment.
- Medical equipment that extracts air from the ambulance unit must be wiped over external parts and transmitted to disinfection of internal parts upon infection. *See Chap. 59 on disinfection of instruments and clean equipment.*
- The equipment/touch points of the patient during transport are washed with soap and water (damp cloth) on the surface, possibly disinfected.
- Disinfectant containers are disinfected outside if used several times (or single-use devices discarded afterwards are recommended).
- Waste containers are disposed as contaminated after each use.
- If work clothes are contaminated, change this before the next transport.
- Spill of small amounts of biological materials may be spot disinfected.

75.4.7.2 Routine Every Day

- Floors and fixtures in the ambulance are washed daily.
- Check the medication box for cleanliness, wipe over with a damp cloth and refill.
- Clean equipment is filled up.

75.4.7.3 Weekly

- Wash the entire ambulance outside and inside with soap and water.
- Medicine container and other containers for equipment are washed inside and outside, and equipment is being controlled.
- All wall-mounted equipment is washed with soap and water.
- Check that infection control equipment is available in the ambulance.
- Set up a wash and disinfection list with date.

75.4.7.4 Monthly

- All cabinets and drawers are cleaned and washed in addition to weekly wash.

75.4.8 Disinfection of the Ambulance

After transport of a patient with possible or defined infection:

- Wash hands thoroughly.
- Remove personal protective equipment (PPE) (surgical mask/cap/eye protection/gown and gloves) according to the defined isolation routine used.
- Learn to undress PPE without contaminating yourself or the environment.
- Change to clean uniform (clean gown/dress) and wash your hands again.

Follow isolation regimes. Depending on the degree of infection (spill, splash) and type of infection (contact, airborne, etc.), the car is thoroughly disinfected and cleaned.

- Contact transmission: spot disinfection or complete disinfection (spray, aerosols).
- Blood-borne pathogens: spot disinfections or complete disinfection (spray, aerosols).
- Airborne transmission: wash with soap and water and wipe over with 70% (+) alcohol.
- Strict isolation (high risk): complete disinfection and wash afterwards with soap and water. Contact infection control personnel for information.

75.4.8.1 Disinfection of the Car's Transport Compartment

Responsibility: *the* head of the department decides the level and extent of disinfection and the means to be used. *See also isolation regimes* Chaps. 14–21.

Procedure: the person who performs the disinfection procedure takes on:

- Surgical mask/eye protection/cap
- Shoe covers/special shoes/boots
- Gown/waterproof/coveralls
- Gloves with long cuff

1. In case of massive contamination, most of the stain is removed with absorbent material, packaged and treated as hazardous waste in yellow solid waste bag. A suitable disinfectant—chloramine 5%—is applied on contaminated surfaces/equipment with a cloth or sponge. Work time 60 min. Close the door. PeraSafe can also be used, working time 30 min.
2. Equipment used, cloths, etc. are packaged and treated as infectious.
3. Buckets, etc. are emptied and disinfected in the decontaminator in the disinfection room.
4. Stretcher is disinfected with the same agent.
5. Protective clothing is removed and packaged/treated as infectious.
6. At the end of the disinfection period, the contaminant is removed, and regular cleaning can be done.
7. The door is open for ventilation.

75.4.8.2 Spot Disinfection

- Limited blood spills and stains of biological material on the car's floor and other surfaces without known infectious hazard.
- Personnel who transport the patient carry out the spot disinfection immediately/as soon as possible in connection with the accident. It is only necessary to disinfect the area contaminated with biological material.

1. Spilled blood and other organic materials are removed with gloves and absorbent material, packaged and treated as hazardous waste.
2. A suitable disinfectant—chloramine 5%—is applied on contaminated surfaces/equipment with a cloth or sponge.
3. Acting—30 min (dried surface) or 60 min (dirty surface).

75.4.8.3 Gas-Mist Disinfection

Chemical gas disinfection of the ambulance before ordinary cleaning is a good disinfection method after transport of patient with a suspected or defined airborne infection, but not used with suspected tuberculosis or other mycobacteria [10, 16–18]. The use of a dry gas/mist of hydrogen peroxide 5% is effective and may be tolerated by corrosion-sensitive equipment [10, 16–18]. The process is defined in cycles, and spore test is used for control of effect on microbes. During the disinfection period, medical-technical instruments may be run to draw the gas through and disinfect the inner parts of the instruments [16–18]. All openings may be closed, and the disinfection may be done in a separate room. Concentration of the gas is recorded. Personnel is not entering the room before the concentration is 1 ppm or lower [16–18].

75.5 Background Information

Ambulance personnel are often the first healthcare personnel who meet and take care of the patient in different situations outside the hospital. Patient may have unknown or known infections or carrier states like MRSA, other resistant microbes, blood-borne viruses or respiratory infections. Most often the infection status is unknown [1–3]. Epidemics of influenza or noroviruses, for example, may be challenging concerning infection control during transport in ambulances. Very seldom, there may be questions about very dangerous infectious agents [4–9].

Organic material and microbes may easily be spread during transport/treatment in the small compartments of the ambulances, especially during a rapid and turbulent transport. Acute treatment during ambulance transport in high speed is a demanding work that may expose personnel and patients to infection if no infection protection is carried out [1–9]. Increasing incidence of dangerous microbes means that knowledge, expertise and resources must be on top [19–24]. Staff must be able to efficiently and easily carry out personal protection with appropriate equipment and ensure that ambulances, instruments and medical devices are cleaned in a proper and regular manner [2–12].

Transport of patient with possible infection

Type of infection (regime)	Infectious agents/disease	Personnel attire
Contact	All gastroenteritis (diarrhoea /vomiting)	H FM
	Hepatitis A (contagious jaundice)	HF
	Skin and wound infections, moderate secretion	HK FK
	Gram-negative rod bacteria with abundant	HK FK
	secretion from respiratory tract or wound	
	Untreated scab and lice	HF
	Other diseases that are spread by contact (e.g. tuberculosis in the intestines, urinary tract or fistula)	HF
Blood	HIV/AIDS uncomplicated	HK
	Hepatitis	HK FK
	Malaria falciparum, *Brucella*, yellow fever	HK FK

Type of infection (regime)	Infectious agents/disease	Personnel attire
Air borne	Pneumonia caused by *Staphylococcus aureus*	M
	Influenza, respiratory infection	M
	Systemic infection with meningococci, *Haemophilus influenzae*, pneumococci first 24 h after treatment starts (meningitis or septicaemia)	HFM
	MRSA (recently or during the past year)	HFM
	Import patient (from healthcare outside country)	HFM
	Other multidrug-resistant bacteria	HFM
	Widespread wounds, a lot of blood spills	HFM
	Widespread wound, skin infections—uncontrolled secretion	HFM
	Suspected infectious pulmonary tuberculosis	HFÅLS
	Known infection – Multidrug-resistant tuberculosis bacteria or—highly infectious tuberculosis with open cavity and expectoration (first 14 days after initiation of treatment, by resistance—longer time). Note: In case of suspicion, contact infection medicine/hospital hygiene/microbiologist *before* the transport	H FXÅLS
Strict isolation	Rare diseases (diphtheria, rabies, pest, anthrax, viral haemorrhagic fever, Ebola) Note: In case of suspicion *before* transport, contact infection medicine/hospital hygiene/microbiologist	Infection protection bag

H gloves, *HK* gloves on contact with the patient
F gown/coverall with hood, *FK* gown/coverall on contact with the patient
M surgical mask, *L* cap, *S* boot cover/special cover
FX bacterial/viral—impermeable/tight gown or coverall with hood
Å respiratory protection P3 (tight mask with hepafilter), or portable respirator (see also "Respiratory protection" Chap. 13, and "Isolation" Chaps. 14–21)
Infection protection bag (for two or more persons): respiratory protection P3 and bacterial/viral impermeable gown, tight goggles, shoe cover and gloves. Instructions for doffing after use are enclosed. This bag should be in preparedness, only used after consultation with departments of infectious disease/infection control/microbiologist. See strict isolation Chap. 19

Patient transport *internally* in hospitals—*to and from*—and *between* hospitals and other institutions increases and can pose a risk of spread of infections [19]. Ambulances may be infected with microbiological agents such as MRSA in *endemic* areas with high levels of MRSA, as shown in England [20]. Among the 21 ambulances tested for MRSA in June 2006, 10 were MRSA positive. In one ambulance, the steering wheel was MRSA positive, and the rest of the positive MRSA samples were found in the patient compartment around handles, etc. [20] A number of other microbes can also live long in the ambulance environment [22–24].

The ambulance coupé is small and narrow and poorly ventilated. The patient comes in close contact with the equipment and personnel when lifting and handling the stretcher or bed.

When arriving at the hospital, the placement of patients in the waiting area must be well planned for both suspected infected patients and patients especially susceptible to infection. Personnel transporting patients should obtain information about current measures.

References

1. CDC Severe Acute Respiratory Syndrome. Infection control in healthcare, home, and community settings. IV Infection control for prehospital emergency medical services. CDC; 8 Jan 2004.
2. Centres for Disease Control and Prevention. Guidelines for the protection of the safety and health of health care workers. CDC; 2007.
3. MCHC. Infection prevention and control guidance for EMS providers. Metropolitan Chicago Healthcare Council; 2012.
4. APIC Implementation Guide. Guide to infection prevention in emergency medical services. APIC; 2013.
5. Interim Guidance for Emergency Medical Services (EMS) systems and 9-1-1 Public Safety Response Points (PSAPs) for Management of Patients Under Investigation (PUIs) for Ebola Virus Disease (EVD) in the United States. Updated: 10 Sep 2015.
6. Guidance on Personal Protective Equipment (PPE) to be used by Healthcare Workers during Management of Patients with Confirmed Ebola or Persons under Investigation (PUIs) for Ebola who are Clinically Unstable or Have Bleeding, Vomiting, or Diarrhea in US Hospitals, Including Procedures for Donning and Doffing PPE. CDC; Aug 2015.
7. WHO. WHO technical advice for case management of influenza A (H1N1) in air transport. Geneva: WHO; 2009.
8. Andersen BM. Microbiology and infection protection. In: Handbook in hygiene and infection control, part 1. Oslo: Fagbokforlaget; 2014.
9. Andersen BM. Infection control guidelines for Ebola. HospitalHealthcare.com; 2015. p. 26–8.
10. Rutala WA, Weber DJ. Disinfection, sterilization, and control of hospital waste. In: Mandell, Douglas, and Bennets principles and practice of infectious diseases, vol. 2. 8th ed. Philadelphia: Elsevier Churchill Livingstone; 2015. p. 3294–309.
11. Madsen P, Syvrud EJ, Hochlin K, Andersen BM. Ambulance and other transport of patients. In: Handbook in hygiene and infection control for hospitals. Oslo: Ullevål University Hospital; 2003. p. 435–41.
12. Karr B, Hochlin K, Andersen BM, Brekke H. Ambulance and other transport of patients. In: Handbook in hygiene and infection control for hospitals. Oslo: Ullevål University Hospital; 2008. p. 618–23.
13. CDC. Infection control guidelines for cabin crew members on commercial aircraft. CDC; 2015.
14. Andersen BM. Transport and admittance of patients between hospitals and nursing homes. In: Handbook in hygiene and infection control for nursing Homes and long-time care institutions. Oslo: Akademika; 2013. p. 411–4.
15. Department of Labour and Administration. Regulations on protection against exposure to biological agents (bacteria, viruses, fungi and more) in the workplace. FOR OSLO: 1997-12-19 nr.1322.
16. Andersen BM, Rasch M, Hochlin K, Jensen JF, Wismar P, Fredriksen JE. Decontamination of rooms, medical equipment and ambulances, using a dry fog or hydrogen peroxide disinfectant. J Hosp Infect. 2006;62:149–55.
17. Andersen BM, Syversen G, Thoresen H, Rasch M, Hochlin K, Seljordslia B, Snevold I, Berg E. Failure of dry fog or hydrogen peroxide 5% to kill *Mycobacterium tuberculosis*. J Hosp Infect. 2010;76:80–3.
18. Andersen BM, Hochlin K, Daling JP. Cleaning and decontamination of reusable medical devices, including the use of hydrogen peroxide dry-fog gas decontamination. J Microbiol Biochem Technol. 2012;4:57–62.
19. Eveillard M, Quenon JL, Rufat P, Mangeol A, Fauvelle F. Association between hospital-acquired infections and patient transfers. Infect Control Hosp Epidemiol. 2001;22:693–6.
20. BBC news. Dirty ambulances infection fear. 2007/11/26 07:37:37 GMT.
21. Schneider J. Ambulance transports. Fire Chief; 1 Mar 2008.

22. Petsas A, Sharma A, Aghadiou O, Abid M, Paranthaman K. A secondary case of meningococcal disease in an ambulance worker, Berkshire, November 2007. Euro Surveill. 2008;13:4.
23. Roline CE, Crumpecker C, Dunn TM. Can methicillin-resistant *Staphylococcus aureus* be found in an ambulance fleet? Prehosp Emerg Care. 2007;11:241–4.
24. News-Medical.Net. Ambulance-weak link in the fight against MRSA. http://www.unison.org.uk.

Part XIII

Hospitals: Areal and Function

Hospital Buildings—Construction Projects

76

Abstract
The development of more advanced medicine and breaking new borders in treatment of serious illnesses may involve poorer and more helpless patients in the hospitals. They will need more personal help with everything and are more bedridden and exposed to infections. Those who are in a better shape will probably be day-treatment patients at the hospital, staying at patient hotels, nursing homes, other homes or at home. The future probably also leads to more resistant and contagious microbes and less effect of antimicrobial agents. Therefore, the hospital buildings, construction, outfit, design and maintenance, are very central elements in the management of modern hospitals with increasing risk of transmitting nosocomial infections. New hospitals, buildings, rebuilding, changed functions and logistic solutions may be well planned and considered thoroughly. Special focus may be placed on effective infection control measures like enough patient beds, single patient rooms and service rooms, design and quality of furniture and the implementation of effective, safe and good hygiene.

Keywords
Hospital buildings · New and rebuilding · Function · Construction · Design Capacity · Logistics · Maintenance · Nosocomial infections · Infection control Hygiene

76.1 Purpose

Prevent hospital infections by ensuring key infection-preventive principles when building new hospitals, upgrading hospital buildings/areas and rebuilding hospital units for other medical use.

B. M. Andersen, *Prevention and Control of Infections in Hospitals*,
https://doi.org/10.1007/978-3-319-99921-0_76

76.2 Comprise

- Infection control competence and local user representations should be included in all plans and implementation of new buildings and changes in use at hospitals.
- This includes current plan solutions, logistics and building quality, aiming at a satisfactory user-friendliness and fulfilments of hygiene requirements and of protection for employees and patients.
- This includes conditions around patients, family and staff located in patient hotels associated with and used by hospitals.

76.3 Responsibility

The granting authority and hospital management provide resources for construction and maintenance that is expected in modern hospital activity. Included are safe conditions for patients, personnel and visitors and a safe working environment. Physical conditions and logistics may not expose patients, employees or visitors to infection [1].

Construction manager/project manager, etc. are responsible for ensuring that all important professional groups are consulted and that long-term, good and flexible solutions are in front of short-term ad hoc solutions.

Architect, user groups, entrepreneurs, etc. shall ensure solutions tailored to the department's needs, requirements for quality of work and materials, requirement of a complete construction budget and plan for annual maintenance costs.

Infection control personnel should attend from the beginning, during the planning phase, the project phase and the implementation phase, to ensure that new buildings, rebuilding and change of use satisfy the requirements for infection protection for patients, visitors and personnel at the hospital [1].

76.4 Practical Measures [2]

- *Hand hygiene*. Access to good hand hygiene in all patient areas. Hand hygiene should be offered to everyone at the entrance of the patient room, at the main entrance, in the elevator, etc. It reduces the spread of infectious microbes. Electronic handwashing is not recommended due to the risk of growth of gram-negative, resistant bacteria and *Legionella* [3].
- *Telephone/computer systems* should not constitute a common source of infection in the environment—between patients, personnel and visitors.
- *Toilet/shower/bathroom* attached to each patient room significantly reduces cross-transmission of microbes. It avoids repeated outbreaks of norovirus, *Clostridium difficile* and other agents. The bathroom should be handicap-designed with plenty of space for a healthcare worker who can help the patient without the risk of being contaminated. The room should not be used by other

patients or visitors. Establishing a throughput decontaminator from the bathroom to the sluice/anteroom may be evaluated.

- *Patient rooms.* Free area around the patient's bed with work access from both sides and at the bed end. There should be at least 2 m clearance on both sides of the bed and at the foot (5 × 4 m) and in addition 2 m clearance from the sink. This is necessary for the use of walking chairs and wheelchairs and effective care of heavy, severely ill patients. The bed should be taken in and out of the room without damaging walls and doors and without contaminating the surroundings.
  - *Good space* simplifies and improves the working environment, increases patient well-being and air volume and reduces patient-to-person transmission of infection. Each patient needs an area of at least 20 m^2 and a separate toilet/shower with entrance from the patient's room.
  - Curtains, rails in the ceiling, etc. must be removed; it collects dust.
- *Single rooms* should replace all double- and multibed rooms in all new buildings. Studies show that single rooms have so many benefits in terms of patient satisfaction, patient safety, privacy, visitor friendliness, silence, efficiency and infection protection and that establishment of such rooms is considered to be cost-effective for hospital operations.
- *Anterooms or sluices* associated with a regular single room are an advantage for visitors to hang out outerwear and wash hands before and after visits and for use with contact or protective isolation.
- *Automatic, silent door opener* for patient rooms will streamline work and prevent cross-contamination.
- *Large, practical and separate service room* in the ward (15–20 beds) for clean textiles (16 m^2), sterile equipment (16 m^2), clean equipment (16 m^2), disinfection room (18–20 m^2), medicine room (14–16 m^2), large equipment (wheelchairs, crutches, etc.) (10–12 m^2) and waste room (10 m^2).
  - Service rooms are arranged in such a way that those who work there do not come too close to the walls and equipment in the room. In a good work area, cross-contamination in the service room is reduced.
  - *Service room properly placed* in relation to patient's rooms and personnel. Adjusted smaller service rooms with little walking distance for the personnel can be most effective. Also smaller service rooms should have ample area for those working there. For a regular ward of 15–20 beds, each such room should have an area of approx. 16 m^2.
- *Treatment rooms and examination rooms*: minimum of 16 m^2.
- *Conference room for 2–3 persons*: approx. 12 m^2.
- *Paper office without patient*: 6–9 m^2.
- *Toilet for personnel*: 3 m, minimum of 1 per 7–14 employees present.
- *Kitchen and disinfection room/cleaning room*—see separate chapters.
- *Stock for sterile equipment*—see separate chapter.
- *Meeting rooms and ward office* adapted to the fixed number of staff during the daytime. Today's ward office is often small, crowded and tidy with many open shelves that collect dust and dirt. There is a great need for access to data and for daily cleaning and more often disinfection of computer keyboard. It should be

facilitated for more good work places and for proper storage of records, other paper and equipment. There should be plenty of room for hand washing and preferably automatic disinfection of hands at the entrance. Do not eat and drink while dealing with patient data due to the risk of cross-contamination (keyboard, journal, etc.).

- *Furniture for patient and visitor* should not be of textile and should be washable, cleaned daily and disinfected regularly.
- *Floors, walls, ceilings and fixtures* should be of good quality, easily washable and robust against daily cleaning and frequent use of disinfectants. The surfaces should be whole and shiny and do not form the basis for microbes. There should not be tiled floors, and floors should be cleaned easily without loosening of the covering. It is recommended to use the floor coverings a little up on the wall to avoid loose mouldings and facilitate cleaning.
- *The ceiling* should be completely robust and slippery and easy to clean without loosening of ceiling panels and without openings for repairs and the like.
- *Light fixture* collects dust and microbes and for that reason should lie evenly with the ceiling, covered with glass.
- *Corridors, wet rooms (toilet, shower, disinfection room,* etc.*) and patient rooms* are especially exposed to contamination of larger amounts of organic materials (excretes, leftovers, etc.) with growth of microbes. This causes bad odour and reduces well-being for both employees and patients and is a contagion in the environment. These areas should have daily cleaning, preferably twice daily, dependent on activity and situation, and must withstand frequent use of disinfectants.
- *Water systems must satisfy monthly* quality controls with regard to germ numbers and particularly unfortunate water bacteria such as *Legionella* and *Pseudomonas.*
- *Ventilation systems* should be checked annually and protected from growth of microbes in water and condense microbes, such as Legionella, gram-negative bacteria and fungi.
- *Cooling and heating of rooms* should not be done by local room systems that are quickly filled with dust and condensation and thus constitute a risk of airborne infection in the room.
- *Ventilation of patient rooms* and other rooms should ensure at least 6–12 fresh air exchanges every hour. This reduces the amount of air contamination in the room by dilution and increases personal well-being.
- *Negative air pressure should be present in waste rooms, disinfection rooms, unclean rooms (toilets* etc.*) and all isolates* for infections so that microbial agents are not spread by air to other rooms. Doors must turn right ways so that the negative pressure is not impaired.
- *Isolation units for infectious patients* should be available in all patient departments and must have negative air pressure and separate ventilation with hepafiltered air exhaust. Contact isolation should preferably be at minus 5–10 pascal negative pressure, while isolates for airborne infections should be at least 25–45 pascal negative pressure. It is an advantage that all isolates get direct access from outside via sluice. See Chaps. 14–21 on isolation regimes.
- *Operation rooms*—see the operation department.

- *Intensive care and postoperative*—see the intensive care unit.
- *Patient logistics* should be facilitated so that the patient is not moved between departments.
- *Flexible solutions*. New building and rebuilding must be carried out in such a way that later change in usage (different specialities) is reasonable and easy to implement.
- *Redecorating* floors, walls and fixtures every 5–7 years should be included in a maintenance plan for the department.

76.5 Background Information

The development of more advanced medicine and breaking new borders in treatment of serious illnesses may involve poorer and more helpless patients in the hospitals. They will need more personal help with everything and are more bedridden and exposed to infections. Those who are in a better shape will probably be day-treatment patients at the hospital, staying at patient hotels, nursing homes, other homes or at home. The future probably also leads to more resistant and contagious microbes and less effect of antimicrobial agents. Therefore, the hospital buildings, construction, outfit, design and maintenance, are very central elements in the management of modern hospitals with increasing risk of transmitting nosocomial infections. New hospitals, buildings, rebuilding, changed functions and logistic solutions may be well planned and considered thoroughly. Special focus may be placed on effective infection control measures like enough patient beds, single patient rooms and service rooms, design and quality of furniture and the implementation of effective, safe and good hygiene [4–14].

76.5.1 Single Room and Area for Patients and Visitors

Modern hospital research has shown an increasing need of area for patients in hospitals. An international study from 2007 of 18 hospitals demonstrated higher activity and shorter hospital stay—from 7 days in 1990 to 3.5 days in 2003 [15]. At the same time, the area per patient has increased in patient wards (not intensive) from 25 to 35 m^2 per bed from 1990, and the entire hospital department area has increased from 60 to over 90 m^2 per bed in 2003, i.e. a total increase of the area of 25% [15].

However, many hospitals having the same total area as 50 years ago still are putting more and more patients in the same room, using more and more rooms for offices and administration and producing overbooked and understaffed hospitals with even higher risk of infection and other patient accidents, than before.

The following advantages are documented for *single room* compared to *two-bed rooms* (and dormitory) [5–23]:

- Reduction of hospital infections.
- Less risk of transmitting infections to roommate [5–14].

- Reduced fall injuries.
- Fewer transfers and medical errors.
- Less cost of transfer.
- Less noise.
- Better sleep quality.
- Better communication with personnel.
- Greater patient discretion, privacy and security for the patient.
- Greater patient satisfaction (very big difference).
- Less costs with regard to daily operations—better utilized room.
- Greater flexibility and ability to fill capacity—especially in medical departments.
- More satisfaction for personnel, nurses and doctors.
- Better conditions around student education.
- Efficiency of personnel.
- Flexibility in hospital planning and change of function.
- Reduced operating costs in the long term due to reduced number of hospital infections. The rooms are easier to clean; there is a shorter patient stay; there is a better compliance with health and safety, etc.; and there is a more flexible use of single rooms—even compared to a four-bed patient room.
- Greater initial construction costs on the other side.

76.5.2 Infections

Twenty to thirty percent of hospital patients have infections, hospital-onset or nonhospital-onset infections, and are given antibiotics while they are hospitalized [24, 25]. Today an increase of resistant bacteria is observed like MRSA and resistant gram-negative bacteria (ESBL, CRE and others) and VRE. *Clostridium difficile* (CD) has changed to become a more serious, dangerous, resistant bacterium, developing chronic diarrhoea with kidney injury, especially in patients with increased susceptibility to infections and on antibiotics. CD spores live for years in the environment if not removed. Outbreaks of gastrointestinal infections are increasing where many or all departments must close for the intake of new patients (see gastrointestinal infections). Norovirus and other gastrointestinal viruses like sapovirus and rotavirus are highly contagious and return year after year and inactivate a significant part of health-related work at hospitals. Influenza and respiratory syncytial virus (RSV) is an annual phenomenon and an increasing global challenge. Common influenza is easily spread in institutions and vaccines do not prevent infection. Modern water and ventilation systems may spread *Legionella and other waterborne bacteria* in health institutions, unless preventive measures are included in building plans.

Emergency preparedness for serious epidemics or accidents with dangerous materials should be developed at all hospitals, not least at the functional level. How a serious lethal epidemic will spread can be demonstrated by the large and inactivating norovirus epidemics that are spread "like fire in dry grass" at older, nonfunctional hospitals.

The hospitalized patient should not be exposed to infection. Also personnel and visitors should be protected against infections in hospitals. The ethical standard around the patient's stay in hospitals is central, concerning hospital infections.

References

1. Ministry of Labor and Administration. Regulations on protection against exposure to biological factors (bacteria, viruses, fungi and more) in the workplace. FOR OSLO: 1997-12-19 nr.1322.
2. Andersen BM. Planning of hospital buildings, reconstruction and change of use. In: Handbook in hygiene and infection control for hospitals. Oslo: Ullevål University Hospital; 2008. p. 654–9.
3. Charron D, Bedard E, Lalancette C, Laferriere C, Prevost M. Impact of electronic faucets and water quality on the occurrence of *Pseudomonas aeruginosa* in water: a multi-hospital study. Infect Control Hosp Epidemiol. 2015;36:311–9.
4. Rutala WA, Weber DJ. Disinfection, sterilization, and control of hospital waste. In: Mandell, Douglas, and Bennets principles and practice of infectious diseases, vol. 2. 8th ed. Philadelphia: Elsevier Churchill Livingstone; 2015. p. 3294–309.
5. Lemmen SW, Hafner H, Zolldann D, Stanzel S, Lutticken R. Distribution of multi-resistant gram-negative versus gram-positive bacteria in the hospital inanimate environment. J Hosp Infect. 2004;56:191–7.
6. Kramer A, Schebke I, Kampf G. How long do nosocomial pathogens persist on the surfaces? A systematic review. BMC Infect Dis. 2006;6:130–8.
7. Yezli S, Otter JA. Minimum infective dose of the major human respiratory and enteric viruses transmitted through food and the environment. Food Environ Microbiol. 2011;3:1–30.
8. Shiomori T, Miyamoto H, Makishima K, Yoshida M, Fujiyoshi T, Udaka T, et al. Evaluation of bed-related airborne and surface methicillin-resistant *Staphylococcus aureus* contamination. J Hosp Infect. 2002;50:30–5.
9. Hamel M, Zoutman D, O'Callaghan C. Exposure to hospital roommates as a risk factor for healthcare-related infection. Am J Infect Control. 2010;38:173–81.
10. Nseir S, Blazejewski C, Lubret R, Wallet F, Courco F, Durocher A. Risk of acquiring multidrug resistant gram-negative bacilli from previous occupants in the intensive care unit. Clin Microbiol Infect. 2011;17:1201–8.
11. Bernard MC, Lanotte P, Lawrence C, Goudeau A, Bernard L. Air contamination around patients colonized with multidrug resistant organisms. Infect Control Hosp Epidemiol. 2012;33:949–51.
12. D'Agata EMC, Venkataraman L, DeGirolami P, Samore M. Molecular epidemiology or ceftazidime-resistant gram-negative bacilli on inanimate surfaces and their role in cross-transmission during nonoutbreak periods. J Clin Microbiol. 1999;37:3065–7.
13. Catalano M, Quelle LS, Jeric PE, Di Martino A, Maimone SM. Survival of *Acinetobacter baumannii* on bed rails during an outbreak and during sporadic cases. J Hosp Infect. 1999;42:27–35.
14. French GL, Otter JA, Shannon KP, Adams NMT, Watling D, Parks MJ. Tackling contamination of the hospital environment by methicillin-resistant *Staphylococcus aureus* (MRSA): a comparison between conventional terminal cleaning and hydrogen peroxide vapor decontamination. J Hosp Infect. 2004;57:31–7.
15. Leach J. Health planning: within your means, 4 Jan 2007. Hospital Development, Aug 2007.
16. Feachem R, Sekhri N, White K. Getting more for their dollar: a comparison of the NHS with California's Kaiser Permanente. BMJ. 2002;324:135–43.
17. Phiri M. One patient room - theory and practice: an evaluation of the Leeds Nuffield Hospital. NHS Estates, January 2004.

18. Ulrich RS. Healthcare design.03. How single versus double patient rooms affect medical outcomes. Texas A & M University. Center for Health Systems and Design; 2007.
19. NHS Confederation. Future proofing buildings for healthcare, 9 June 2005.
20. NHS Estates. Ward layouts with single rooms and space for flexibility. Discussion document. Evidence of evidence, 1 Feb 2005.
21. Winning ways: working together to reduce healthcare related infection in England. Department of Health; 2003.
22. Behrendt MD. Single rooms: the perspective of infection prevention. Infection Control Unit, Dep With Microbiol and Infect Dis, Erasmus MC, Rotterdam (unpublished).
23. Herr CEW, Heckrodt TH, Hofmann FA, Schnettler R, Eikmann F. Additional costs for preventing spread of methicillin-resistant *Staphylococcus aureus* and a strategy for reducing these costs on a surgical ward. Infect Control Hosp Epidemiol. 2003;24:9.
24. Andersen BM, Holta Ringertz S, Gullord Petersen T, Hermansen W, Lelek M, Norman BI, Næs B, Tilrem Nystad M, Andersen Rød K, Røed RT, Solheim N, Smidesand IJ, Tandberg S, Halsnes R, Høystad MW. A three-year survey of nosocomial and community-acquired infections, antibiotic treatment and re-hospitalization in a Norwegian health region. J Hosp Infect. 2000;44:214–23.
25. Andersen BM, Andersen BM, Rasch M, Hochlin K, Tollefsen T, Sandvik L. Hospital-acquired infections before and after healthcare reorganization in a tertiary university hospital in Norway. J Public Health. 2009;7:1–7.

Hospital Kitchen

77

Abstract

In the hospital kitchens, food and drink are stored especially for providing food between meal times, for patients under examination/treatment when regular food service is in progress and for patients with poor appetite/special food, etc. Food and beverages are well-known vehicles for the spread of infectious diseases in hospitals. The following chapter is focused on areal and outfits of hospital kitchens to avoid transmittance of infections between patients, personnel and environment.

Keywords

Hospital kitchen · Food and beverage · Building and outfit · Infection control Hygiene

77.1 Purpose

Protect patients, staff, visitors and the environment from infections by establishing a hygienic and well-outfitted kitchen for patients [1–6].

77.2 Comprise

Personnel who works in the kitchen or supplies goods, food, etc. to and from the kitchen and includes all types of serving, dishwashing, cleaning and cooking.

B. M. Andersen, *Prevention and Control of Infections in Hospitals*,
https://doi.org/10.1007/978-3-319-99921-0_77

77.3 Responsibility

The hospital management shall provide hygienic guidelines regarding the serving of food and drink to the patients and for all food services to be carried out in accordance with the country's Food Safety Authority's guidelines (like in Norway) [1–6].

The department's management is responsible for the training and controlling of good kitchen hygiene.

Staff working with foodstuffs should follow guidelines regarding personal and general hygiene.

77.4 Practical Measures [7, 8]

Hand hygiene is a prerequisite before and after handling food and beverages. The post kitchen must have a good sink.

Clean equipment and clean storage for equipment. The post kitchen should be spacious with clear distinction between clean and unclean (used) equipment.

Dishwasher that at least reaches 85 °C in the goods during the washing process. No open washing process in the kitchen area that creates splashes and aerosols and spreads contaminants.

Clean plates, cups, glasses and cutlery should be stored in a clean cupboard with a door, not near a dishwasher or unclean equipment.

Standard for post kitchen (on a ward) with serving food on a tray to each patient

Methods for serving heated food vary and must be set according to local conditions and needs.

77.4.1 Kitchen Area

A minimum of 16 m^2 areal is necessary for a post kitchen to serve a regular bed post (ward) with 15–20 patients.

77.4.2 Function of the Kitchen

- The food is brought on separate trays or in bulks from the central kitchen.
- Storage of beverages and dry foods such as biscuits, soups, tea, coffee, etc., for patients who need food and drink. The storage needs plenty of space in cupboard with clear glass doors in the kitchen.
- Storing a limited amount of cutlery and crockery and various kitchen utensils. Equipment needed for extra serving may be cleaned at the kitchen in a closed dishwasher.
- All used dinnerware, plates, etc. are sent back to the central kitchen in separate transport trolleys or other local solutions.

77.4.3 Furnishings

- *The bench space* should be shared in *clean and unclean zones*—plenty of space.
- *Unclean zone* should have a *dishwasher* (min. 85 °C for 5–10 min).
- *Sink unit* with long touchless arm.
- *Washbasin* with falling height on the water not exceeding 30 cm. Hot water should be at least 75 °C, after a few minutes. Check with thermometer a few times a year.
- Do not use electronic wash at fixed temperature; there is a risk of increased growth of gram-negative bacteria like *Pseudomonas aeruginosa* and *Legionella* due to low temperature [9–13].
- Hand disinfectants, preferably automatic dispenser.
- Separate washbasin with large washroom—optionally two, depending on the need for use, 50 × 40 cm, and a depth of 15 cm. The hot water should be at least 75 °C, after a few minutes [9–13].
- Waste rack with pedal lock.
- Lockable cabinet for storage of detergents.
- Space for transport trolleys that may return to the central kitchen. Local solutions.
- Clean zone with stove and bench space on both sides. Cabinets/drawers are easy to keep clean.
- Adequate refrigerator, preferably two, to relieve temperature changes; minimum 4 L per person per day, with freezing facilities.
- Good space for microwave.
- Ice machine should be on the clean side, easily accessible for cleaning of the inner and outer parts, and a good distance of 50 cm for other equipment on both sides.
- Space for storage of clean transport trolley for food.
- Room for refrigerator for employees.

77.4.4 Surfaces

- *Unclean side:* Continuous stainless steel worktop and edge to the wall.
- *Clean side:* Worktop of durable, water resistant, smooth surface (laminate) that can withstand satisfactory cleaning and which is not made of wood material.
- Cabinets and drawers should have a smooth surface, laminated or painted with min. gloss 20.
- Floors should have a durable surface (high quality) and be waterproof and easy to clean, for example, vinyl with vinyl hole lists, 75 mm on the wall, glued with contact adhesive.
- Walls should be smooth, water repellent and easy to keep clean. Painted surfaces must have minimum gloss 20 (acryl proof 20). If "reinforcement" is required due to the nature of the wall, glass fibre cloth must be used. Over the benches there should be suitable tiles on the wall, good standard 15 × 15 cm with smooth epoxy

joints. Use of moving joints should be used with polyurethane with good adhesion and which contain fungicides. Optional vinyl coating over kitchen bench.
- Roofs should be constructed with a minimum of potential for dust and impurities accumulation. Painted ceiling must have a minimum of shine 20 (acrylic).

77.4.5 Traffic

- The kitchen should not be used as a thoroughfare room. Wide door, if possible, turns out into the corridor.
- The post kitchen is placed as centrally as possible in relation to the bed rooms. Daylight if possible and a good working light.
- Patients, relatives and others have no access to the kitchen.
- See also the health institution's food procedures.

77.5 Background Information

At the kitchen, food and drink are stored especially for patients under examination/treatment when regular food service is in progress and for patients with poor appetite/special food, etc. Ice cubes from a contaminated ice machine can be a source of infection in the environment.

Dishwashers at post kitchen shall meet the requirements for hot water, >85 °C, and hot water from sink must have a temperature of 75 °C or higher. This is to avoid heat-resistant microbes, biofilm formation and growth of legionella and gram-negative environmental bacteria such as *Pseudomonas aeruginosa* [9–13] (*see also* Chap. 70).

References

1. Nutrition hygiene regulations. November 12, 1997, no. 1239, Oslo.
2. The large kitchen project 1997. Environmental Protection Agency and food Safety Agency. Oslo Municipality; 1997.
3. Regulations for hygiene and foodstuffs of 8 July 1983, no. 1253, Oslo.
4. Operating conditions in food business. NMT info D1 17.11.1995, Oslo.
5. Approval of food business. NMT info G1 30.05.1995, Oslo.
6. Premises, décor and equipment in food business. NMT info L1. 09/29/1995, Oslo.
7. Laugerud F, Akre O, Arnesen V, Solheim N, Andersen M. Postkitchen interior design and use. In: Handbook in hygiene and infection control for hospitals. Oslo: Ullevål University Hospital; 2003. p. 466–9.
8. Akre O, Arnesen V, Rasch M, Andersen BM, Laugerud F. Postkitchen - interior design and use. In: Handbook in hygiene and infection control for hospitals. Oslo: Ullevål University Hospital; 2008. p. 646–9.
9. Charron D, Bedard E, Lalancette C, Laferriere C, Prevost M. Impact of electronic faucets and water quality on the occurrence of *Pseudomonas aeruginosa* in water: a multi-hospital study. Infect Control Hosp Epidemiol. 2015;36:311–9.

10. Moore G, Walker J. Presence and control of *Legionella pneumophilia* and *Pseudomonas aeruginosa* biofilms in hospital water systems. In: Percival SL, Williams DW, Randle J, Coioper T, editors. Biofilms in infection prevention and control. Boston: Academic; 2014. p. 311–37.
11. Assadian O, El-Madani N, Seper E, et al. Sensor-operated faucets: a possible source of nosocomial infection? Infect Control Hosp Epidemiol. 2002;23:44–6.
12. Andersen BM. Gramnegative rod bacteria in the intestine and/or environment. In: Microbiology and infection protection. Handbook in hygiene and infection protection part 1. Norway: Fagbokforlaget; 2014. p. 85–94.
13. Andersen BM. Legionella. In: Microbiology and infection protection. Handbook in hygiene and infection control part 1. Norway: Fagbokforlaget; 2014. p. 116–9.

78 Disinfection Room: Cleaning Room

Abstract

The disinfection room is central to all operations and is a multifunctional room. Here, all contaminants and organic materials are taken care of and removed. Contaminated textiles are sorted and ordinary waste from infectious waste. Used syringes and other stabbing/cutting waste, glass, etc. are collected as hazardous waste. Used wheelchairs and other major patient aids are usually washed here. The bedpan, urine bottles, etc. are disinfected in the decontaminator. The room has a large load of dirt and microbial agents where the personnel may perform many space-demanding tasks. A large and efficient area with good separation between clean and unclean work tasks, good ventilation and negative pressure ventilation and good methods for cleaning and disinfection are necessary. The following chapter is focused on areal and outfit of the disinfection room to avoid transmittance of infections between patients, personal and environment.

Keywords

Disinfection room · Waste room · Used equipment · Decontaminator · Instrument washing-machine · Bedpans · Urine bottles

78.1 Purpose

To protect patients, personnel and the environment against infection [1–4].

78.2 Comprise

All staff who use the disinfection room. All equipment, textiles, waste, etc., which are treated/stored/collected and sorted in the disinfection room.

B. M. Andersen, *Prevention and Control of Infections in Hospitals*,
https://doi.org/10.1007/978-3-319-99921-0_78

78.3 Responsibility

The hospital's management ensures that disinfection rooms are adapted to the function and patient beds of the individual department. The disinfection unit may, according to area, outfit, structure and routines, protect personnel, patients and environment against infections [1]. Written procedures for work and control in disinfection rooms shall be available.

The department's management complies with hygienic guidelines, ensures that staff are educated and reports to the director if the disinfection system may present a risk to patients and personnel.

The personnel follow guidelines for personal and general hygiene and procedures for the disinfection room.

78.4 Practical Measures [5, 6]

78.4.1 Location, Size and Design of the Disinfection Room

- The disinfection room must be easily accessible, centrally located in the department/ward and with direct access from the corridor. Do not throughput to the corridor because of the fire department's rules.
- The disinfection room must have a negative air pressure so that airborne contaminants are kept mostly within the room. Keep the door closed. Keep all throughput openings closed. The ventilation should be good, at least 8 fresh air exchanges/hour.
- Separate extracts/hoods may be established if using special chemical disinfectants.
- Large enough area for the department/patient beds activities; at least 3 m between clean and unclean sides (due to splash and aerosol formation). The area required is usually 18–20 m [2]. The work must be carried out efficiently and risk-free even if the doors to the decontaminator are opened.
- Floors and walls must withstand strong disinfectants and frequent cleaning.
- Drain in the floor may be correct.
- There should be a large enough area for cleaning of wheelchairs, aids, etc., if the hospital does not have a separate cleaning facility or system for large equipment between patients.
- The disinfection unit may have its own clean storage room for cleaned and ready-to-use bedpans, urine bottles, flower glasses, cleaned walking chairs and other noncritical aids. This store room should **not** be used for clean textiles, sterile equipment, etc.!

78.4.2 Equipment and Fixtures

- Sink with single-grip battery and with long touchless arm.
- There should be plenty of space for one to two machines (decontaminator, instrument washing machine) with the position of the soap system well above the floor.

The area requirement for machines may be approximately 4–6 m [2]. It should be easy to carry out cleaning around/under the machines.

- Hand washbasin with soap and hand disinfectant at the door with plenty of space for washing and tiled wall down to the floor. Fall height of the water should not exceed 30 cm (avoid splash).
- The hot water should be at least 75 °C, after a few minutes. Check with thermometer a few times a year. Discuss the use of electronic wash at fixed temperature because of risk of increased growth of gram-negative bacteria such as *Pseudomonas aeruginosa* and *legionella* due to low temperature [7–11].
- Hand disinfectants, preferably automatic dispenser.
- Collecting racks for laundry, waste, special waste, etc. (unclean side)—area requirement approximately6 m [2]. Racks with pedal lock.
- Benches for unloading equipment for clean and unclean side.
- Separate washbasin with large rinsing basin—possibly two, depending on usage needs and other benches for storage.
- Throughput closet for optional drying after wash in a drying cabinet. Note that the doors in the drying cabinet must not stand open! In such cases, the negative air pressure may disappear, and possibly infectious agents may spread to other rooms via the air.
- Lockable closet for disinfectants.
- Cabinet for storage of clean equipment for waste management.
- All important procedures must be in writing in protected, washable plastic.

78.4.3 Control Functions

- Daily check that machines are working properly. Check daily that there is soap on the container of the decontaminator. Report to medical-technical department if leakage, suspicion of low temperature or if the equipment is unclean after washing.
- Daily check that all waste, including infectious, cans with cutting/stinging contaminants and the laundry, is properly handled and removed by appointment and before it gets overcrowded.
- Unauthorized personnel are not allowed to stay in the room. No access for relatives or patients.
- Daily check of cleaning of floors and benches. Daily washing of floors, surfaces and around wash all day of the week; *see Chap. 65 on cleaning of rooms.*
- Equipment not belonging to the disinfection room system shall not be placed on the disinfection room.
- Temperature control of decontaminator and instrument washing machine every 14days. Register in the list.

78.5 Background Information

To the disinfection room, a number of potentially infectious agents are brought daily, which—if not properly treated—exposes personnel and patients to infection.

Microbiological agents brought into the disinfection room can cause serious infections via:

- *Blood-borne infection*: hepatitis A, B, C, D, E, HIV, HTLV, etc.
- *Contact-transmitted infection*: *Staphylococcus aureus*, streptococci, *Salmonella*, *Shigella*, *Clostridium difficile*, hepatitis A, norovirus, rotavirus, etc.
- *Airborne infection (including contact)*: tuberculosis, MRSA and other resistant bacteria, influenza, respiratory syncytial virus—RSV, norovirus, sapovirus, bocavirus, coronavirus, etc.

78.5.1 Good Hygiene Prevents Infection Risk

In the disinfection room, both *clean and unclean* material is treated, often at the same time during a busy day in the ward. It is important to distinguish between clean and unclean sides of the room and carry out good hand hygiene between work tasks. Risk processes that cause splash/contamination of biological material must be avoided. Everything must be treated with care. No contamination or misunderstanding may occur that exposes personnel or patients to infection risk.

See also Chap. 66 on disinfection.

References

1. The Norwegian State Drug Control: chemical disinfectants for technical use in health- and nursing. Oslo: Statens Legemiddelverk, Sosial- og Helsedepartementet; 2012.
2. Ministry of Labor and Administration. Regulations on protection against exposure to biological factors (bacteria, viruses, fungi and more) in the workplace. FOR OSLO: 1997-12-19 nr.1322.
3. Sehulster LM, Chinn RYW, Ardunio MJ, et al. Guidelines for environmental infection control in health-care facilities. CDC. MMWR. 2003;52:1–42.
4. Rutala WA, Weber DJ. Disinfection, sterilization, and control of hospital waste. In: Mandell, Douglas, and Bennets principles and practice of infectious diseases, vol. 2. Philadelphia: Elsevier Churchill Livingstone; 2015. p. 3294–309.
5. Hochlin K, Solheim N, Rasch M, Laugerud F, Andersen BM. Disinfection room/cleaning room - fitting and use. In: Handbook in hygiene and infection control for hospitals. Oslo: Ullevål University Hospital; 2003. p. 470–3.
6. Laugerud F, Hochlin K, Rasch M, Andersen BM. Disinfection room/cleaning room - fitting and use. In: Handbook in hygiene and infection control for hospitals. Oslo: Ullevål University Hospital; 2008. p. 650–3.
7. Charron D, Bedard E, Lalancette C, Laferriere C, Prevost M. Impact of electronic faucets and water quality on the occurrence of *Pseudomonas aeruginosa* in water: a multi-hospital study. Infect Control Hosp Epidemiol. 2015;36:311–9.
8. Andersen BM. *Legionella*. In: In: microbiology and infection control. Handbook in hygiene and infection control part 1. Bergen: Fagbokforlaget; 2014. p. 116–9.

9. Moore G, Walker J. Presence and control of *Legionella pneumophilia* and *Pseudomonas aeruginosa* biofilms in hospital water systems. In: Percival SL, Williams DW, Randle J, Coioper T, editors. Biofilms in infection prevention and control. Boston: Academic; 2014. p. 311–37.
10. Assadian O, El-Madani N, Seper E, et al. Sensor-operated faucets: a possible source of nosocomial infection? Infect Control Hosp Epidemiol. 2002;23:44–6.
11. Andersen BM. Gram-negative rod bacteria in the intestine and/or environment. In: Microbiology and infection control. Handbook in hygiene and infection control part 1. Bergen: Fagbokforlaget; 2014. p. 85–94.

Internal Infection Control: Checklist

79

Abstract

Internal control is an important and time-saving way of reviewing the department's standard with regard to hygiene and infection control. Internal control is carried out by the department's own employees and is an internal matter. Results of the check often result in a note/report that is then used as a document for improvement measures. The following chapter is focused on hygienic control and check routines that may protect against the spread of infections between patients, personal and environment.

Keywords

Internal control · Hygienic checklist · Patient ward · Infection control

79.1 Purpose

- To ensure good hygienic routines for the department.
- To detect defects, unfortunate routines, procedures and measures that may be of major importance for infection control and hygiene at the department.

79.2 Comprise

- Patients, visitors and healthcare personnel at the department.

79.3 Responsibility

The hospital's management should provide a written infection control programme including a procedure for internal control.

B. M. Andersen, *Prevention and Control of Infections in Hospitals*,
https://doi.org/10.1007/978-3-319-99921-0_79

Department management should implement internal controls with regard to hygiene and infection control, twice per year, and with written report to the Director and to the infection control personnel.

Hygiene contact is responsible for participating in internal control work.

The safety deputy is responsible for protection issues that must be submitted to the safety overseer.

The cleaning manager is responsible for the feedback to the workplace and the head of the service department regarding deviations according to hygiene and infection protection.

All personnel are responsible for ensuring that current procedures and guidelines are implemented and followed up.

79.4 Practical Measures

Internal controls regarding hygiene and infection protection are carried out at all departments at least twice a year. The control should be performed by the department's management (manager), hygiene contact, safety representative and cleaning manager. Department nurses attend at their wards; the kitchen manager participates in the ward kitchen. Technical department is contacted concerning technical internal control, i.e. control of technical equipment.

The department's responsible physician should, if possible, participate in internal control, especially during periods of problems with hospital infections.

Prevalence and incidence of all infections and hospital infections at the department should be included as documentation.

Inspection reports from the hospital hygiene/infection protection personnel are used as the basis for internal control.

79.4.1 The Department Management Is Responsible for

- Hand hygiene training for all department employees (including extra duty, night duty, etc.)
- Adequate washbasins with liquid soap and disinfectant dispensers, paper towels and waste bin with bag and placement of this.
- Good personal hygiene among the staff, patient hygiene and use of the hospital's work uniform.
- The quality and cleaning of patient beds, mattresses, bed linen, toilet chairs, wheelchairs, other chairs, textiles and other equipment.
- Proper cleaning of patient room, toilet room, washroom, laundry room, storage for clean/sterile equipment, other storage room, dining room, corridor and living room.
- Good hygienic conditions for newly operated patients.
- Proper wound care and treatment of wound infections.
- Measures for epidemics or outbreaks of communicable diseases, according to hospital routines.

- Responsibility for proper use of isolation regimes.
- Knowledge of guidelines concerning resistant microbes.
- Good hygienic conditions in nutrition, fluid treatment and care.
- Distribution, storage and handling of drugs.
- Training in correct treatment and separation of clean versus unclean items: patient clothes, waste, equipment, etc.
- Distribution, storage, inspection and expiry date of disinfectants.
- In case of purchasing new equipment, disposable equipment, etc., contact infection control personnel/medical technical units for advice and approval.
- Errors and deviations are reported to the hospital's management, quality selection and infection control nurse.

79.4.2 Responsibilities in the Ward Kitchen (Kitchen Chef)

- Proper cleaning, preventing microbes from spreading in the environment and causing infections in patients and personnel. This applies to daily cleaning and main cleaning.
- To comply with procedures and regulations of the Ministry of Social Affairs—the country's Food Safety Authority to ensure that staff have good practices for personal hygiene and hand hygiene.
- To arrange washbasins with liquid soap, paper and hand disinfection container.
- Make sure the kitchen has trash cans with pedal lock.
- To ensure proper storage of clean equipment.
- That all sorts of foods are kept in a hygienically satisfactory manner.
- That the dishwasher has a satisfactory temperature and that the machine has a proper flush/cleaning and disinfecting effect.
- Checking the temperature of the dishwasher according to plan.
- To distinguish clear between clean and unclean equipment.
- To clean equipment in a satisfactory way.
- Daily cleaning and order in the kitchen.
- Cleaning of food trays, trolleys and containers.
- Main cleaning of kitchen and storage rooms once a year—or more often if needed.
- Equipment replacement and maintenance (of the equipment).
- Errors and deviations are reported to the department's management; the kitchen chef reports to the hospital's management.
- Conditions of importance for hygiene and infection control are reported to the hospital's management, quality committee and infection control unit.

79.4.3 Responsibilities for Cleaners (Cleaning Management)

- Hand hygiene training (including temporary staff).
- Personal hygiene and uniform.
- Current procedures for cleaning are followed.

- Proper cleaning of patient room, toilet room, washroom, laundry room, storage for clean/sterile equipment, other storage rooms, dining room, corridor and living room.
- Proper cleaning of patient beds, mattresses, toilet chairs, wheelchairs, other chairs, etc.
- Proper methods and soaps are used, according to plan. This applies to daily cleaning of the department and main cleaning once a year or more often.
- Storage, checking and shelf life of disinfectants.
- Training in current infection control procedures and practical review of disinfection and cleaning of contaminated rooms and furniture.
- Errors and deviations are reported to the department's management and hospital management via the hospital's reporting system for deviations.
- Conditions of importance for hygiene and infection control are reported to the hospital's management, quality committee and infection control unit.

79.4.4 The Safety Deputy Is Responsible for Controlling

- That the staff are not exposed to infection.
- That technical equipment and aids work appropriately, to avoid strain injuries.
- Disinfectants/chemicals are stored and used in accordance with the regulations.
- Error and deviations are reported to the safety overseer, the department's management, the hospital's management, the quality committee and the infection protection unit.

79.4.5 Technical Department Is Responsible for Controlling

- Maintenance of windows, ceilings, walls and floors, as well as all technical installations.
- That the ventilation filter is checked and replaced by agreement with the supplier of the hospital ventilation system and that there is no leakage between the filter and the ventilation duct.
- That in some departments, filter change is advised twice a year.
- Cleaning of valves for air intake and extraction.
- That hot water from the crane has at least 75 °C.
- Temperatures of dishwashers (at least 85 °C) and decontaminators (at least 85 °C).
- That logbook is kept to document temperatures in decontaminators, washing machines, dishwashers and filters.
- Error and deviations are reported to the department's management and to the hospital's management, quality selection and infection control unit.

79.4.6 Responsible for the Textile Department Must Check

- Hand hygiene training (including temporary staff).
- Textile personnel's personal hygiene and working suit.

- Training of personnel in washing procedures and proper treatment and separation between clean and unclean textiles.
- Adequate washbasins with liquid soap dispensers, paper towels, hand disinfectants and waste bin with bag and placement of this.
- Purchasing, transportation and use of all fabrics at the institution.
- Internal control in the laundry.
- Washer/dryer and other laundry equipment.
- Storage of clean textiles.
- Laundry of different textile fabrics.
- Laundry of regular hospital textiles.
- Laundry of infected textiles.
- Storage and sorting of used textiles.
- Storage and sorting of infectious textiles.
- Cleaning of laundry trolleys.
- Cleaning of laundry containers.
- Daily cleaning in the laundry unit and dust removal.
- Main cleaning of the laundry unit at least once a year.
- Errors and deviations are reported to the hospital's management, quality selection and infection control unit.

79.4.7 Checklist for Internal Control: A Regular Patient Ward

This is a checklist for a regular patient ward. It is recommended that special departments (laboratory medicine, radiology departments, internal service, surgery and intensive care unit) should make their own checklists, even contact the infection control unit.

79.4.7.1 Patient Rooms

- Beds/mattresses/bedding, storage, placement and cover of clean beds.
- Washbasins, liquid soap, paper towels, hand disinfectants.
- Waste bin with bag.
- Cleaning of fixtures and rooms.
- Cleaning of call button, telephone, light switches, door handles.
- Cleaning of wardrobe, curtain and display board.
- Light.
- No storage of clean clothes, bandages, ointments, etc. in the patient room.
- Check the number of patients/m^2 area in the patient room (at least 16 m^2 per patient); furthermore the distance between beds (at least 130 cm) and between beds and washbasin (at least 130 cm) and between bedside and wall (at least 130 cm).
- Check that beds do not stand against the wall with long sides.
- Check cleaning/disinfection of medical devices used by patients.
- Everything up from the floor.
- Hygienically safe toilet/shower.

79.4.7.2 Isolation Unit (Patient Room, Sluice, Toilet/Shower/Decontamination)

- Check routines for isolating patients with infection.
- Check that the department's cleaner can provide decontamination and isolation routines.
- Check negative air pressure in airborne isolation unit and check logbook for measurements of pressure.
- See also patient rooms.

79.4.7.3 Toilet-Bathroom Conditions

- Handwash, hand disinfection.
- Liquid soap, paper towels, waste bin with bag.
- Hanging for toilet paper.
- No storage space for equipment.
- Cleaning twice a day.
- Control of toilet, lid, cleaning.
- Check the silicone at the floor around the toilet.
- Cleaning of toilet seats, seat higher (also below).
- Check that the correct cleaning routine is followed (how to clean the toilet).

79.4.7.4 Shower

- Daily cleaning of the sink and shower room.
- Cleaning in showers between each patient.
- If a shower cabinet is used by several patients, an infected patient will shower as the last person. Disinfect the shower afterwards.
- Check the wall and floor coverings.
- Disposable bag for textile rack.

79.4.7.5 Bathroom

- Check cleaning procedures of bath/handwash, hand disinfection.
- Cleaning and disinfection procedures for patients with and without infection.
- Bubble bath should preferably not be used.
- Waste bin with bag.
- Cleaning of shelves.
- Stand for unclean laundry/towels.
- No storage space for clean textiles, bandages, ointments, etc.

79.4.7.6 Textile Storage

- Order.
- Cleaning.
- Everything up from the floor.
- No unauthorized effects.

79.4.7.7 Disinfection Room

- Handwash.
- Liquid soap/paper towels/hand disinfectants.
- Disinfectants and strong detergents in locked cabinets.
- Own stand for waste and laundry.
- Cleaning of shelves and cabinets.
- Cleaning of all surfaces, floors daily.
- Strong distinction between clean/unclean.
- Temperature control and function control of the decontaminator and instrument washing machine.
- Container with tight fitting lid for disinfectant, if used.
- Collection of waste.
- Collection of laundry.
- Do not wash or dry laundry in the disinfection room.
- Order.
- Everything up from the floor.
- Negative air pressure compared to other rooms and corridor.

79.4.7.8 Clean Storage

- Order.
- Hand hygiene.
- Check daily cleaning and cleaning of cabinets.
- Everything up from the floor.
- Only clean equipment on clean storage.
- No unauthorized effects.
- No office space.

79.4.7.9 Post (Ward) Kitchen

- Handwash.
- Liquid soap, paper towels, hand disinfection.
- Sink, sufficient washbasins.
- Cleaning of cabinets and drawers weekly.
- Cleaning of floors daily.
- Replacement of worn-out equipment.
- Waste container with pedal lock for food residue.
- Waste bin with a waste bag.
- Check that the Foodstuffs Act with regulations is followed.
- Cleaning of cookers, etc., daily.
- Weekly cleaning of ice machine.
- Cleaning of refrigerator once a week.
- Freezer compartment/cupboard twice a year.
- Main cleaning twice a year.

- Temperature control on the fridge every day.
- Temperature control on dishwasher (measured in the basket) every 14 days.
- Temperature control of hot food.
- Check storage of food.
- Daily cleaning of the food trolley.

79.4.7.10 Ward Office

- Check training in hand hygiene.
- Are written routines for infection control and hygiene easily accessible?
- Is the staff familiar with the routines?
- Washbasin with soap dispenser/paper towels/hand disinfectant/lotion and waste bin with bag
- Daily cleaning of all surfaces/phone/floor/data and keyboard.
- Weekly cleaning of chairs and fixtures.
- Make sure that there is no food or drink when working with patient journals, patient samples or medicines.
- No equipment or wires on the floor.

79.4.7.11 Medicine Room/Medicine Cabinet/Unit

- Daily cleaning of all surfaces.
- Weekly cleaning of all shelves/drawers/cabinets and carts.
- Main cleaning of the room twice a year.
- Check the hood.
- Check opened vials/ampoules/medicines for durability and storage.
- Check the handling of medications.
- Check cleaning of medicine boards, trays, trolleys, etc.

79.4.7.12 Storage Room of Washing Equipment

- Sink.
- Liquid soap, paper towels, hand disinfection.
- Sufficient shelf space.
- Peg for hanging equipment, etc.
- Daily wash of the sink/bucket rack.
- Daily disinfection of the buckets.
- Cleanliness and order.
- Floor space free of equipment and supplies.
- No private laundry.
- Waste bin with bag.

79.4.7.13 Dining Room and Living Room

- Washing tables after each meal.
- Cleaning of floors daily, possibly twice a day and when needed.
- Washing of seats, window frames, lists and fixtures weekly.

79.4.7.14 Corridors on Wards

- Cleaning once a day.
- Cleaning of railings twice a week.
- Wash the door handles daily.
- All furniture is vacuum cleaned and cleaned weekly.
- Dirty/broken furniture is sent for cleaning/repair.

79.4.7.15 Elevator

- Daily cleaning of floors, railing and pushbuttons.
- Check cleaning.
- Light conditions.

79.4.7.16 Waste Disposal

- Proper treatment of waste.
- All surfaces easily washable.
- Drain to water in the floor.
- Check routines for removal and transport of waste.
- Cleaning once a week.
- Negative air pressure relative to the corridor.
- Check any shafts for dropping.

79.4.7.17 Physiotherapy

- Handwash, soap dispenser, paper towels, hand disinfection.
- Waste bin with bag.
- Adequate closet space for all equipment.
- Cleaning procedures for equipment are followed.
- Daily cleaning of all tables/benches/floors.
- Hygiene rules for physiotherapists are followed.
- Check cleaning.

79.4.7.18 Ergo-therapy Room

- Handwash, soap dispenser, paper towels, hand disinfection.
- Waste bin with bag.
- Daily cleaning of all tables/benches/floors.
- Regular cleaning and order in the cabinets.
- Check cleaning.

79.4.7.19 Ventilation Valves

- Cleaning/cleaning of all valves every 3 months.
- Note! Fungi are growing in valves, especially in bathroom/shower room/kitchen/laundry and waste room.

79.4.7.20 Ventilation Filter

- Regular check of filter, eventually shift.

79.4.7.21 Wardrobe for Employees

- Handwash, soap dispenser, paper towels, hand disinfection.
- Waste bin with bag.
- Clean storage room for clean uniforms/clothes.
- Proper storage of used clothes and good emptying routines.
- No equipment, shoes, clothes on the floor.
- Check cleaning of available wardrobes.
- Check cleaning under and on top of the wardrobe.

79.4.7.22 Shower

- Daily cleaning of washbasin, shower room and toilet.
- Check walls and floor coverings.
- Disposable bag for used clothes and rack.

79.4.7.23 Toilet

- Handwash.
- Liquid soap, paper towels, waste bin with bag.
- Hanging for toilet paper.
- No storage space for equipment.
- Cleaning daily.
- Control of toilet, lid, cleaning.
- Check the silicone at the floor around the toilet bowls.
- Check that the correct cleaning routine is followed (how to clean the toilet).

79.5 Background Information

Internal control: to ensure compliance with requirements stipulated in or in compliance with the law or regulation.

79.5.1 Law/Regulation/Guidelines: Example from Norway

- Regulations on internal control. Determined by kgl res. 22 March 1991 pursuant to Act 4 February 1977 No. 4 Section 16a on Workers protection and Work Environment, etc.
- Regulations on infection protection in healthcare institutions—hospital infections. Established by the Ministry of Social Affairs and Health on 5 July 1996 pursuant to Sections 4–7 and 7–11 of Act No. 5 of 5 August 1994 on protection against communicable diseases.
- Infection control programme for each hospital, updated locally.
- Hygiene Regulations for production and marketing, etc., of foodstuffs, determined by kgl, 8 July 1983, No. 1253, changed by kgl. of 29 April 1988 No. 312, pursuant to paragraphs 1 and 3 of the Act of 19 May 1933 No. 3 on supervision of foodstuffs, etc. with later changes.

- Internal control in foodstuffs—businesses IK—Food at NMT, INFO G 3 7 October 1997.
- Working Environment Act published by the Directorate for Labour Inspection.

Internal control is an important and relatively little time-consuming way of reviewing the department's standard with regard to hygiene and infection control. Internal control is carried out by the department's own employees and is an internal matter. Results of the check often result in a note/report that is then used as a document for improvement measures.

Part XIV

High-Risk Microbes

Dangerous Microbes 80

Abstract

The most dangerous microbes for humans are those that are easily transmitted, virulent and invasive to central organs like the blood and lung, robust survivors in the environment, have a low infection dose and are without any specific treatment or vaccine. Most of them are zoonoses transmitted from animals and often with insects as vectors. The most dangerous microbes cause a very high mortality, are identified as high-risk agents or "biohazard-level 4" agents and are treated at the highest level of infection protection with strict isolation measures. Dangerous microbes occur as a problem mostly in countries with low hygiene standards/high population density and in tropical-subtropical areas. Infection control must always be based on hygienic measures and strict infection protection.

This chapter is a short information about the most virulent and pathogenic agents, geographic area and severity of disease.

Keywords

Microbes · Dangerous microbes · Geographic area of virulent agents · Dangerous virus and bacteria · Zoonosis · VHF · Anthrax · Plague · Biosafety level 4 Infection control · Survivors · High-risk microbes · Severity of disease

80.1 Dangerous Microbes

New, emerging or re-emerging infectious diseases and agents still appear. More than 15 new potential human pathogenic microbe types may be registered every year. New infectious diseases and emerging virulence properties still appear, for

---

Current agents are described in more detail in: Andersen BM. Part 1. Microbiology and infection protection. Fagbokforlaget 2014.

B. M. Andersen, *Prevention and Control of Infections in Hospitals*,
https://doi.org/10.1007/978-3-319-99921-0_80

example, avian influenza viruses (H5N1 and others), HTLV and other retroviruses, HPV, Sindbis virus, Parvovirus, Bocavirus, Coronavirus, or bacteria like *Legionella*, *Borrelia*, group A streptococci and meningococci [1–5].

Virus not vaccine preventable or without specific treatment option, low infection dose and high capacity to survive in the environment will be a major problem if associated with incurable disease, disability or death. Virulent and dangerous microbes occur as a problem mostly in countries with low hygiene standards/high population density and in tropical-subtropical areas. Infection control must be based on hygienic measures and proper infection protection [2–7].

The most dangerous microbes for humans are those that are easily transmitted, virulent and invasive to the central organs like the blood and lung, robust survivors in the environment, have a low infection dose and are without any specific treatment or vaccine [2–5]. Most of them are zoonosis transmitted from animals and often with insects as vectors [8–12]. Dangerous microbes have also been used as biological weapons like anthrax, plague, botulism, *Coxiella*, *Brucella*, viral haemorrhagic fever (VHF) viruses, poxviruses and a number of other unusual agents [4, 13–25]. In the United States, there was an anthrax bioterrorism attack in 2001 [18, 19].

If the infectious agent and transmission ways are unknown and the situation is uncontrollable, it is important to follow pre-planned practical measures like strict isolation in negative air pressure isolation, registering of all contacts and the use of personal protective equipment (PPE) for air- and contact-borne infection [4, 8–13, 17, 20, 24, 26–29].

80.1.1 Dangerous Virus

During the last 20 years, there have been several large outbreaks of new and re-emerging viruses. Examples are systemic acute respiratory syndrome (SARS) (2002–2003), avian influenza viruses (H5N1, 2005), pandemic influenza (2009), Middle East respiratory syndrome (MERS) (2012) and Ebola (2014 and 2016) [1, 4, 5, 8, 11, 12].

VHF virus and a number of other special viruses are considered to cause the world's most dangerous infections with very high mortality, lack of therapeutic possibilities and often absence of effective vaccines. Such viruses are identified as high-risk agents or "biohazard-level 4" agents and are treated at the highest level of infection protection with strict isolation measures [4, 11, 12, 26–28].

- Virus families, with members especially dangerous to humans, are *Arenaviridae*, *Filoviridae*, *Flaviviridae*, *Bunyaviridae*, *Togaviridae* and *Paramyxoviridae* (Nipah encephalitis virus, etc.) and several others. They are mostly vector borne by insects and animals (zoonosis), dependent on a tropical-subtropical climate and temperature. Therefore, the colder zones in Europe, America, Asia and Australia are nearly free from more such serious infectious agents (see the table below) [1, 2, 4, 11, 12].

- Some very virulent viruses may be spread on all continents: TBE, RSSE, CCHF, rabies virus (*Rhabdoviridae*), avian influenza virus (AH5N1) and other high-pathogenic influenza viruses (*Orthomyxoviridae*). SARS and MERS (*Coronaviridae*) may be spread globally as nosocomial infections. MERS is a newly discovered coronavirus-zoonosis (dromedaries, bats, etc.) and acts as SARS, also with a tendency for nosocomial spread in hospitals, still going on in the Middle East. [30] These and other viruses are adapted to the climate and spread by direct transmission person-to-person, by increased mobility in the population and/or spread via new vectors, like animals, birds and insects [1, 4].
- A few of these dangerous viruses are vaccine preventable, and specific antiviral therapy is lacking in most cases.

80.1.1.1 Other New Virulent Viruses

- *Zika* virus—newly discovered flavivirus in South America, with mild to serious symptoms and teratogenic effect [11].
- *Polio-like illnesses*, especially among children, discovered in August 2014 in the United States. Probably caused by enterovirus D68 [31].
- *HIV aggressive variants* (CRF19) have been detected in Cuba in 2015 and earlier in Africa, with a faster course from infection to AIDS development [32].

80.1.2 Dangerous Bacteria

Bacteria resistant to antibacterial drugs have developed rapidly among staphylococci (MRSA), enterococci (VRE), tuberculosis bacilli (multidrug-resistant mycobacteria) and gram-negative rods (ESBL) in the last 30–50 years. From 2009 to 2010 onwards, super-resistant gram-negative rods (CRE, CPE) have increased rapidly with transmission of genes with total drug resistance (NDM-1) [1–5]. Bacteria sensitive to common antibacterial agents will probably not be a major problem in the future, unless changed antibacterial sensitivity.

- Anthrax is still endemic or hyperendemic on all continents in the world, mainly as a zoonosis among unvaccinated cattle [1–6, 13, 33]. It has been known for more than 4000 years and was earlier called “Black bane”. Natural anthrax in human is associated with contact with sick animals and animal products. The bacterium *Bacillus anthracis* is producing lethal toxins and spores that can survive in the environments for 100 years or more. Minimum infectious dose is 1–3 spores, and toxin-producing anthrax may cause skin, lung or intestinal anthrax, dependent on the transmission via contact, air or food. The non-skin anthrax has a very high lethality. Today, about 2000 people are infected each year, from eating or handling infected meat. During peace time, there are few incidents of threats using bioterror weapons like anthrax. However, autumn 2001 anthrax was spread in the United States by “powder letters” [18, 19].
- Plague, caused by *Yersinia pestis* (*Enterobacteriaceae*), is a zoonotic disease, vector-transmitted from infected rodents to humans via infected insects (fleas and lice)

[1–5, 8]. It is one of the great historical diseases. In the last 1500 years, plague has killed more than 200 million people during large epidemics (Black Death), especially from the year 1347. Still, plague causes bubonic-glandular pest, lung pest and/or septicaemia in 2000–3000 cases each year, and more than 10 outbreaks (Africa, Asia, Australia, Madagascar) have occurred since the year 2000 [8, 34].

- Cholera caused by *Vibrio cholera* is one of the great quarantine diseases, called "mother of all epidemics", still very active in Asia and Africa. Cholera is associated with contaminated water, war and nature catastrophes, like in Haiti 2010, with 670,000 cholera cases (profuse diarrhoea) [1–5, 35].
- *Brucella* species (*Brucellaceae*) are one of the most important zoonotic diseases both for animals and humans all over the world. They easily spread via contact and air from animals and food, survive in the environment for months especially during colder seasons, are very easily transmitted and may cause nosocomial infections, chronic febris undulans, septicaemia and lung diseases. Vaccination of animals may eradicate the zoonotic disease [15]. *Brucella* are particularly related to laboratory outbreaks but are easily transferable outside the laboratory and are considered highly infectious [36].
- *Francisella tularensis* (zoonosis) is defined as a category A bioterrorism agent, highly infectious and increasing in the society, has low infection dose (one to ten bacteria) and can be inhaled or infected via food and water [1–5, 8]. Occasionally, such patients are detected in hospitals, even in the operating department [37]. Tularemia is a zoonotic disease or colonization among wild animals as rodents and hares and may survive at colder seasons for long periods in water, amoebas, birds and insects like ticks. The infection (skin, lung, intestine) is transmitted via contact with infected animals, inhalation of airborne bacteria, contaminated water and ticks.
- *Botulism* is caused by a bacterial-produced toxin (*Clostridium botulinum*) that causes paresis and is common in soil as spores [1–5]. The disease can be associated with toxin formation in contaminated and poorly canned foods, shrimp fish, bacon, etc. under anaerobic conditions and randomly affects both healthy people and vulnerable groups, such as infants who have had honey infected with the bacterium, which has happened repeatedly [38]. The toxin is the most dangerous we know and is on the list of bioterrorism.
- Family *Rickettsiaceae* is associated with many different types of small, intracellular microbes that are zoonotic and survive for a long time in the nature and in infected animals, birds, insects, water and amoeba [2, 3, 10]. *Coxiella burnetii* is a global zoonosis among animals like sheep and goats and may be airborne for several kilometres, causing frequent outbreaks of Q-fever in Europe in more than 4000 cases in the Netherlands during 2007–2010 [10]. *Rickettsia* species are more than 25 types, and many of them, especially the typhus group, are causing severe diseases. Humans are mostly infected by insects, including ticks from infected wild animals and rodents usually found in tropical or subtropical areas, but climatic changes, lack of good hygiene, war and natural catastrophes may spread these infections. During the period 1881–1920, 30 million people got epidemic typhus, and three million died in East Europe and Russia [2, 3, 10].

80.1.3 Other Bacteria That Are Causing Concern

- *Borrelia* (*Spirochetaceae*) has an increasing number of species that may infect human cases all over the world. The disease may cause chronic infections in the skin, muscles, heart, nerve tissue and brain. Borreliosis is a typical emerging zoonosis, spread via different ticks from animals and birds over large geographic areas and with large climatic variations [9].
- *Syphilis* (*Spirochetaceae*) and *Treponema pallidum* are old, historical diseases, transmitted via sex, from mother to child during pregnancy and via blood products. Now re-emerging and increasing worldwide [9].
- Other spirochetes or the like may cause zoonosis, like *Borrelia recurrentis* and *Leptospirosis* [9].
- *Burkholderia pseudomallei* is causing melioidosis, pneumonia, septicaemia, disseminated infection and shock. Incubation period may be up to 20–40 years. It is a long survivor in the environment (2–10 years), robust at tropical-subtropical temperatures >25 °C and is very dangerous. Endemic in Southeast Asia and may be spread by increasing globalization [1–5].

80.1.4 Other Infective/Dangerous Agents

- *Fungi and mould*—different types are especially related to floods, water damage, etc. and to contamination of medical products and equipment [39, 40]. Especially, the newly defined *Candida auris* may be very virulent.
- *Prion disease-new Shy-Drager syndrome* is rediscovered in 2015; Multiple-system atrophy (MSA) [5, 41].
- *Ricin* is a plant-derived toxin that is still used for bioterrorism in letters to, among others, President Obama [42].

Serious and unusual microbial infections

Microbes	Geographic area	Disease
Virus		
Arena virus		
Lassa	West Africa	Severe, often fatal
Guanarito	Venezuela	Severe
Junin (Argentine haemorrhagic fever-HF)	Argentina	Severe
Machupo (Bolivian haemorrhagic fever)	Bolivia	Severe
Sabia	Brazil	Severe
LCM	Global	Mild to severe
Filovirus		
Marburg	Africa	23–100 % fatal
Ebola	Africa	20–100 % fatal

Microbes	Geographic area	Disease
Bunyaviridae (over 60 viral types from asymptomatic to fatal)		
Rift Valley fever	Africa	1 % develops HF
California enceph	United States, Europe	2 % fatal
Crimean-Congo haemorrhagic fever (CCHF)	Africa, Asia, Europe	Severe
Hantaan group	North and South America, Europe, Asia	Moderate to severe
Arbovirus (Togaviridae and Flaviviridae)		
Tick-borne (TBE) encephalitis virus complex	All continents	Moderate to fatal
Russian spring and summer encephalitis (RSSE)		
Omsk haemorrhagic fever		
Central European encephalitis viruses		
Venezuelan equine encephalitis virus		Moderate to severe
Yellow fever virus	Africa, America	Moderate to severe
Semliki Forest virus	Africa, epidemic	Mild to fatal
Dengue virus	All tropical-subtropical areas	Mild to fatal
Japanese B encephalitis	Asia; Korea, Japan, Philippines	Often fatal
Rabies	In all parts of the world	100% fatal without tr.
Monkey pox (B)	Animal experiments	Severe, often fatal
Smallpox Virus	Eradicate, but kept	Severe, often fatal in unvaccinated
Avian influenza A H5N1	Asia, Africa, Europe	80% fatal without treat
Nipah encephalitis virus (paramyxovirus)	Asia, Malaysia, India, Bangladesh	75% fatal
Corona Virus		
Systemic acute respiratory syndrome (SARS)	Asia, Canada, proliferation	Severe, 10% fatal
Middle East respiratory syndrome (MERS)	Middle East, emerging	Severe, 30–40% fatal
Bacteria		
Richettsiaceae		
Rickettsia	All continents	Many types, severe
Orientia	Asia, Australia	Moderate to severe
Bartonellaceae	All continents	Moderate to severe
Coxiella burnetii	All continents	Moderate to severe
Bacillus anthracis	All continents	Moderate to severe
Brucella	All continents	Mild to severe
Burkholderia pseudomallei	Asia	Mild to severe
Francisella tularensis	All continents	Mild to severe
Vibrio cholera	Asia, Africa and South America	Mild to severe
Bacillus anthracis	All continents	Moderate to severe
Yersinia pestis	Africa and Asia	Moderate to severe

References

1. Mandell D. Bennet's principles and practice of infectious diseases. 8th ed. Philadelphia: Churchill Livingston; 2015.
2. Andersen BM. Pathogenic bacteria-diagnostic, treatment and infection control. Oslo: Gyldendal Akademisk; 2000.
3. Andersen BM. Bacteria and disease. Oslo: Gyldendal Academisk; 2005.
4. Andersen BM, Lereim I, Hochlin K. Serious, unusual dangerous infections. In: Handbook in hygiene and infection control for hospitals. Oslo: Ullevål University Hospital; 2008. p. 550–91.
5. Andersen BM. Handbook in hygiene and infection control for hospitals. Part 1. Microbiology and infection control. Norway: Fagbokforlaget; 2014.
6. European Parliament and Council Directive 2000/54/EC of 18 September 2000 on the protection of workers from the risks related to exposure to biological agents at work.
7. Ministry of Labour and Administration. Regulations on protection against exposure to biological factors (bacteria, viruses, fungi and more) in the workplace. FOR OSLO: 1997-12-19 nr.1322.
8. Andersen BM. Zoonosis-transmitted from animals, insects and environment. In: Handbook in hygiene and infection control for hospitals. Part 1. Norway: Fagbokforlaget; 2014. p. 144–53.
9. Andersen BM. Borreliosis and other spirochetes-zoonosis. In: Handbook in hygiene and infection control for hospitals. Part 1. Norway: Fagbokforlaget; 2014. p. 154–62.
10. Andersen BM. Coxiella, rickettsia and other small bacteria – often intracellular – zoonosis. In: Handbook in hygiene and infection control for hospitals. Part 1. Norway: Fagbokforlaget; 2014. p. 163–6.
11. Andersen BM. Other serious viral infections - zoonosis. In: Handbook in hygiene and infection control for hospitals. Part 1. Norway: Fagbokforlaget; 2014. p. 278–90.
12. Andersen BM. Ebola, Lassa, and other haemorrhagic viruses. In: Handbook in hygiene and infection control for hospitals. Part 1. Norway: Fagbokforlaget; 2014. p. 291–9.
13. Andersen BM. Anthrax and emergency routines at Ullevål University Hospital. Tidsskr Nor Legeforen. 2002;122:852–5.
14. Borio L, Inglesby BL, Peters CJ, et al. Haemorrhagic fever viruses as biological weapons: medical and public health management. JAMA. 2002;287:2391–405.
15. Jernigan JA, Stephens DS, Ashford DA, Omenaca C, Topiel MS, Galbraith M, et al. Bioterrorism-related inhalation anthrax: the first 10 cases reported in the United States. Emerg Infect Dis. 2001;7:933–44.
16. Inglesby TV, O'Toole T, Hendersen DA, et al. Anthrax as a biological weapon, 2002: updated recommendations for management. JAMA. 2002;287:2236–52.
17. Yakupogullari Y, Koroglu M. Nosocomial spread of *Bacillus anthracis*. J Hosp Infect. 2007;66:401–40.
18. Dull PM, Wilson KE, Kournikakis B, Whitney EAS, Boulet CA, Ho JYW, et al. *Bacillus anthracis* aerosolization associated with a contaminated mail sorting machine. Emerg Infect Dis. 2002;8:1044–7.
19. Weis CP, Intrepido AJ, Miller AK, Cowin PG, Durno MA, Gebhart JS, et al. Secondary aerosolization of viable *Bacillus anthracis* spores in a contaminated US Senate office. J Am Med Ass. 2002;288:2853–8.
20. Peters CJ, Hartley DM. Anthrax inhalation and lethal human infection. Lancet. 2002;359:710–1.
21. Byrne D. Bioterrorism: crime and opportunity. Eurosurveillance. 2001;6:157–8.
22. Coignard B. Bioterrorism preparedness and response in European public health institutes. Eurosurveillance. 2001;6:159–66.
23. Levy-Bruhl D, Guerin N. The use of smallpox virus as a biological weapon: the vaccination situation in France. Eurosurveillance. 2001;6:171–8.
24. Rebman T. Infectious disease disaster: bioterrorism, emerging infections, and pandemics. In: APIC text of infection control and epidemiology. St. Louis: APIC, St. Louis University; 2014. p. 1201–22.

25. English JF, Cundiff MY, Malone JD et al. Bioterrorism readiness plan: a template for healthcare facilities. APIC, CDC; 13 April 1999.
26. Promed mail September 14, 2014. Andersen BM. Infection control is not working.
27. Andersen BM. International infection control guidelines for Ebola. Hospital Healthcare Europe. Facilities management; April 2015. www.hospitalhealthcare.com.
28. CDC. Guidance on personal protective equipment to be used by Healthcare Workers during management of patients with Ebola virus disease in US hospitals, including procedures for putting on (donning) and removal, 20 October 2014.
29. McKay I, Sax H, Harbarth S, Bernard L, Pittet D. Multi-resistant infections in repatriated patients after natural disaster: lessons learned from the 2004 tsunami for hospital infection control. J Hosp Infect. 2008;68:1–8.
30. Promed-mail August 28, 2015. MERS-COV: Jordan, Saudi Arabia, Nosocomial.
31. Pastula DM, Aliabadi N, Haynes AK, et al. Acute neurological disease of unknown etiology in children - Colorado, August-September 2014. MMWR. 2014;63:1–2.
32. Promed-mail February 14, 2015. HIV-Cuba: New aggressive variant, CRF19.
33. Andersen BM. Anthrax. Bacteria and disease. Epidemiology, infections and infection protection. Oslo: Gyldendal Akademisk; 2005. p. 9–44.
34. Promed mail November 21, 2014. Plague - Madagascar.
35. Andersen BM. Cholera (*Vibrio cholerae*). In: Handbook in hygiene and infection control for hospitals. Part 1. Norway: Fagbokforlaget; 2014. p. 105–7.
36. Lowe CF, Showler AJ, Perera S, et al. Hospital-associated transmission of *Brucella melitensis* outside the laboratory. Emerg Infect Dis. 2015;21:150–2.
37. Becker SL, Splettesteesser WD, Kim YJ, et al. Potential risk of aerosol-borne *Francisella tularensis* transmission in the operating room. Infect Control Hosp Epidemiol. 2015;36:490–1.
38. Valley ML, Bye K, Nilsen KB, Rørvik LM, Tessem GAG. An infant with acute paresis. Tidsskr Nor Legeforen. 2015;135:1455–8.
39. CDC. Brandt M, Brown C, Burkhart J, et al. Mould-preventing strategies and possible health effects in the aftermath of hurricanes and major floods. MMWR. 2006;55:1–27.
40. Andersen BM. Fungi-human pathogenic. In: Handbook in hygiene and infection control for hospitals. Part 1. Norway: Fagbokforlaget; 2014. p. 393–9.
41. Promed-mail September 17, 2015. Prion disease updated: novel prion disease - SHY-DRAGER syndrome.
42. Promed-mail April 17, 2013. Ricin-USA: Washington, DC, Letters.

Emergency Preparedness

81

Abstract
Outbreaks of infectious diseases during peacetime or in disaster/war-related conditions, may most often need an effective crisis management in the hospital. The emergency preparedness in hospitals may vary within, and between countries, dependent on endemic and epidemic conditions, capacity, knowledge and economy. Lack of preparedness may result in a high risk of disease burden and death and cause a high economic impact on the health care.

Keywords
High-risk microbes · Lassa/Ebola/SARS/MERS/Nipah/avian influenza and other viruses · Anthrax/pest/cholera/diphtheria and other bacteria · Emergency Preparedness · Crisis management · Infection control · Isolation · Disinfection

81.1 Purpose

- Protect the healthcare institution and the society in general:
  - Against spread of infection during outbreak of unusually infectious and universal very dangerous disease
  - Unusually high number in the society of transmitted contagious disease in peacetime, in disasters, and when the country is in war or when war threatens
- Have an emergency plan for how to act in situations of such outbreaks.

81.2 Comprise

- All persons responsible for the emergency plan and for implementation of the plan
- Determined by epidemic situation and the type of infectious agent

B. M. Andersen, *Prevention and Control of Infections in Hospitals*,
https://doi.org/10.1007/978-3-319-99921-0_81

81.3 Responsibility

The hospital's management/crisis management in cooperation with the emergency response team for infection control supervises the work at the hospital in cooperation *with national health authorities and county governor* [1–7].

The Directorate for Social Security and Preparedness is responsible for the national risk image and for follow-up. (DSB, Norway 2014)

Law on Health and Social Preparedness for Infectious Diseases may be present and implemented in some countries, like in Norway [1].

Emergency Plans, Guidelines and Reports are made for outbreaks of infections like anthrax, SARS, avian influenza, pandemic influenza, MERS, Ebola, etc, see Table 80.1 [1–64], Chap. 80.

- **National**—example Norway [1–15]
- **Local**—example Ullevål University Hospital, Oslo [16–34, 52, 53]
- **International**—WHO, ECDC, CDC, UK, etc. [35–51]

81.4 Practical Measures [23]

Epidemiological conditions—concerning infectious diseases:

81.4.1 "Normal" Conditions

Globally, there are endemic and epidemic conditions that may vary by time, localisation and use of antibiotics and still be perceived as "normal" for this actual country [65–77]. Special infections, like resistant microbes, are increasing in most countries in the world, and WHO made in 2017 a priority list of 12 families of bacteria ("nightmare" bacteria) that agency experts say "pose the greatest threat to human health and kill millions of people every year" (WHO 27 Feb 2017) [67]. In 2017 CDC identified more than 220 samples of these "nightmare" bacteria containing unusual resistance genes in the United States and more than 1400 isolates from clinical samples of 32 states during the first 9 months of 2017 [66–70]. The endemic and epidemic conditions of these resistant bacteria vary between countries and are associated with risk of deaths, a high disease burden and death and an overall economic impact, reducing the gross domestic product (GDP) up to 1.6% [70].

Resistant microbes usually follow patients and personnel with "import status" (from other countries or areas with endemic conditions) and are caught early in the process by good routines and preliminary investigations [52, 53, 73–77]. Import routines (testing for MRSA, ESBL, CRE, CP, VRE, TBC, etc.) work usually well at the hospital, both for patients and for personnel (MRSA and TBC) [52, 53, 71–75]. Resistant microbes create even larger problems in primary care.

Healthcare professionals are generally exposed to infection if relevant precautions are not used. About 5–10% of MRSA-exposed healthcare persons may be infected or carriers with MRSA, and 10–20% of infected may need treatment, long-term sick leave, etc. [74–76] Screening of healthcare contacts of patients infected with carbapenemase-producing, very resistant bacteria with super-resistant genes in the United States found that one in ten was colonized with these bacteria [66].

Annual norovirus epidemics occupy the isolation capacity and lead to high sickness absence among infected healthcare professionals. Winter epidemics of RS virus and rotavirus in infants and flu outbreaks in all age groups occur each year. These are normal epidemiological conditions.

See also pre-examinations of patients, Chap. 47 and different isolation procedures, Chaps. 14–19.

81.4.2 Sporadic Outbreak of Serious Infectious Disease: Import Disease

Preparedness measures depend on the agent, extent and rate of development. As a rule, such infections are far from most countries in Europe, such as SARS, bird flu and Ebola, and are usually taken care of where they occur. It may rarely lead to import, for example, Ebola-infected healthcare personnel transported to actual homeland for treatment, in 2014.

81.4.3 Disasters: Natural or Inflicted—and Bioterrorism

The hospital emergency preparedness plan/disaster plan must be available and followed after adaptation to the current situation.

A number of natural disasters lead to increased risk of outbreaks of serious epidemics in society such as earthquakes; floods; tsunami in holiday paradises; earth, stone or clay landslides; snow avalanches; extreme heat; radiation damage; hurricane/tornado; fire over large areas; volcanic eruptions; explosions; etc. The disasters may cause a heavy load on the healthcare system in general [54]. This may happen in own country or harm own citizens abroad [1, 3, 4, 12].

War-related or disaster-related measures at terrorist attacks against the population often cause major damage and spread of infections due to a paralysed infrastructure. Bioterrorism, for example, by anthrax can cause uncontrolled epidemic outbreaks in the population; *see separate chapter.*

The result could be a massive destruction or paralysis of infrastructure such as water and sewage, energy supply, transport system, access to food and water, healthcare systems, broken hospitals and communications networks, etc.

In such statements it is important to have both disaster plans and infection control plans in place, like the examples published from CDC [54–64, 78–82].

Proposal for a mandate for the emergency response group for infection control/crises team [23]:

- The director at the hospital has overall responsibility and determining authority and leads the emergency group.
- The emergency group shall advise on unusually large outbreaks, particularly dangerous microbes, in an uncontrollable epidemic and in disasters/state of war/ suspected biological sabotage.
- The emergency group shall be adviser before, during and after the situation described above and shall propose preventive measures and guidelines in the current situation.
- Infection control leader coordinate the infection protection according to what is determined, in the same way as under normal conditions.
- Under normal circumstances, the emergency group meets once a year with ongoing updating of the action plan. The director summon for the meeting.
- In case of epidemic outbreak, particularly dangerous microbe or uncontrollable situation, the director summons the hospital's disaster leader in cooperation with the infection control leader for emergency group meetings. The group meets so often it is necessary to come up with updated recommendations and measures.

81.4.4 Suggestions to Members of the Emergency Response Group

81.4.4.1 Permanent Members

- The director (manager)
- Assistant hospital director
- Head of disaster committee or equivalent (deputy head)
- Emergency chief
- Information officer
- Head of Infection Control Department (coordinator for disease prevention) [82]
- Head of the Department of Infectious Diseases
- Head of the Department of Medical Microbiology
- Head of the Department for Internal Service, prehospital service (ambulances), etc.
- Hospital medical officer

81.4.4.2 Situational Members

Head of the department(s) with the problem(s), external participants from the state and municipal health authorities, safety overseer, HR representative.

81.4.5 Work Tasks at Situation of Increased Preparedness

The emergency preparedness group assesses the situation on a continuous basis and checks that:

- Competent infection control personnel (hygiene nurses, infection control doctor, epidemiologist, etc.) are available and can provide advice and guidance as well as carry out preparatory control measures regarding:

  - Isolation regime and routines for the actual patient group
  - Written infection control procedures for patients, personnel and visitors
  - Personnel access to and use of personal protection equipment (PPE)
  - Control of isolates (air pressure and function)
  - Triage—practical plan
  - Patient logistics, to avoid spreading to other patients
  - General infection control at the hospital, including cleaning and disinfection
  - Other prophylactic measures such as vaccines and drugs
  - Special measures for infection-exposed persons and especially susceptible persons (patients, personnel and visitors)
- *Infection isolates*: A written updated overview must be available for all types of isolates and single rooms at the hospital. The required number and quality must be calculated. The isolates must be routinely checked for ventilation and negative pressure—by the technically responsible at the hospital.
- *Cohort treatment and mobilization*: There should be a feasible plan for cohort treatment of patients that have the same diagnostic type of infection, mobilization and relocation of other patients and an escalation plan for more beds in cooperation with other hospitals, health institutions, etc.
- *Competent hospital staff* (doctors, nurses, cleaners, porters, ambulance staff, service units, etc.) must be available for the appropriate infection control work, in addition to treatment staff. Resources must be considered.
- *Infection control equipment* should be available and sufficient (respirators, tight-fitting goggles, double gloves, infection gown, cap/hood, coverings of the head/neck, room-bound shoes/shoe coverings, decontamination equipment/machines and chemical disinfectants, including hand disinfectants) and in accordance with the actual infectious agent (see isolation procedures).
- *Vaccines* that are currently preventive should be made available from defined stocks within a certain time limit (flu, rabies, anthrax, plague, smallpox, diphtheria, tetanus, polio, BCG, haemorrhagic viruses, etc.).
- *Drugs and specific immunoglobulins* should be made available from defined stocks as needed.
- *The escalation plan* must be available for further treatment and isolation of patients and exposed personnel, including healthcare professionals.

81.4.6 Intentional Infection: Bioterror and High-Risk Science Laboratories [79–83]

The Norwegian biotechnology community has warned about inadequate preparedness—easy to spread disease and hazardous agents in drinking water, air or food [83]. This is a well-known phenomenon for many other countries. Biosafety level 4 is the strictest level of safety where dangerous infection is identified and worked on. Nonetheless, infection occurs, and biologically dangerous and living agents have—by misunderstanding—been sent from such laboratories [84]. Work in high-risk laboratories is complicated and not everyone is equally well-trained [85].

There is a great variety in Europe in terms of quality of how high risk-infected patients become isolated [86, 87]. Checklists for infection control at high-level isolation have been designed and tested for five special units in Europe: in France, Germany, Italy, England (London) and Sweden (Linköping) [88]. The isolation unit was checked for separate entry for healthcare personnel and infected patient, safety control and security personnel, constant power and throughput autoclaves. The isolation room was checked for internal communication system, negative air pressure indicators, self-closing doors and separate/private bathroom/toilet. It is also checked for medical technical devices for intensive treatment and diagnostics and infection control procedures such as the use of PPE, hand hygiene, disinfection and waste management, external and internal transport, training in infection control and post-mortem treatment [88].

Guidance for outbreak response and incident management is recently made for acute care hospitals in the United States [89].

References

1. Law on Health and Social Preparedness 23 June 2000, No. 56. Oslo: Royal Health and Social Affairs; 2000.
2. Ministry of Social Affairs and Health. National emergency plan for pandemic flu. Oslo: 1999, 2001, 2006, 2009.
3. Ministry of Health and Care Services. Superior national health and social preparedness plan. Norway; 2007.
4. Regional plan for health and social preparedness in health region east, Norway; 2005.
5. Norwegian Health Directorate. Pandemic planning in municipal health services. Organization, Processing, Logistics. Draft 26 April 2009.
6. Norwegian Health Directorate. Pandemic planning in the specialist health service. Organization, Patient Reception and Treatment Draft 27 April 2009.
7. Directorate for Civil Protection and Emergency. Continuity planning—pandemic flu. *DSB* 5.6.2009.
8. National Institute for Public Health. Plan for mass vaccination against pandemic influenza in healthcare enterprises. Oslo 1.11.2008.
9. National Institute for Public Health. Report on recommended order for vaccination against new influenza A (H1N1), September 2009.
10. Norwegian Medicines Agency. Adverse reaction reported at Pandemrix—week 11; 03/18/2010.
11. Norwegian Medicines Agency. Annual report 2012. Vaccine effects. Reported side effects of vaccine against pandemic flu; 2012. p. 12–3.
12. Directorate for Civil Protection and Emergency. National risk image 2014. *DSB* 15 December 2014.
13. Blystad H. Preparedness/infection control plans and asylum reception. National Institute for Public Health, 2014.
14. Guldvåg B, Stoltenberg C. National Emergency Plan against Ebola. Interim plan. December 2014. Norwegian Directorate of Health/National Institute of Public Health December 2014.
15. Ebola guideline—from the Norwegian Institute of Public Health. November 2014.
16. Dalgard R, Espinoza R, Levy F, Rustung Jemtland AL, Røed R, Andersen BM. Emergency preparedness for outbreaks of serious, common infectious disease—import infection. In: Handbook in hygiene and infection control. Oslo: Ullevål Hospital; 1996. p. 170–80.
17. Dalgard R, Brubakk O, Levy F, Rustung Jemtland AL, Røed R, Andersen BM. Emergency preparedness for outbreaks of serious, common infectious disease—import infection. In: Handbook in hygiene and infection control. Oslo: Ullevål Hospital; 1999. p. 254–64.

18. Emergency preparedness at Ullevål University Hospital in connection with biological weapons. http://www.ulleval.sykehus.oslo.kommune.no/default.asp?page=/News&Id=23370. Accessed 25 Oct 2001.
19. Andersen BM. Anthrax and emergency routines at Ullevål University Hospital. Tidsskr Nor Legeforen. 2002;122:852–5.
20. Kjersem H, Lereim I. Emergency preparedness group at Ullevål University Hospital. Outbreaks of particularly infectious diseases during peacetime and in disasters/war related conditions. In: Handbook in hygiene and infection control for hospitals. Oslo: Ullevål University Hospital; 2003. p. 325–7.
21. Hafstad AM, Brubakk O, Madsen P, Rustung Jemtland AL, Levy F, Hochlin K, Andersen BM. Emergency preparedness plan for outbreak of serious infectious diseases—import disease. In: Handbook in hygiene and infection control for hospitals. Oslo: Ullevål University Hospital; 2003. p. 310–23.
22. Lereim I, Madsen P, Hylen Ranhoff A, Brubakk O, Melby K, Andersen BM. Preparedness for Ullevål University Hospital in connection with biological weapons. In: Handbook in hygiene and infection control for hospitals. Oslo: Ullevål University Hospital; 2003. p. 328–30.
23. Lereim I, Andersen BM. Emergency Response Group. In: Handbook in hygiene and infection control for hospitals. Oslo: Ullevål University Hospital; 2008. p. 550–2.
24. Andersen BM, Lereim I, Hochlin K. Serious, public infection scenarios. In: Handbook in hygiene and infection control for hospitals. Oslo: Ullevål University Hospital; 2008. p. 553–62.
25. Andersen BM, Hochlin K, Lereim I. Serious infections. Isolation. In: Handbook in hygiene and infection control for hospitals. Oslo: Ullevål University Hospital; 2008. p. 563–6.
26. Andersen BM. Severe infection. Use of personal protective equipment—PPE. In: Handbook in hygiene and infection control for hospitals. Oslo: Ullevål University Hospital; 2008. p. 567–8.
27. Andersen BM, Lereim I. General information and advice. In: Handbook in hygiene and infection control for hospitals. Oslo: Ullevål University Hospital; 2008. p. 569–70.
28. Andersen BM, Lereim I. Triage-treatment. In: Handbook in hygiene and infection control for hospitals. Oslo: Ullevål University Hospital; 2008. p. 571–2.
29. Andersen BM, Hochlin K, Lereim I. Patient management—logistics for serious infectious disease. In: Handbook in hygiene and infection control for hospitals. Oslo: Ullevål University Hospital; 2008. p. 569–70.
30. Andersen BM, Hochlin K, Rasch M. Viral haemorrhagic fever (VHF) and other serious viral diseases. In: Handbook in hygiene and infection control for hospitals. Oslo: Ullevål University Hospital; 2008. p. 575–82.
31. Andersen BM, Lereim I. Suspected use of biological weapons—for example anthrax. In: Handbook in hygiene and infection control for hospitals. Oslo: Ullevål University Hospital; 2008. p. 583–5.
32. Andersen BM, Lereim I. Preparedness for biological weapons. In: Handbook in hygiene and infection control for hospitals. Oslo: Ullevål University Hospital; 2008. p. 586–7.
33. Andersen BM, Lereim I. Contamination of dangerous agents/chemical substances. In: Handbook in hygiene and infection control for hospitals. Oslo: Ullevål University Hospital; 2008. p. 588–91.
34. Andersen BM. Pandemic preparedness 2010—evaluation of the pandemic 2009 at OUS-Ullevål. 20/12/2010. Attachment to the evaluation report to HSØ from OUS.
35. WHO. Hospital infection control guidance for severe acute respiratory syndrome (SARS) revised 24 April 2003.
36. WHO. Avian influenza, including influenza A (H5N1) in humans: WHO interim infection control guidelines of health care facilities, 2006.
37. WHO Infection prevention and control of epidemic—and pandemic- prone acute respiratory disease in healthcare. WHO/CDS/EPR/2007.6.
38. WHO. Infection prevention and control in health care for confirmed or suspected cases of pandemic (H1N1) 2009 and influenza-like conditions. WHO 25 June 2009.
39. WHO. Human infection with pandemic (H1N1) 2009 virus: updated interim WHO guidance on global surveillance. WHO 10 July 2009.

40. WHO. Patient care checklist. New influenza A (H1N1) 15 May 2009.
41. CDC. H1N1 Flu. Interim recommendations for facemask and respiratory use in certain community settings where H1N1 influenza virus transmission has been detected, 27 April 2009.
42. CDC. H1N1 Flu. Interim guidance for emergency medical services (EMS) systems and 9-1-1 Public Safety Response Points (PSAPs) for management of patients with confirmed or suspected swine-origin influenza A (H1N1) infection, 29 April 2009.
43. CDC. H1N1 Flu. Interim guidance for infection control for care of patients with confirmed or suspected swine influenza A (H1N1). Virus infection in a healthcare setting, 3 May 2009.
44. CDC. Vaccine safety. CDC statement on narcolepsy following Pandemrix influenza vaccination in Europe. CDC 27 March 2013.
45. Council of Europe: influenza vaccination a scandal. *Aftenposten* 27 Jan 2010.
46. ECDC. New ECDC technical report on "Narcolepsy in association with pandemic influenza vaccination—a multi-country European epidemiological investigation ", 20 Sep 2012.
47. WHO. Global alert and response. Middle East respiratory syndrome coronavirus (MERS-CoV)—update. 11 March 2014.
48. WHO. Interim-infection prevention and control guidance for care of patients with suspected or confirmed filovirus haemorrhagic fever in health-care settings, with focus on Ebola, Sep 2014.
49. CDC. Infection prevention and control recommendations for hospitalized patients with known or suspected Ebola haemorrhagic fever in US hospitals, Aug 2014.
50. UK, Department of Health. Management of hazard group 4 viral haemorrhagic fevers and similar human infectious diseases of high consequences, Sept 2014.
51. CDC. Guidance on personal protective equipment to be used by healthcare workers during management of patients with Ebola virus disease in US hospitals, including procedures for putting on (donning) and removing (doffing), 20 Oct 2014.
52. Andersen BM. Preliminary examination of patients. In: Handbook in hygiene and infection control for hospitals. Osla: Ullevål University Hospital; 2008. p. 405.
53. Andersen BM. Prevention of import infection and unknown infection. In: Handbook in hygiene and infection control for hospitals. Osla: Ullevål University Hospital; 2008. p. 406–15.
54. CDC. Health and safety concerns for all disasters/natural disasters and severe weather.
55. CDC. Preparation and planning.
56. CDC. Be ready! Earthquakes.
57. CDC. Prevent illness after a disaster, 8 Aug 2014.
58. CDC. Medical management of ill disaster evacuees, 20 June 2014.
59. CDC. Infection control guidance for community evacuation centres following disasters, 20 June 2014.
60. CDC. Infectious diseases after a disaster, 21 Aug 2014.
61. CDC. Remedication and infection control considerations for reopening healthcare facilities closed due to extensive water and wind damage, 20 June 2014.
62. CDC, Brandt M, Brown C, Burkhart J, et al. Mould-preventing strategies and possible health effects in the aftermath of hurricanes and major floods. MMWR. 2006;55:1–27.
63. Sehulster LM, Chinn RYW, Ardunio MJ, et al. Guidelines for environmental infection control in health-care facilities. CDC MMWR. 2003;52:1–42.
64. Rutala WA, Weber DJ. Disinfection, sterilization, and control of hospital waste. In: Mandell, Douglas, and Bennets principles and practice of infectious diseases. 8th ed. vol. 2. Philadelphia: Elsevier Churchill Livingstone; 2015. p. 3294–309.
65. CDC. Antibiotic resistance threats in the United States, 2013.
66. CDC Vital signs report, 3 Apr 2018.
67. Promed-mail 27 Febr 2017. Antibiotic resistance: WHO, priority pathogens.
68. Promed-mail 3 April 2018. Antibiotic resistance: USA, CDC coordinated containment strategy.
69. Woodworth KR, Walters MS, Weiner LM, Edwards J, Brown AC, Huang JY, et al. Vital signs: containment of novel multidrug-resistant organisms and resistance mechanisms—United States, 2006-2017. Morbid Mort Wkly Rep. 2018;67:1–7.
70. WHO. Antimicrobial resistance global report on surveillance, 2014.

71. ECDC. Summary of the latest data on antibiotic consumption in the European Union. ESAC-Net surveillance data, November 2017.
72. ECDC. Summary of the latest data on antibiotic resistance in the European Union. EARS-Net surveillance data, November 2017.
73. Andersen BM, Sørlie D, Hotvedt D, Almdahl SM, Olafsen K, George RC, Gilfillian A. Multiply beta-lactam resistant *Enterbacter cloacae* infections linked to the environmental flora in a unit of cardiothoracic and vascular surgery. Scand J Infect Dis. 1989;21:181–19.
74. Andersen BM, Bergh K, Steinbakk M, Syversen G, Magnæs B, Dalen H, Bruun JN. A Norwegian nosocomial outbreak of methicillin-resistant *Staphylococcus aureus* resistant to fusidic acid and susceptible to other anti-staphylococcal agents. J Hosp Infect. 1999;41:123–32.
75. Andersen BM, Lindemann R, Bergh K, Nesheim B-I, Syversen G, Solheim N, Laugerud F. Spread of methicillin-resistant *Staphylococcus aureus* in a neonatal intensive unit associated with understaffing, overcrowding and mixing of patients. J Hosp Infect. 2002;1:1–7.
76. Andersen BM, Tollefsen T, Seljordslia B, Hochlin K, Syversen G, Jonassen Ø, Rasch M. Rapid MRSA test in exposed persons: costs and savings in hospitals. J Infect. 2010;60:293–9.
77. Andersen BM, Seljordslia B, Hochlin K, Rasch M, Syveren G. A predicted outbreak in an overcrowded, administratively neglected and run-down haemo-dialysis unit as an offer of "New Public Management" in Norwegian hospitals. J Hosp Admin. 2013;2:15–24.
78. American Nurses Association. Adapting standards of care under extreme conditions. ANA, March 2008.
79. Rebman T. Infection prevention and emergency management. Institute for Biosecurity, Saint Louis University School of Public Health. (slides).
80. Rebman T. Infectious disease disaster: bioterrorism, emerging infections, and pandemics. APIC text of infection control and epidemiology 2014, chapter 120: 1–22.
81. English JF, Cundiff MY, Malone JD et al. Bioterrorism readiness plan: a template for healthcare facilities. APIC, CDC, 4/13/99.
82. Rebman T, the 2008 APIC Emergency Preparedness Committee, St. Louis, Missouri. APIC state-of-the-art report: the role of the infection preventionist in emergency management. Am J Infect Control. 2009;37:271–81.
83. Gjerding ML. Warns against bio terrorism in Norway. VG net, 23.10.2012.
84. CDC Lab incident: Anthrax. CDC. Updated 19 July 2014.
85. LeDuc JW, Anderson K, Bloom ME, et al. Framework for leadership and training of biosafety level 4 Laboratory workers. Emerg Infect Dis. 2008;14:1685–8.
86. Merens A, Cavallo JD, Thibault F, et al. Assessment of the bio-preparedness and of the training of the French hospital laboratories in the event of biological threat. Eurosurveillance. 2012;17:20312.
87. Maltezou HC, Fusco FM, Schilling S, et al. Infection control practices in facilities for highly infectious diseases across Europe. J Hosp Infect. 2012;81:184–91.
88. Fusco FM, Schilling S, Puro V, et al. EuroNHID checklists for the assessment of high-level isolation units and reference centers for highly infectious diseases: results from the pilot phase of a European survey. Clin Microbiol Infect. 2009;15:711–9.
89. Banach DB, Johnston BL, Al-Zubeidi D, Bartlett AH, Bleasdale SC, Deloney VM, et al. Outbreak response and incident management: SHEA Guidance and resources for healthcare epidemiologists in United States acute-care hospitals. Infect Control Hosp Epidemiol. 2017;38

82 Scenarios: Serious, Infectious Diseases

Abstract

Scenarios for serious, infectious diseases are important procedures used to understand the special microbe's behaviour (clinical illness, spread of infection, etc.) and how to act most rational during special dangerous outbreaks. Furthermore, scenarios describe how to handle patients, personnel and others possibly exposed to infections,- outside and inside the hospital- to stop spread of the infection as soon as possible. Today, it is not acceptable to place a patient with a known high-risk, serious infection in the same hospital room as other patients with not the same disease (WHO). In this chapter, some seldom but realistic scenario is described to better understand how to react and treat patients to stop spread of microbes during the primary phase of dangerous transmittable diseases.

Keywords

High-risk microbes · Scenarios · Transmittable dangerous agents · Lassa/Ebola/SARS/MERS/Nipah/avian influenza and other viruses · Anthrax/pest/cholera/diphtheria and other specific dangerous bacteria · Emergency · Preparedness Crisis management · Infection control · Isolation · Disinfection

82.1 Purpose

- Describe some rare but not unthinkable scenarios in the primary phase of dangerous transferable diseases.
- Describe certain important scenarios and practical measures to avoid spread of life-threatening disease among roommates, other patients or personnel, equipment or environment [1–3].

Current agents are described in more detail in: Andersen BM. Part 1. Microbiology and infection protection. Fagbokforlaget 2014.

B. M. Andersen, *Prevention and Control of Infections in Hospitals*,
https://doi.org/10.1007/978-3-319-99921-0_82

82.2 Comprise

- All personnel who are the first in contact with the infected/exposed person, relatives, other contacts and environment.
- *It is not acceptable to place a patient (with not defined same disease) in the same room with a patient with known high-risk infectious disease (WHO).*

82.3 Responsibility

The hospital's management provides written plans for how to react in situations where personnel and others may be exposed to known/unknown serious communicable disease and a practical arrangement for how to handle the situation.

The *infection control officer* at the level of where the problem occurs, and at the departments/ward where the infection may spread, is responsible for following local emergency plans.

Personnel who unprotected have come in a seriously contagious situation and may have been exposed to infectious agents are responsible for contacting the nearest responsible/infectious unit for advice and of following written guideline and practical advice.

82.4 Practical Measures [4]

- *The patient* (infected/suspected infected) is usually relatively easy to deal with since there are guidelines for preventing spread of infection and treating the patient for the current disease; *see isolation routines.*
- *Contacts exposed to infection* are often worse to handle since it may be larger numbers of people (travel company, etc.) and because fear of being infected itself creates uncertainty. Therefore, some imaginable scenarios are made that deal with infected contacts.
- *Transport by ambulance.* All transport of infectious patients from the place of arrival to the hospital should take place in ambulances using the same infection control regime as for the individual infectious disease (contact infection, airborne infection, strict isolation); see *isolation regimes; Chaps. 14–19 and chapter on transport of patients; 75. The infection regime should be in accordance with information/suspected findings and contact infection control personnel to ensure that this is the correct isolation level.*
- Always use respiratory protection and PPE in case of suspected pulmonary tuberculosis and other highly infectious, severe diseases, and use a surgical face mask or respiratory protective device (P2-P3 mask without valve) on all patients with respiratory symptoms.

82.5 Scenarios

82.5.1 Suspected *Viral Haemorrhagic Fever* (VHF) or Similar High-Risk Infection [4–6]

(Lassa, Ebola, Marburg, Machupo, Guanarito, Junin, Sabia, Nipah, Congo-Crimean, etc.)

82.5.1.1 Patient: Strict Isolation Airborne Infection in Isolate with Negative Air Pressure

Example: person from Liberia visiting relatives in Oslo in spring 2014. Sick 10 days after arrival in Oslo. He attended a number of family gatherings. At the onset of disease (*fever, respiratory symptoms and skin bleeding*), he lived with a family of eight people in Oslo. Medical contact was taken after 3 days of illness. In all, there had been 20 contacts with the patient after he became ill, and before Ebola virus, infection was suspected. He was admitted directly to the isolate for airborne infections with direct access from outside. Ambulance staff was pre-equipped (PPE) for transport of patients suspected of VHF. The municipality's infection control doctor is notified and takes responsibility for the message, measures and follow-up outside the hospital together with the emergency preparedness group for the municipality.

- *Unlikely in countries like Norway.* However a verified Ebola patient was imported autumn 2014. The patient came to the country as a high-risk infection patient and treated as such at Ullevål University Hospital, Oslo.
- *Quarantine disease.* Usually no more than one to two cases that (unexpectedly) get symptoms in Norway or while travelling to Norway. It is most likely that the symptoms come after arriving to Norway (2–21 days of incubation).
- *Registration.* Close contacts (name, address, telephone number and contact level with the patient). If sick on plane/boat/train, etc. to Norway, fellow passengers (same cabin/room/flight) must be registered.
- *Ambulance* personnel and other personnel use—*in suspicion*—infection control routines for VHF on contact and transport of the patient (see serious viral disease and personal infection prevention). Use respiratory equipment (P3 mask) and personal protective equipment (PPE), and put on a surgical mask on the patient.
- *Remember! Once too much is better than once too little!*
- *Risk of spread of VHF.* There is no significant risk of infection in Norway if the proper use of protective equipment is used when handling such patients. The Ebola outbreak in 3 African countries in 2014 showed that almost 30,000 were registered ill, more than 11,000 died, 800 health professionals became ill and more than half of them died. Lack of use of PPE and proper infection control led to escalation of the epidemic. The staff used only 1 m distance from the patient

as a zone of infection, as recommended by the WHO and CDC, and lacked protection for the head, hair and neck when within the 1 m zone and used only ordinary masks [7–10]. This occurred despite the fact that Ebola is defined as a high-risk, biosafety level 4 infection in which airborne infection could be relevant [11–14]. The epidemic declined from 14 September 2014, following the introduction of more proper use of personal protection equipment and infection control routines [11, 12, 15].

Contacts are differentiated after infection risk:

1. *High-risk contact*: physical contact with VHF, or with blood secretion or excretion. Healthcare staff, ambulance staff, laboratory staff, family or others who have treated the patient before admission.
2. *Low-risk contact*: been in the same room with the patient after the onset of the disease, but not in direct contact with the patient, equipment or others in the room. Examine the contacts; measure temperature two times for 3 weeks.
3. *Transmission from healthy contacts is considered unlikely.* However, everyone who has been in the same place at the same time with a VHF sick patient should be informed and followed up.

82.5.1.2 Monitor Contacts at Home

If probable or verified VHF, inform the contacts—low chance of infection:

- The contacts keep calm at home and measure the temperature daily two times for 3 weeks after the last contact with the index patient. No crowding with many people and no use of collective traffic.
- If temperature 38 °C or more, or rash/flu symptoms/sickness, contact the infection medical department.
- If this cannot be achieved at home, the contact may come to defined outpatient clinic for temperature measurement by appointment or is admitted to hospital.
- Served with food, etc. brought out from store to door, possibly, while isolated at home.

82.5.2 Multidrug-Resistant Bacteria: Outbreak of Infection

MRSA (methicillin-resistant *Staphylococcus aureus*), vancomycin-resistant MRSA, penicillin-resistant pneumococci, super-resistant gram-negative bacteria (ESBL, CRE,CP, NDM-1 bacteria), multidrug-resistant tubercle bacteria (tuberculosis), vancomycin-resistant enterococci (VRE), etc. evaluated in collaboration with microbiological laboratory. This was especially observed during the major tsunami disaster in 2004 [16]. Serious problems can occur in areas with melioidosis and other highly virulent bacteria.

82.5.2.1 Patient: Isolated in Accordance with Bacterial Type and Routines (Contact and/or Air Isolated)

In hospital, not usually many at the same time, but dependent on endemic situation. The patient can be contact or air isolated, depending on the infectious agent.

- *Registering* of direct contacts—depending on the infectious agent (name, address), and include where the patient have been earlier (information).
- *Ambulance* personnel and other personnel use routines for the relevant infection type according to *isolation procedures* and in accordance with emergency department's report. In case of doubt, contact infection control personnel.
- Use respiratory protection, P3 mask, if suspecting pulmonary tuberculosis, and put a surgical mask or P2/P3 mask without a valve on the patient in case of suspected pulmonary tuberculosis or respiratory tract infection.

Contacts/carriers—differentiated follow-up—low chance of getting sick:

1. Treated/controlled by the municipal infection control team in collaboration with infection protection personnel according to the type of infection.
2. Carriers live at home with eventually contact infection restrictions as defined and followed up by the Municipal Infection Surveillance Authority.
3. During stays at nursing homes, other hospitals, and in home nursing, these are followed up by the municipal infection physician/institution's physician in collaboration with infection control personnel.
4. In case of pulmonary tuberculosis, follow the defined guidelines for the control and follow-up of unprotected contacts according to defined routines (tuberculin test, screen check, clinical examination; *see separate chapter*).

82.5.3 Notification of Air Passengers with "Cholera" at Oslo Airport

82.5.3.1 Patient Is Contact Isolated

Example: Three people in a Norwegian travel company get voluminous, watery, painless diarrhoea on return from Bangladesh, just before landing at Oslo Airport, Gardermoen. Due to a loss of fluid, they were transported with an ambulance equipped for "import infection" and admitted directly into contact isolation. Municipal infection control doctor is notified and is responsible for reporting, measures and follow-up outside the hospital together with the municipal emergency response group.

This is one of the old, major quarantine diseases. Only a few get sick (top of the iceberg), i.e. 1–4 patients out of 1000 infected. There is a low mortality by proper treatment (<5%). The transmission risk is relatively low due to good hygiene and good sanitation in today's Norway and other developed countries. Most patients are shedding bacteria in large amounts and are also carriers without symptoms. Patients are isolated with contact isolation regimens.

The infection can reach unmanageable heights in disaster areas, by hunger, contaminated water supply and destroyed infrastructure. Following the natural disaster in Haiti, cholera was introduced with infected helper crew from Asia (carriers), and an epidemic started in 2010, which in 2013 had increased to 670,000 cholera patients, 370,000 hospitalized and 8200 deaths [17].

- *Registering of* contacts and remaining passengers in the airplane and from same travel company (name, address, telephone number).
- *Ambulance staff* and other personnel use the contact regime. If risk of spills, etc., use also surgical mask, visor and cap in addition to gloves and gown/overall.

Contacts/carriers of infection—low chance of getting sick:

1. Sampling (feces sample) from close contacts—those that may have the same source of infection as the index case (same travel company).
2. Enhance hand hygiene and personal hygiene for all.
3. Contact outpatient clinic for infections directly by gastrointestinal symptoms—contact by phone in advance.

82.5.4 Diphtheria After a Bus Trip to Moscow

82.5.4.1 Patient: Strict Isolation—Airborne Disease Isolation with Negative Air Pressure

Example: An elderly woman who recently attended a bus trip to Moscow became sick 2 days after returning to Oslo. She had sore throat, fever, cough and eventually a white, firm-sitting "plaque" in the throat. She was hospitalized after 3 days because of suspected diphtheria. Contact persons and other close contacts were contacted for follow-up and treatment with erythromycin (according to resistance pattern).

Municipal infection control doctor is notified and is responsible for reporting, measures and follow-up outside the hospital together with the municipal emergency response group.

Diphtheria may still be periodic problems in Eastern Europe and many places in the world. Vaccination status is good in children in most countries but more uncertain in elderly, especially in women. This is a contact and airborne infection, relatively highly infectious. There are probably few cases in an outbreak due to herd immunity. Patients are isolated with air and contact isolation regime until free from bacteria (negative culture). A historically serious infectious disease also in Norway, with high mortality rates until the middle of the last century [18]. Ullevål Hospital, Oslo, introduced treatment with the diphtheria serum in 1914 and achieved an impressive response—from 20–35% mortality to 3–5% [19].

- *Registering:* All exposed persons (name, address, telephone number) and follow-up; see below.

- *Ambulance staff* and other personnel use the contact and airborne infection regime when picking up and transporting a patient. Use respiratory protection, visor and cap in addition to gloves and gown/overall, and put a surgical mask on the patient.

Contacts/carriers of diphtheria are differentiated—vaccination protects against disease:

1. Sampling (nasopharynx samples) of *all* exposed persons (even if vaccinated and are not sick, you may be a carrier).
2. Prophylactic/therapeutic treatment with erythromycin may be initiated rapidly.
3. If living at home, others should not be exposed to infection/carrier state.
4. Short-time airborne isolation may be relevant for carrier or exposed to infection until the infection state is clarified/effect of antibacterial therapy.
5. Booster vaccine against diphtheria is considered for all contacts.

82.5.5 Lung Pest Plague After Stay in Madagascar, Sick on the Plane Home

82.5.5.1 Patient: Strict Isolation—Negative Air Pressure Isolation

Example: A person of a family of five who has stayed in Madagascar for a month got sick on his way home to Norway. He coughs, has fever and develops skin rashes that resemble big boils, especially in the groin. He was admitted directly to strict isolation in hospital and suspected of serious import infection.

The municipal infection control doctor is notified and is responsible for reporting, measures and follow-up outside the hospital together with the municipal emergency response group.

- *Quarantine disease*: Periodic problem in the East Asia, especially India, and ongoing outbreaks in Africa, Namibia and Madagascar. Pest may be a war-related disease (biological warfare). Untreated dies more than 50% of the cases while, with streptomycin treatment, less than 5%. This is a typical airborne disease, relatively highly infectious when respiratory tract symptoms. There is usually small outbreak with few cases (1–2). Air and contact infection regime until free for bacteria. In November 2014, new pest outbreaks were reported in Madagascar. About 120 patients got sick, of whom 40 died of bubonic plague [20]. The infection spread rapidly between humans and "killed quickly" [20]. Multidrug-resistant *Yersinia pestis* is described in this country [20].
- *Registering:* All infected persons (same travel company, all in the same flight home) are registered (name, address, telephone number) and followed up.
- *Ambulance staff* and other personnel use the contact and airborne isolation regime when picking up and transporting a patient. Use respiratory protection (P3 mask), visor and cap in addition to gloves and gown/overall, and put a surgical mask on the patient.

All close contacts/carriers are isolated to infection state is clarified—little chance of getting sick:

1. Sampling from all exposed persons
2. Prophylactic/therapeutic treatment, eventually vaccine
3. Short-time airborne isolation of exposed cases until the infection state is clarified/effect of antibacterial therapy

82.5.6 Anthrax After Staying in Turkey, Sick on the Plane Home

82.5.6.1 Patient: Strict Isolation—Air Pressure Isolate with Pressure [21, 22]

Example: Two out of six people who have been on family visits in Turkey for a week, on farms with goats and skin production, are acutely ill on the plane home with cough, shortness of breath and fever. Upon arrival, the emergency outpatient clinic was contacted by the patients who were immediately transferred to intensive care unit for airway symptoms and suspected import infection. At the hospital, anthrax is suspected, and patients are strictly isolated in air isolate and treated.

Municipal infection control doctor is notified and is responsible for reporting, measures and follow-up outside the hospital together with the municipal emergency response group.

- *Endemic problem in* several places (Asia, Africa, Middle East, North and South America), war-related (biological warfare). Varying number of cases of anthrax at outbreaks during peacetime, depending on how many people have eaten, for example, infected food, etc.
- *Symptoms*: 95% are cutaneous, 5% are respiratory, and a few cases are gastrointestinal anthrax. The latter two are two-phasic and almost always fatal.
- *The bacterium Bacillus anthracis is* a spore-forming, resistant, gram-positive rod that survives nearly infinity in the environment if not removed. The bacteria are usually penicillin-sensitive.
- *Infection:* Person-to-person infection is unlikely, but hospital infection is described. Air and contact regime is conducted around such patients in hospitals until free of bacteria (ca 24 h treatment); however spores may survive for a long time.
- *Registering*: All directly exposed persons are registered (name, address, telephone number) and followed up.
- *Ambulance* personnel use contact and airborne regime for patient pickup and transport. Use respiratory protection (P3 mask), visor and cap in addition to gloves and gown/overall, and put a surgical mask on the patient.

Contacts/carriers—low risk of getting sick:

1. Sampling and antibacterial treatment are offered to all contacts that may have a common source of infection with the index patients (travel company, co-passenger). Person-to-person transmission is unlikely.

2. Vaccine may, in addition to antibacterial treatment, be applicable to people with a common source of infection with the index patients—when risk of large outbreaks (note that vaccination should be discussed due to some serious adverse reactions).
3. While waiting for result of the sampling, close contacts live at home with contact isolation restrictions.
4. In case of detected anthrax in contact (incubation phase for disease 3–7 days), the person is isolated and treated, and vaccination may be assessed for close contacts.

82.5.7 Rabies

82.5.7.1 Patient Is Isolated

This is an endemic problem among wild animals in most countries. Person-to-person transmission is unlikely. It is almost never reported more than one case at a time, infected by animal bites or licking but occasionally without known exposure. Close contacts/exposed persons are registered.

- *Registering:* All exposed persons are registered (name, address, telephone number) and followed up.
- *Ambulance staff* and other personnel use the contact and airborne regime when picking up and transporting a patient. Use respiratory protection and PPR; put a surgical mask on the patient.

  Contacts/exposed—low chance of getting sick:

1. Close contacts/exposed persons are assessed for vaccine and rabies immunoglobulin.
2. Followed up at the infection outpatient clinic.

82.5.8 SARS and MERS: See Separate Chapter

Patients and contacts are treated just like at VHF.

82.5.9 Avian: Pandemic Flu (API) (See Separate Chapter)

Patients and contacts are treated mainly like VHF.

82.5.10 New Contagious Severe Disease: Unknown Agent and Pathway

See also SARS and bird flu.

New infectious diseases and agents still appear, for example, SARS, avian viruses (H5N1), HTLV and other retroviruses, HPV, sindbis virus, parvovirus, bocavirus, coronavirus, etc., or bacteria like *Legionella* and *Borrelia*, or agents with virulence changes, like group A streptococci, meningococci, etc.

- *Biological terrorism* made anthrax, plague, botulism, *Coxiella*, *Brucella*, VHF, poxviruses and a number of other unusual agents more appropriate as biological weapons [21–41].
- *Bacteria* sensitive to common antibacterial agents will probably not be a major problem.
- *Viruses* with no vaccine or treatment against low infection dose and high capacity to survive will be a major problem if associated with incurable disease, disability or death.
- It is probable that this will be a problem first in countries with low hygiene standards/high population density.

If the infectious agent is unknown, transmission ways are unknown and the situation is uncertain or uncontrollable, this practical measure may be followed:

Patient and contacts: strict isolation—negative air pressure isolation

1. Serious illness: isolation of index case and all contacts
2. Less severe disease: isolation of index case and close contacts
   - *Registering:* All exposed persons are registered (name, address, telephone number) and followed up.
   - *Ambulance* personnel use contact and airborne regime for patient pickup and transport. Use respiratory protection (P3 mask), visor and cap in addition to gloves and gown/overall/shoe covers/dedicated shoes, and put a surgical mask on the patient.

82.5.11 Other Dangerous Agents/Infections

- *Botulism* is caused by a bacteria-produced toxin (*Clostridium botulinum*) that causes paresis and is common in soil as spores. The disease can be associated with toxin formation in contaminated and poorly canned foods, shrimp fish, bacon, etc. under anaerobic conditions and randomly affects both healthy people and vulnerable groups, such as infants who have had honey infected with the bacterium, which has happened repeatedly [42]. The toxin is the most dangerous we know and is on the list of bioterrorism.
- *Brucella* bacteria (zoonosis) are particularly related to laboratory outbreaks but are easily transferable outside the laboratory and are considered highly infectious. [43]
- *Francisella tularensis* (zoonosis) is defined as a category A bioterrorism agent, highly infectious and increasing in the society, has low infection dose (10–25

bacteria) and can be inhaled or infected via food and water. Occasionally, such patients are detected in hospitals, even in the operating department [44].

- *MERS—Middle East respiratory syndrome*—newly discovered coronavirus zoonosis (dromedaries, bats, etc.) and acts as SARS, also with a tendency for nosocomial spread in hospitals. In 2015 there were 1100 cases, of which 40% died [45].
- *Polio-like illnesses*, especially among children, were discovered in August 2014 in different states in the United States. Probably caused by enterovirus D68 [46].
- *HIV—aggressive variants* (CRF19) have been detected in Cuba in 2015 and earlier in Africa, with a faster course from infection to AIDS development [47].
- *Prion disease—new Shy-Drager syndrome* is rediscovered in 2015; multiple-system atrophy (MSA) [48].
- *Ricin* is a plant-derived toxin that is still used for bioterrorism in letters to, among others, President Obama [49].
- *Fungi and mould*: different types that are especially related to floods, water damage, etc. and to pollution of medical products [50–53]. In Norway, a recent overview of candida in blood cultures showed a stable state for the past 22 years [54].
- *Zika* virus: newly discovered flavivirus with mild to serious symptoms and teratogenic effect [5].

References

1. Ministry of Labour and Administration. Regulations on protection against exposure to biological factors (bacteria, viruses, fungi and more) in the workplace. FOR OSLO: 1997-12-19 nr.1322.
2. Sehulster LM, Chinn RYW, Ardunio MJ, et al. Guidelines for environmental infection control in health-care facilities. CDC MMWR. 2003;52:1–42.
3. Rutala WA, Weber DJ. Disinfection, sterilization, and control of hospital waste. In: Mandell, Douglas, and Bennets principles and practice of infectious diseases. 8th ed. vol. 2. Philadelphia: Elsevier Churchill Livingstone; 2015. p. 3294–309.
4. Andersen BM, Lereim I, Hochlin K. Serious, common contagious scenarios. In: Handbook in hygiene and infection control for hospitals. Olso: Ullevål University Hospital; 2008. p. 553–62.
5. Andersen BM. Other serious viral infections—zoonoses. In: Handbook in hygiene and infection control for hospitals. Part 1 Fagbokforlaget; 2014. p. 278–90.
6. Andersen BM. Ebola, Lassa, and other haemorrhagic viruses. In: Handbook in hygiene and infection control for hospitals. Part 1. Fagbokforlaget; 2014. p. 291–9.
7. WHO. Interim-infection prevention and control guidance for care of patients with suspected or confirmed filovirus haemorrhagic fever in health-care settings, with focus on Ebola, September 2014.
8. CDC. Infection prevention and control recommendations for hospitalized patients with known or suspected Ebola haemorrhagic fever in US hospitals, August 2014.
9. UK, Department of Health. Management of hazard group 4 viral haemorrhagic fevers and similar human infectious diseases of high consequences, September 2014.
10. Ebola guideline—from the Norwegian Institute of Public Health 09/11/2014.
11. Promed mail 14 September 2014. Andersen BM Infection control is not working.

12. Andersen BM. International infection control guidelines for Ebola. Hospital Healthcare Europe. Facilities management. April 2015. www.hospitalhealthcare.com.
13. Weingartl HM, Embury-Hyatt C, Nfon C. Transmission or Ebola virus from pigs to non-human primates. Scientific Rep. 2012; 2:article number: 811.
14. Bourouiba L, Dehandschoewerker E, Bush JWM. Violent expiratory events: on coughing and sneezing. J Fluid Mech. 2014;845:537–63.
15. CDC. Guidance on personal protective equipment to be used by healthcare workers during management of patients with Ebola virus disease in US hospitals, including procedures for putting on (donning) and removal, 20 Oct 2014.
16. McKay I, Sax H, Harbarth S, Bernard L, Pittet D. Multi-resistant infections in repatriated patients after natural disaster: lessons learned from the 2004 tsunami for hospital infection control. J Hosp Infect. 2008;68:1–8.
17. Andersen BM. Cholera (Vibrio cholerae). In: Handbook in hygiene and infection control for hospitals. Part 1. Fagbokforlaget; 2014. p. 105–7.
18. Breivik E, Gradmann C. Tonsillitis in Europe's outskirt—when the diphtheria toxin came to the county of Romsdal. Tidsskr Nor Legeforen. 2014;134:732–5.
19. Linnestad P. "Blood is a very special juice"—introduction of serum therapy for diphtheria in Norway. Tidsskr Nor Legeforen. 2014;134:1780–1.
20. Promed Mail November 21, 2014. Plague—Madagascar.
21. Preparedness at Ullevål University Hospital in connection with biological weapons. http://www.ulleval sykehus.oslo.kommune.no/default.asp?page=/Nyheter&Id=23370. Accessed 25 Oct 2001.
22. Andersen BM. Anthrax and emergency routines at Ullevål University Hospital. Tidsskr Nor Legeforen. 2002;122:852–5.
23. Siegrist DW. The threat of biological attack: why concern now? Emerg Infect Dis. 1999;5:505–8.
24. Borio L, Inglesby BL, Peters CJ, et al. Haemorrhagic fever viruses as biological weapons: medical and public health management. JAMA. 2002;287:2391–405.
25. Jernigan JA, Stephens DS, Ashford DA, Omenaca C, Topiel MS, Galbraith M, et al. Bioterrorism-related inhalation anthrax: the first 10 cases reported in the United States. Emerg Infect Dis. 2001;7:933–44.
26. Inglesby TV, O'Toole T, Hendersen DA, et al. Anthrax as a biological weapon, 2002: updated recommendations for management. JAMA. 2002;287:2236–52.
27. Sirisanthana T, Brown AE. Anthrax of the gastrointestinal tract. Emerg Infect Dis. 2002;8:649–51.
28. Yakupogullari Y, Koroglu M. Nosocomial spread of *Bacillus anthracis*. J Hosp Infect. 2007:401–40.
29. Andersen BM. Anthrax. Bacteria and disease. Epidemiology, infections and infection protection. Oslo: Gyldendal Akademisk, Gyldendal Norsk Forlag AS; 2005. p. 9–44.
30. Høiby N. Can anthrax infect from patient to patient? Ugeskr Leger. 2001;163:6606–7.
31. Dull PM, Wilson KE, Kournikakis B, Whitney EAS, Boulet CA, Ho JYW, et al. *Bacillus anthracis* aerosolization associated with a contaminated mail sorting machine. Emerg Infect Dis. 2002;8:1044–7.
32. Weis CP, Intrepido AJ, Miller AK, Cowin PG, Durno MA, Gebhart JS, et al. Secondary aerosolization of viable *Bacillus anthracis* spores in a contaminated US Senate office. J Am Med Assoc. 2002;288:2853–8.
33. Kournikakis B, Armor SJ, Boulet CA, Spence M, Parsons B. Risk assessments of anthrax threat letters. Defense research establishment suffield. DRES technical report 2001–038. September 2001. http://www.dres.dnd.ca/Meetings/FirstResponders/tr01-048_annex.pdf.
34. Peters CJ, Hartley DM. Anthrax inhalation and lethal human infection. Lancet. 2002;359:710–1.
35. Byrne D. Bioterrorism: crime and opportunity. Euro Surveill. 2001;6:157–8.
36. Coignard B. Bioterrorism preparedness and response in European public health institutes. Euro Surveill. 2001;6:159–66.

37. Harling R, Twisselmann B, Asgari-Jirhandeh, Morgan D, Lightfoot N, Reacher M, Nicoli A, Deliberate Releases of Biological Agents. Initial lessons for Europe from events in the United States. Euro Surveill. 2001;6:166–71.
38. Levy-Bruhl D, Guerin N. The use of smallpox virus as a biological weapon: the vaccination situation in France. Euro Surveill. 2001;6:171–8.
39. Desenclos JC. Are there «new » and «old » ways to track infectious diseases hazards and outbreaks ? Euro Surveill. 2006;11:206–7.
40. Rebman T. Infectious disease disaster: bioterrorism, emerging infections, and pandemics. APIC text of infection control and epidemiology; 2014. p. 1–22 (Chapter 120).
41. English JF, Cundiff MY, Malone JD et al. Bioterrorism readiness plan: a template for healthcare facilities. APIC, CDC. 4/13/99.
42. Valley ML, Bye K, Nilsen KB, Rørvik LM, Tessem GAG. An infant with acute paresis. Tidsskr Nor Legeforen. 2015;135:1455–8.
43. Lowe CF, Showler AJ, Perera S, et al. Hospital-associated transmission of *Brucella melitensis* outside the laboratory. Emerg Infect Dis. 2015;21:150–2.
44. Becker SL, Splettesteesser WD, Kim YJ, et al. Potential risk of aerosol-borne *Francisella tularensis* transmission in the operating room. Infect Control Hosp Epidemiol. 2015;36:490–1.
45. Promed-mail 28 August 2015. MERS-COV. Jordan, Saudi Arabia, Nosocomial.
46. Pastula DM, Aliabadi N, Haynes AK, et al. Acute neurological disease of unknown etiology in children—Colorado, August-September 2014. MMWR. 2014;63:1–2.
47. Promed-mail 14 February 2015. HIV-Cuba: new aggressive variant, CRF19.
48. Promed-mail 17 September 2015. Prion disease updated: novel prion disease—SHY-DRAGER syndrome.
49. Promed-mail 17 April 2013. Ricin-USA: Washington, DC, Letters.
50. CDC, Brandt M, Brown C, Burkhart J, et al. Mould-preventing strategies and possible health effects in the aftermath of hurricanes and major floods. MMWR. 2006;55:1–27.
51. Andersen BM. Fungi-human pathogenic. In: Handbook in hygiene and infection control for hospitals. Part 1. Fagbokforlaget; 2014. p. 393–9.
52. Promed-mail 17 November 2014. Mucormycosis—USA: fatal, premature infant, probiotic supplement, recall, alert.
53. Promed-mail 1 September 2014. Sporotrichosis-Australia: Northern Territory.
54. Hesstvedt L, Gaustad P, Andersen CT, et al. Twenty-two years of candidaemia surveillance: results from a Norwegian national study. Clin Microbiol Infect. 2015;21:938–45.

Isolation: Serious, Infectious Diseases 83

Abstract

All persons staying in hospitals should be protected against exposure to infectious agents, and especially to high-risk, dangerous agents - that pose a risk to health and life. It is not acceptable to place a patient with a known high-risk, serious infection in the same hospital room as other patients (WHO). In this chapter, the preparedness of isolation capacity and escalation of hospital beds for patients with dangerous infections are described.

Keywords

Isolation capacity · Cohort isolation · Contact isolation · Airborne isolation Escalating increased need of beds

83.1 Purpose

- Describe the need for preparedness concerning isolation capacity in case of serious outbreaks and escalating need for isolation beds.
- Evaluate in cooperation with other hospitals (regional, national) the acute need for isolation capacity.
- Evaluate measures to handle outbreaks during normal epidemiological situation, smaller outbreaks and large outbreaks [1–3].

83.2 Comprise

- The hospital' management, infection control personnel and all persons responsible for the emergency plan and for implementation of the plan.

B. M. Andersen, *Prevention and Control of Infections in Hospitals*,
https://doi.org/10.1007/978-3-319-99921-0_83

83.3 Responsibility

The hospital's management, emergency group and infection control personnel provides updated written information concerning isolation capacity and types in the hospital and the actual region.

The decision of increased need of isolates, more special trained personnel and equipment is made in cooperation with emergency team and with regional and national infection control coordinators.

Department management has the overall responsibility for ensuring that isolates are functioning as they should and that routines are followed.

83.4 Practical Measures [4]

83.4.1 Patients with Infections: Need for Isolation Units in Hospitals

Normal situation—concerning infectious diseases caused by bacteria—is dependent on endemic situation, use of antibiotics and development of resistance.

- In Scandinavian countries like Norway, at least 20% of hospitalized patients may have infections—community or institutional associated—and 20–30% receive antibacterial agents, prophylactically or therapeutic [4–8]. Approximately 20% of all admitted patients need at minimum a single room due to risk of transmission of infections. At least 10% of nosocomial infections are transmitted via droplets—airborne [4–8].
- At least 5% of invasive *Escherichia coli* in Scandinavia were resistant to third-generation cephalosporins in 2016, while up to 50% were resistant in countries in the south of Europe [9]. The EARS-Net surveillance data for 2016 showed a pattern of more resistant, invasive bacteria in the south than north of Europe, for *Klebsiella pneumonia*, *Acinetobacter* sp., MRSA and *Enterococcus faecium* [10].
- The consumption of antibiotics in the community was up to 20 DDD per 1000 inhabitants per day in Scandinavia, while up to 36 DDD per day in the south of Europe in 2016 [10].
- The consumption of antibiotics for systemic use in the hospital sector was 1.4–2.1 DDD per 1000 inhabitants per day, in Norway, Sweden and Denmark and higher, up to 2.9 DDD, in Finland that included remote primary healthcare centres and nursing homes [10]. The population-weighted mean consumption of antibiotics for systemic use in the hospital sector in Europe/EEA was 2.0 DDD per 1000 inhabitants per day [10].

Local outbreaks of, for example, norovirus, rotavirus, influenza virus, metapneumovirus, respiratory syncytial virus (RSV) or resistant bacteria from home and abroad double the need for isolates or single rooms in hospitals in periods.

Influenza pandemics it has previously been estimated that in larger outbreaks, 0.3% of the population will need hospitalization, and approximately 13% need outpatient treatment. Capacity and readiness for escalating—if needed—should be calculated and included in emergency preparedness plans in and outside hospitals. In such cases it may be appropriate to request *predefined*, newer hotels or healthcare institutions.

For example, the need in the Oslo region with about 800,000 inhabitants would be 2400 additional hospitalizations of isolation-needing patients over a short period of 1–2 months. If the average stay would be 10 days and the patients were equally distributed over this period (which is not the situation), the need at any time would be approximately 400 extra isolate beds.

83.4.2 Pandemic Flu AH1N1 2009: Experience from Norway

The pandemic flu AH1N1 came quickly and disappeared relatively rapidly—from spring to autumn of 2009—in Norway [5, 6, 11–17]. There was a tendency for a two-phase epidemic development, with a slight top during weeks 28–32 [11]. Microbiological detection of virus (AH1N1) was quickly established but never exceeded 2800 positive findings on a weekly basis in a population of ca. five million inhabitants; see Fig. 83.1 [11].

On a national basis, the number of hospitalized patients per day in the peak period was approximately 90 patients, and 20–30 patients were in intensive care units (Fig. 83.2).

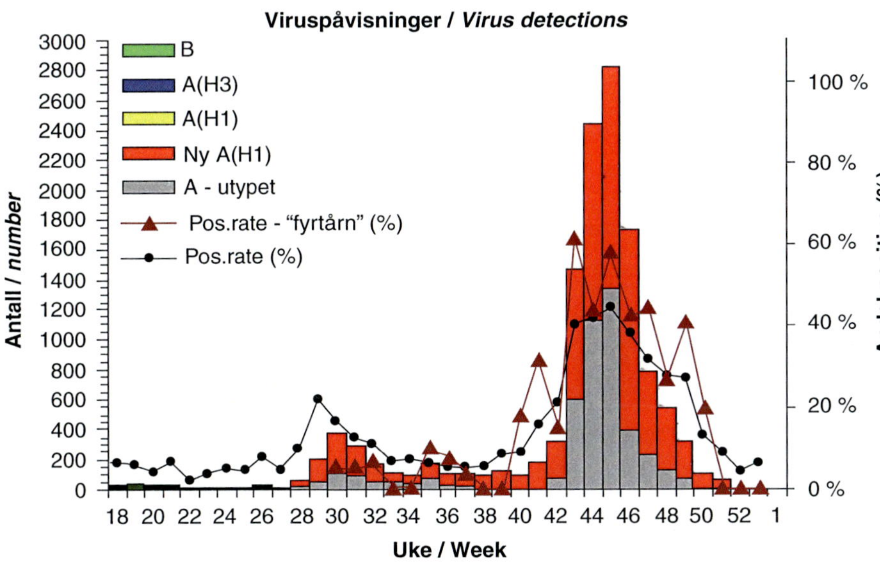

Fig. 83.1 Pandemic influenza had a two-phase development from spring to autumn 2009. Source: National Public Health Norway [11]

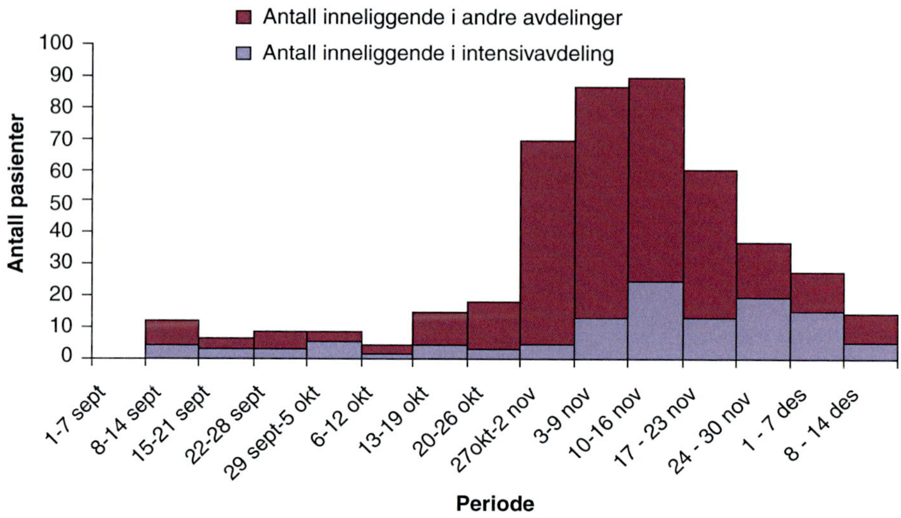

Fig. 83.2 Number of hospitalized patients with laboratory-detected pandemic influenza A H1N1 from 1 September 2009. Patients: blue admitted to ICUs and red to other departments. Source: National Public Health Norway [11]

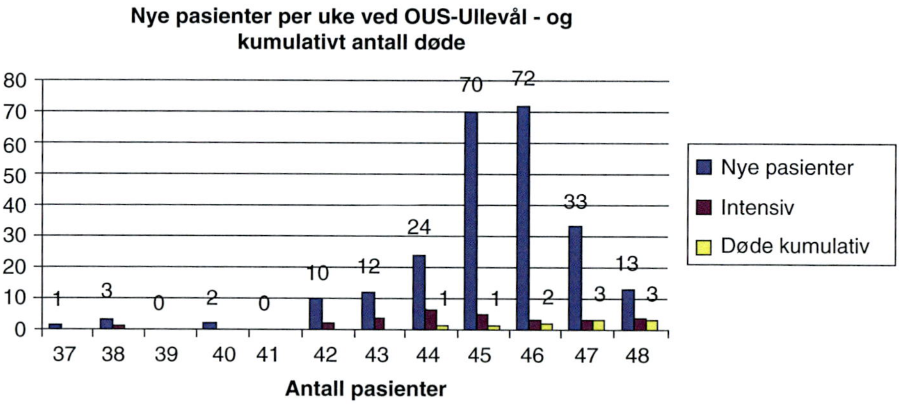

Fig. 83.3 Number of new patients with influenza AH1N1 (blue), admitted to OUS—Ullevål University Hospital per week; number of patients in intensive units (red)—and cumulatively number of deaths (yellow). Source: BM Andersen, OUS—Ullevål University Hospital 2009 [5, 6]

OUS—Ullevål University Hospital, Oslo, is the main hospital for about 800,000 inhabitants in the southeast of Norway. There were a maximum of 72 patients admitted to the hospital per week (46), because of influenza AH1N1, including ca. 10 patients at the intensive care units per week (Fig. 83.3) [5, 6]. There was no capacity shortage due to a ready distribution system for patients, as well as a plan for cohort isolation at a separate hospital building [5, 6]. Three patients were registered dead because of the pandemic at Ullevål; one of them was dead on arrival [5, 6].

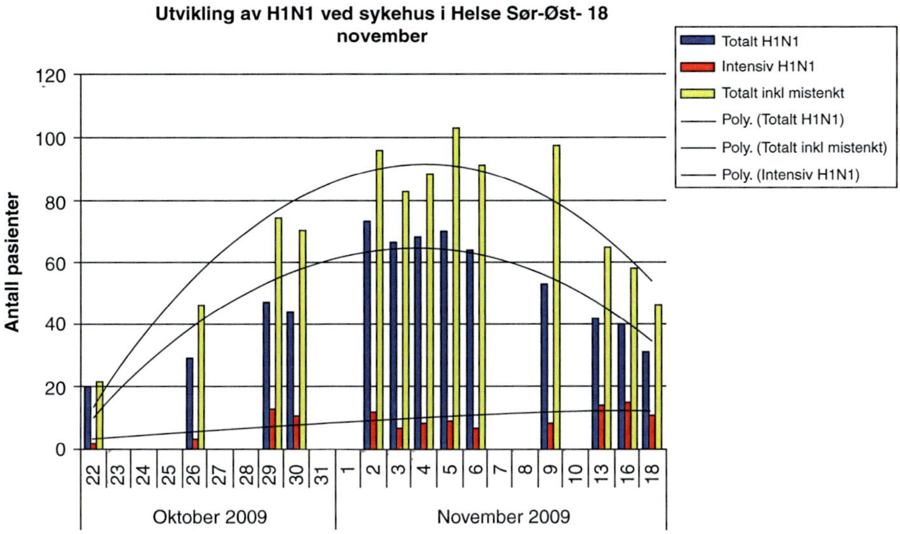

Fig. 83.4 Number of patients with influenza AH1N1 (blue), admitted to hospitals in the health region southeast of Norway (ca 2.5 million inhabitants) per week; number of patients in intensive units (red)—and total number, included suspect cases (yellow) from October to November 2009. Source: BM Andersen, OUS—Ullevål University Hospital 2009 [5, 6]

Including all hospitals in the health region southeast of Norway (2.5 million inhabitants), there were around 100 hospitalized influenza patients daily during the period 2–9 November and then a rapid decline (Fig. 83.4) [4, 5]. Between 10 and 18 intensive patients were treated for pandemic flu each day during this period.

Experiences from this pandemic showed that the calculated scenarios did not agree with the facts, either regarding the number of infected (probably), hospital admissions, intensive care or death rate.

83.4.3 Isolates: Capacity

83.4.3.1 Number and Status [5, 6, 11–17]

It is important to have an overview of the number and types of isolates for infectious diseases in a radius of at least 100 km around densely populated areas. The isolates should be checked at least once a year that they function according to the mode of use. Isolates for airborne infectious agents should have a negative air pressure, sluice and separate bathroom disinfection room with decontaminator, and contact isolates should also have a separate bathroom disinfection room with decontaminator and through-put and should have some degree of negative air pressure in relation to corridor, etc.

Single room with toilet/shower. It is essential to have a list available on the number of well-equipped rooms that can be used for contact isolation.

A large hospital like Ullevål University Hospital with approx. 800 somatic beds have 41 (5.1%) isolation units for airborne infections (of which 20 for children), 25 contact isolates (3.1%) and 74 single beds (9.3%).

Isolation requirement in case of minor outbreaks under normal epidemiologically situations:

- *Patients*: Under normal circumstances, the number of satisfactory isolates should cover the usual needs of the population, if also included the use of other hospitals in the area, flexible. Most outbreaks of serious epidemics are related to a few patients, 1–5.
- *Close contact/exposed/carriers*: Short-term isolation may be applicable to persons exposed to infection by diphtheria (adults, elderly), plague and possibly anthrax. In some cases, isolation is applicable to infected persons or carriers who cannot take care of themselves/do not follow preventive measures or other conditions that require isolation (e.g., exposure/carrier status of cholera and other intestinal pathogenic microbes, multidrug-resistant bacteria, VHF).

Isolates needed for major outbreaks—serious epidemic in the population—exceeds capacity:

- *Escalating situation.* An escalation plan must be available, with an overview of hospitals, other health institutions, hotels, etc. that can be predefined and staffed by appointment. Fixed, annual technical control must be carried out. It should not be far away from core areas but sheltered.
- If *cohort treatment of* patients with the same microbiological diagnosis—put patients in the same room; it will facilitate the care situation and save personal protection equipment (PPE). In case of major outbreaks, the entire departments or hospitals can be dedicated to patients with laboratory-diagnosed infection (see SARS outbreaks in China and Singapore 2003 where they had their own SARS hospitals).
- *Avoid long transportation of infection patients.* Isolate units should not be far from hospitals that take care of the epidemic (where most cases are occurring). Long transport takes large resources and time and can cause fear in the population.

How to increase the capacity if the outbreak escalates:

Depending on the *number of* people involved in an outbreak of infection, it should be planned as follows:

- Patients with identical microbiological agent and increased need of hospital treatment—escalate:
  - Infection disease wards or intensive units with isolates
  - Other suitable departments (area shielded/the building is closed for other patients)
  - Other suitable hospitals in the region.
  - If necessary—a complete hospital, entire nursing home or pre-arranged/requested hotel

- Carriers/exposed/close contacts
  - Isolation at home, if possible.
  - Isolation at designated buildings, at hospital or at predesignated hotel.
  - Note! Nursing homes and similar buildings with common ventilation are not suitable for airborne isolation of exposed, close contacts or infectious carriers because of risk of transmission via air.
  - It is assumed that the general minimum requirements for emergency response/mass isolation are met (see below).

Isolate need for major epidemics/disasters:

In case of war with for instance biological weapons or an unusual epidemic extent/condition, the need for isolates will be large. Here it will probably be relevant for cooperation between states and countries. In such cases it may be appropriate to request *predefined*, newer hotels, cf. the Norwegian Health and Social Preparedness Act, §3-1 Requisition [12–17]. A report of 22 February 1984 to the Director General of Health, under review, "Proposal for Planning of Epidemiological Preparedness" by a reference group set up by the Directorate of Health on 30 March 1982. The report states that after the "nature and extent of the disaster," different measures may be needed for the isolation, treatment and care of patients with infectious diseases. "In *all* these cases, one must assume that the best suited for these purposes are our many and good *hotels*." It is emphasized that in all parts of the country, *preferentially*, *new hotels* should be *pre*designated for this purpose. Most hotels have a high quality of the building and hygienic standard. They have single and double rooms, most of them with separate bathrooms and toilets, which is of the utmost importance as it facilitates isolation and care. They also have laundry facilities and kitchens, and most have wings that can be shut down. These are qualities that are approaching the requirements of an isolation department. The ventilation should be considered turned off. Ventilation can be done via windows if not large passage of people directly outside (WHO).

General requirements for emergency response/mass isolation—area:

- Fast, mobilizable and flexible.
- Preferably direct access from outside or via closed corridor.
- Preferably one bedroom with a high hygienic standard; sink, bath/shower.
- Access to kitchen or other cooking facilities.
- Can be closed to other parts of the building.
- Preferably not in densely populated areas.
- If situated outside the main hospital, it should be so close that it can be operated from the hospital departments (infectious medicine, intensive, lung, X-ray, sampling, cleaning, textile, purchasing, kitchen, transportation and a number of other service functions).

Need for personnel, equipment, service, transport, etc.:

- An estimate of needed qualified personnel in an escalation plan must be available.

- Requirements for specific equipment such as respirator, other ventilation equipment, etc.—escalation plan must be available.
- Service plan of service (food, water, laundry, consumables, etc.).
- Plan for cleaning, disinfection and disposal.
- Transport plan (patients, equipment, vehicles, etc.) must be available.

References

1. Ministry of Labour and Administration. Regulations on protection against exposure to biological factors (bacteria, viruses, fungi and more) in the workplace. FOR OSLO: 1997-12-19 nr.1322.
2. Sehulster LM, Chinn RYW, Ardunio MJ, et al. Guidelines for environmental infection control in health-care facilities. CDC MMWR. 2003;52:1–42.
3. Rutala WA, Weber DJ. Disinfection, sterilization, and control of hospital waste. In: Mandell, Douglas, and Bennets principles and practice of infectious diseases, vol. 2. 8th ed. Philadelphia: Elsevier Churchill Livingstone; 2015. p. 3294–309.
4. Andersen BM, Hochlin K, Lereim I. Serious infections—isolation. In: Handbook in hygiene and infectious diseases for hospitals. Oslo: Ullevål University Hospital; 2008. p. 563–6.
5. Andersen BM. Pandemic flu. In: Handbook in hygiene and infection control for hospitals. Part 1. Fagbokforlaget; 2014. p. 212–36.
6. Andersen BM. Pandemic preparedness 2010—evaluation—pandemic 2009—OUS-Ullevål. 20/12/2010. Attachment to the evaluation report to HSØ from OUS.
7. Andersen BM, Holta Ringertz S, Gullord Petersen T, Hermansen W, Lelek M, Norman BI, Næs B, Tilrem Nystad M, Andersen Rød K, Røed RT, Solheim N, Smidesand IJ, Tandberg S, Halsnes R, Høystad MW. A three-year survey of nosocomial and community-acquired infections, antibiotic treatment and re-hospitalization in a Norwegian health region. J Hosp Infect. 2000;44:214–23.
8. Andersen BM, Rasch M, Hochlin K, Tollefsen T, Sandvik L. Hospital-acquired infections before and after healthcare reorganization in a tertiary university hospital in Norway. J Public Health. 2009;7:1–7.
9. ECDC. Summary of the latest data on antibiotic resistance in the European Union. EARS-Net surveillance data, November 2017.
10. ECDC. Summary of the latest data on antibiotic consumption in the European Union. ESAC-Net surveillance data, November 2017.
11. National Public Health of Norway. Pandemic reports 2009.
12. Law on Health and Social Preparedness 23 June 2000, No. 56. Oslo: Royal Health and Social Affairs; 2000.
13. Ministry of Social Affairs and Health. National emergency plan for pandemic flu. Oslo; 1999, 2001, 2006, 2009.
14. Ministry of Health and Care Services. Superior National Health and Social Preparedness Plan. Norway; 2007.
15. Regional Plan for Health and Social Preparedness in Health Region East, Norway; 2005.
16. Norwegian Health Directorate. Pandemic planning in municipal health services. Organization, processing, logistics. Draft 26 April 2009.
17. Norwegian Health Directorate. Pandemic planning in the specialist health service. Organization, patient reception and treatment. 2009.

84 Personal Protective Equipment (PPE)

Abstract
It is not acceptable to work with patients with dangerous infections without using, knowing and implementing adequate personal protective equipment—PPE. Personnel, patients and visitors should not be exposed to infectious agents by patients, others, equipment or the environment—which may be serious to health or life (ECDC). It is not acceptable to place a patient with undefined infectious disease in the same room as a patient with known high-risk disease (WHO). In this chapter the need and use of PPE are described, to stop spread of infections in the hospital during outbreaks.

Keywords
Personal protective equipment · PPE · Infection control · Hygiene · Disinfection

84.1 Purpose

- To describe necessary capacity and types of PPE - personal protective equipment -needed for protection of health care personnel during epidemics.
- Describe the need for PPE in case of serious, dangerous outbreaks in hospitals [1–3].

84.2 Comprise

- Personnel in contact with infected/exposed patients and/or equipment used on such patients.
- Special trained personnel in work with high-risk, infectious patients.
- Emergency groups and infection control personnel.

B. M. Andersen, *Prevention and Control of Infections in Hospitals*,
https://doi.org/10.1007/978-3-319-99921-0_84

84.3 Responsibility

The hospital's management is responsible for written procedures for the use of PPE in the actual situation, provide plans for necessary supply of PPE, storage and use.

Infection control doctor and emergency team are responsible for practical advice and training in taking on and off PPE and infection risk around these procedures.

Personnel follows written routines and contacts nearest responsible for advice if unprotected exposed to dangerous agents.

84.4 Practical Measures [4–7]

84.4.1 Need for Personal Protection Equipment in Case of Serious, Dangerous Infection Outbreaks

A survey was conducted in Australia with regard to the need for disposable sets of personal protective equipment recommended by the WHO (disposable gown, respiratory protection, gloves and eye protection—PPE kit), if a patient with suspected avian influenza was hospitalized [4–7]. Healthcare staff went through training in advance. At an unknown time, a patient—an actor—was admitted with "clinical symptoms" as if he had bird flu [7]. The symptoms were clear for suspicion of bird flu (avian pandemic influenza—API): *3-day high fever, cough, shortness of breath, severely impaired general condition and recent return from countries in Southeast Asia and had handled diseased poultry in an area of bird avian influenza.* The course was recorded by observers who followed what happened around the patient for the first 6 h after admission to the emergency department [7].

Each incoming API patient led to a consumption of 20–25 sets of PPEs—already *the first 6 h after the admission* [7]. However, more than 40% of healthcare professionals would need post-exposure treatment with antivirals in this situation due to lack of or incorrect use of PPE! In the absence of access to PPE, the need for antiviral treatment would increase with 12–13 treatment schedules per API patient. A real event would expose many more people over a longer period of time with a high need for additional PPE resources per API patient.

The emergency preparedness exercise in Australia is an important alert to show the need for more thoughtful preparations for personal protection for healthcare professionals and others who are going to take care of patients with severe pandemic influenza. During the SARS epidemic, it was after a short time—impossible to get PPE from a number of key and major manufacturers. The same must be considered if a serious pandemic should occur.

84.4.2 Under Norwegian Conditions, the Australian Experiment would give the Following Results

Estimated need for personal protection equipment (PPE) in case of severe pandemic outbreak [4–7]

	Norway Need of PPE set	Oslo region Need of PPE set
Hospitals (0.3% of the population)[a]		
1. First 6 h in hospital (20 PPE/patient)	2,700,000	50,000
2. Addition for average 10 days in hospitals; 10 PPE/day/patient	1,350,000	250,000
Primary health services (13% of the population)[b]		
1. Policlinic/primary health service—*first contact*; 3PPE/contact	1,560,000	312,000
2. Supplement for others[c]; about 10 PPE set/patient	5,200,000	1,040,000
Total estimated PPE sets needed	8,380,000	1,652,000

[a]ca. 13,500 admissions on a national basis, 2500 in Oslo
[b]ca.520,000 additional contacts on a national basis, 104,000 in the Oslo region
[c]Family/contacts, transport, service, home care, nursing homes, public services, etc., ca. 10 PPE sets/patients

This scenario demonstrates that the earlier a strict, comprehensive and proper intervention is done to stop a serious epidemic, the faster it may stop and the less need for PPE.

84.5 Emergency Preparedness Stocks

Emergency preparedness stocks for PPE and disinfectants in hospitals and primary care must be reassessed. Continuous consumption and rotation must be ensured in today's infection control work so that the equipment does not become outdated, at the same time as the personnel are training in the use of PPE. Stocks should be controlled by infection control personnel responsible for training and protection against improper or wrong use of PPE.

PPE is particularly important in cases where there is delayed or lack of access to an effective vaccine and in the absence of antiviral/antimicrobial agents such as SARS, MERS and Ebola. PPE is of particular importance for healthcare professionals and other service providers to feel safe and to work effectively during serious epidemics/pandemics.

References

1. Ministry of Labour and Administration. Regulations on protection against exposure to biological factors (bacteria, viruses, fungi and more) in the workplace. FOR OSLO: 1997-12-19 nr.1322.
2. Sehulster LM, Chinn RYW, Ardunio MJ, et al. Guidelines for environmental infection control in health-care facilities. CDC MMWR. 2003;52:1–42.
3. Rutala WA, Weber DJ. Disinfection, sterilization, and control of hospital waste. In: Mandell, Douglas, and Bennets principles and practice of infectious diseases, vol. 2. 8th ed. Philadelphia: Elsevier Churchill Livingstone; 2015. p. 3294–309.
4. Andersen BM. Severe infection - personal protective equipment - PPE. In: Handbook in hygiene and infection control for hospitals. Oslo: Ullevål University Hospital; 2008. p. 567–8.
5. Andersen BM. Bird flu with pandemic potential. In: Handbook in hygiene and infection control for hospitals. Part 1, vol. 2014. Norway: Fagbokforlaget. p. 300–9.
6. Andersen BM. Scenario pandemic influenza and pandemic bird flu. In: Handbook in hygiene and infection control for hospitals. Part 1, vol. 2014. Norway: Fagbokforlaget. p. 310–8.
7. Swaminathan A, Martin R, Gamon S, et al. Personal protective equipment and antiviral drug use during hospitalization for suspected avian or pandemic influenza. Emerg Infect Dis. 2007;13:1541–7.

Communication, Information and Advice 85

Abstract

Information and communication are central measures during serious outbreaks of infections, especially concerning high-risk, dangerous microbes. A thorough and clear information about how to act in the society to protect against infection may calm and reduce the panic among people. It is important to have enough people to answer all who is asking about the outbreak and to react rapidly to information of disease-suspected cases.

Keywords

High-risk infections · Communication · Information · Infection control · Hygiene Disinfection

85.1 Purpose

- To inform leaders in the hospital, municipal health service, (eventually regional and national) when detecting suspect dangerous infection in the hospital or in the community [1–3].
- To inform the population, media etc. concerning how to act during outbreaks.
- To inform each person/patient/family that asks for advice about a possible dangerous outbreak.

85.2 Comprise

- All personnel who are the first in contact with the infected/exposed person, relatives, other contacts and environment.
- All who are predefined to do the information work during serious outbreaks.

B. M. Andersen, *Prevention and Control of Infections in Hospitals*,
https://doi.org/10.1007/978-3-319-99921-0_85

85.3 Responsibility

The hospital's management provides written plans for how to react in situations where personnel and others may be exposed to known/unknown serious communicable disease and a practical arrangement for how to handle the situation.

The *infection control officer* at the level of where the problem occurs, and at the departments/ward where the infection may spread, is responsible for following local emergency plans.

Personnel who unprotected have come in a seriously contagious situation and may have been exposed to infectious agents are responsible for contacting the nearest responsible/infectious unit for advice and of following written guideline and practical advice.

85.4 Practical Measures [4–6]

85.4.1 Hospital

Telephone/Internet centre with registration of all hospitalized patients. Information telephone for advice and measures, staffed with healthcare personnel and in close cooperation with emergency services, ambulances and municipal health services.

85.4.2 The Municipal Health Service

Telephone/Internet centre with registration of patients in homes, nursing homes, home nursing, etc. Information telephone for advice and measures, staffed with healthcare professionals and in close cooperation with hospital, emergency room, ambulances.

Important general information in case of major epidemic outbreaks and high risk of infection:

- Most homes, apartments, etc. with own shower and toilet are really very good isolates.
- Avoid gatherings, meetings, etc.
- In case of major outbreaks, children should be home from school/nursery—there will be a large spread of infection if someone is infected.
- Stay home if exposed to severe infectious disease (been in the same room, cared for a patient). Measure temperature × 2 every day—usually for 10-14-21 days—depending on the infectious agent.
- Good hand hygiene with alcoholic wipes, hand washing.
- In case of respiratory symptoms, cough/sneeze in disposable wipers that are disposed of in waste bag. Hand hygiene afterwards. Do not use your clothes like "handkerchief"!

– If you think you are ill, call your doctor/hospital/hospital's telephone for advice.
– If you are to be examined by a doctor/admitted to hospital, you will be notified of where to come or if you are being picked up in an ambulance. Use surgical mask and wash hands.
– Avoid public transport if you are ill—and avoid other people. You can drive your own car.

- Listen to the radio regarding reasonable measures.
- If contaminated via water or food, boil the water and cook current food (possibly throw the food away).
- Do you have a dog/cat that needs to be aired—keep the animal in a strap and wipe off the paws with an alcoholic wipe afterwards.
- Food, etc. can be ordered from the store and brought to your home, possibly other solutions in cooperation with the civil defence.
- Handle waste trash in a safe manner so that collector workers and others are not unnecessarily exposed to infection.
- Listen to the radio, TV, etc. for advice and messages.

References

1. Ministry of Labour and Administration. Regulations on protection against exposure to biological factors (bacteria, viruses, fungi and more) in the workplace. FOR OSLO: 1997-12-19 nr.1322.
2. Sehulster LM, Chinn RYW, Ardunio MJ, et al. Guidelines for environmental infection control in health-care facilities. CDC MMWR. 2003;52:1–42.
3. Rutala WA, Weber DJ. Disinfection, sterilization, and control of hospital waste. In: Mandell, Douglas, and Bennets principles and practice of infectious diseases. 8th ed. vol 2. . Philadelphia: Elsevier Churchill Livingstone; 2015. p. 3294–309.
4. Andersen BM. Severe infections—personal preventive equipment—PPE. In: Handbook in hygiene and infection control for hospitals. Ullevål University Hospital; 2008. p. 567–8.
5. Andersen BM. Bird flu with pandemic potential. In: Handbook in hygiene and infection control for hospitals. Part 1. *Fagbokforlaget*; 2014. p. 300–9.
6. Andersen BM. Scenario pandemic influenza and pandemic bird flu. In: Handbook in hygiene and infection control for hospitals. Part 1. *Fagbokforlaget*; 2014. p. 310–8.

Triage: Serious Infections 86

Abstract
Triage is a system used to avoid spread of serious infections between infected and noninfected persons seeking help and advice at hospitals or other healthcare institutions. It is usually one way in (all) to a place for examination and two ways out (suspected infected or not infected). It is especially important to protect non-infected persons during the way into the triage, using surgical mask, hand hygiene and no contact between people.

Keywords
High-risk infections · Triage · Information · Infection control · Hygiene Disinfection

86.1 Purpose

- Triage is a system to select sick or exposed patients from healthy people or patients with other disease.
- The purpose is to protect and isolate infected patients or exposed persons from others and to stop spread of infection between infected and non-infected persons [1–3].
- Triage is also used for vaccination, giving prophylactic medicaments, use of PPE and other protection advice.

86.2 Comprise

- All persons with or without symptoms on actual illness.
- All who may have been exposed to the actual infection and all who are worried of being infected.

B. M. Andersen, *Prevention and Control of Infections in Hospitals*,
https://doi.org/10.1007/978-3-319-99921-0_86

- The triage separates between not infected, maybe infected, and infected - and gives advice, vaccination, medicaments, use of PPE and other protection.

86.3 Responsibility

The hospital's management and emergency group provides written plans for using the triage system at the hospital, when it is to be used, technical supply, vaccines, prophylactic medicaments, enough trained personnel, etc.

Departments management is following routines for triage treatment in the hospital.

Predefined trained personnel are working in the triage situation.

86.4 Practical Measures [4, 5]

86.4.1 Definition

A three-parted system:

- One input and two outputs (home or further diagnostics/treatment/vaccination, etc.).
- A good triage system in primary and specialist health services is an important factor in stopping epidemic development.
- Triage must be used in such a way that it does not constitute an epidemic spreading factor.
- Triage can be used for diagnostics, categorization of persons with symptoms, vaccinations, drug delivery, infection protection equipment, information, etc.

86.4.2 Triage for Personnel at the Hospital

- Vaccination/medication—as needed and available—is provided by the corporate health service in cooperation with health authorities.
- Respiratory equipment—as required and available—is provided by the infection control staff.
- Use of PPE—training and control—is provided by infection control staff.

86.4.3 Triage for Patients at the Hospital

- Diagnostics, categorization of patients and information at the hospital are planned in advance.
- Preliminary examination to determine admittance or provide information (separate house, etc.).

- Avoid queue (increase spread of infection). Delivery of surgical mask and information to all who are waiting.

86.4.4 Triage for the Municipal Health Service Personnel

- Vaccination/medication—as needed and available
- Respiratory equipment—as needed and quantity available
- Use of PPE—training and control

86.4.5 Triage for Patients in the Municipality

- Diagnostics and preliminary examination—to determine admittance to hospital or provide information
- Avoid queue (increase spread of infection).
- Delivery of surgical mask and information to all who are waiting.
- Vaccination and/or delivery of drugs.

References

1. Ministry of Labour and Administration. Regulations on protection against exposure to biological factors (bacteria, viruses, fungi and more) in the workplace. FOR OSLO: 1997-12-19 nr.1322.
2. Sehulster LM, Chinn RYW, Ardunio MJ, et al. Guidelines for environmental infection control in health-care facilities. CDC MMWR. 2003;52:1–42.
3. Rutala WA, Weber DJ. Disinfection, sterilization, and control of hospital waste. In: Mandell, Douglas, and Bennets principles and practice of infectious diseases, vol. 2. 8th ed. Philadelphia: Elsevier Churchill Livingstone; 2015. p. 3294–309.
4. Andersen BM, Lereim I. Triage – serious infection. In: Handbook in hygiene and infection control for hospitals. Oslo: Ullevål University Hospital; 2008. p. 571–2.
5. Andersen BM. Severe infection – personal preventive equipment - PPE. In: Handbook in hygiene and infection control for hospitals. Oslo: Ullevål University Hospital; 2008. p. 567–8.

Patient Management: Logistic 87

Abstract
During outbreak of very dangerous and/or easily transmittable infections, the handling of infected patients in the hospital is both difficult and important when the hospital at the same time has to take care of other acute patients - like road accidents or heart infarct etc. Dangerous infections may cause paralysis of all hospital activity if the infection is out of control. A written consensus plan for how to act when high-risk patients are admitted to hospitals is therefore important.

Keywords
High-risk infections · Patient-logistic · Information · Infection control · Hygiene Disinfection

87.1 Purpose

- To handle seriously infected patients in such a way in the hospital that transmission of infection to others is avoided.
- To take care of other emergency activities at the same time in the hospital by using logistic and infection control.

87.2 Comprise

- All patients with suspected high-risk, dangerous /easily transmitted infectious disease admitted to hospitals [1–5].
- *All health care personnel handling infectious high-risk patients.*

B. M. Andersen, *Prevention and Control of Infections in Hospitals*,
https://doi.org/10.1007/978-3-319-99921-0_87

87.3 Responsibility

The hospital's management provides written plans for how to react in situations where personnel and others may be exposed to known/unknown serious communicable disease and a practical arrangement for how to handle the situation.

The *infection control officer* at the level of where the problem occurs, and at the departments/ward where the infection may spread, is responsible for following local emergency plans.

Personnel who unprotected have come in a seriously contagious situation and may have been exposed to infectious agents are responsible for contacting the nearest responsible/infectious unit for advice and of following written guideline and practical advice.

87.4 Practical Measures [4, 5]

87.4.1 Patients: Admission to Hospital

1. Admission priority in relation to outbreak and epidemic situation:
   - Calculated by the extent of the outbreak, symptoms and need for treatment and how quickly the epidemic develops; see SARS.
   - *First phase—minor outbreak*: Only sick, treatment-needing patients are admitted. Patients with laboratory-confirmed diagnosis may be cohort treated (in the same room).
   - *Second Phase—large outbreak:* Only patients who need intensive or other life-saving treatment are admitted to the hospital. Patients with laboratory-confirmed diagnosis or a reliable clinical diagnosis can be cohort treated; however, a laboratory-confirmed diagnosis is needed for children and adolescents.
2. Release of isolation space for high-risk infections:
   - *Isolates are emptied and clarified.* Local isolates are prepared for the intake of high-risk patients. Other (previous) isolation patients are transferred to other departments or hospitals—preferably with infection-medical expertise.
   - *Normal bed wards are emptied as needed.* Patients that were admitted are sent home or transferred to other hospitals/nursing homes, freeing of beds and staff.
   - *Elective treatment is* reduced or stopped, freeing of patient beds, postoperative treatment, intensive beds and staff.
   - *Intensive personnel are* displaced to relevant isolates as needed.
   - *Emergencies and loops for other patients* (caesarean surgery, traffic accident surgery, myocardial infarction, etc.) are established in a separate unit or at another hospital with the possibility of isolation of the infected patient with another emergency disease (like pregnant with high-risk infection).
   - *Transfer of treatment—needing* patients with epidemic disease to a dedicated, separate hospital/unit with adequate competence and capacity.

- *All transport of infectious patients* between hospitals and from the place of arrival to the hospital must be based on the infection control routines determined for the individual infectious disease (contact, airborne, high-risk isolation); *see isolation regimes.*
- *Disinfection of the ambulance used for high-risk infection patients is* carried out partially after each transport and once a day or more often if possible—a complete disinfection (dependent on outbreak and severity). The ambulance is not used for noninfected patients.
- *See Chap. 75 on ambulance and transport.*

87.4.2 Infectious Carriers, Close Contacts and Persons in Incubation Phase of High-Risk Disease

Carriers of high-risk agent. Healthy carriers can mostly be taken care of outside hospitals. This should be done in cooperation with and under the supervision of the municipal infectious healthcare provider. In case of doubt, infection control persons should be contacted. Carriers of intestinal bacteria, MRSA, VRE, and other multidrug-resistant microbes—MDRO, etc.—are usually not defined as high-risk carriers.

In a possible incubation phase of illness, most people may be at home. Serious infectious diseases are most commonly contagious *after* disease outbreaks (but not all). The case should be followed up in cooperation with and under the supervision of the municipality's infection control. In case of doubt, contact infection control personnel.

References

1. Ministry of Labour and Administration. Regulations on protection against exposure to biological factors (bacteria, viruses, fungi and more) in the workplace. FOR OSLO: 1997-12-19 nr.1322.
2. Sehulster LM, Chinn RYW, Ardunio MJ, et al. Guidelines for environmental infection control in health-care facilities. CDC MMWR. 2003;52:1–42.
3. Rutala WA, Weber DJ. Disinfection, sterilization, and control of hospital waste. In: Mandell, Douglas, and Bennets principles and practice of infectious diseases, vol. 2. 8th ed. Philadelphia: Elsevier Churchill Livingstone; 2015. p. 3294–309.
4. Andersen BM, Lereim I. Triage – serious infection. In: Handbook in hygiene and infection control for hospitals Ullevål University Hospital; 2008. p. 571–2.
5. Andersen BM. Severe infection – personal preventive equipment - PPE. In: Handbook in hygiene and infection control for hospitals Ullevål University Hospital; 2008. p. 567–8.

Viral Haemorrhagic Fever (VHF) and Other Serious Viral Infections

88

First contact - how to act and protect

Abstract

Viral haemorrhagic fever—VHF—virus and a number of other special viruses are considered to cause the world's most dangerous infections with very high mortality, lack of therapeutic possibilities and often absence of effective vaccines. Such viruses are identified as "biohazard-level 4" agents and are treated at the highest level of infection protection with strict isolation measures. At least 14 patients with Ebola disease were transported to Europe and the United States (11 patients) for hospital treatment during the African epidemic in 2014. There were no secondary spread of VHF import cases in Europe and the United States from 1999 until the Ebola outbreak in 2014. Then there were three cases of nosocomial spread to personnel in hospitals, two in the United States and one in Spain, despite alleged use of strict containment routines. This indicates a high risk of spread of infection through intensive treatment and handling of very sick persons with VHF like Ebola. In most cases vaccines are not available or specific antiviral drugs. Therefore, infection control must be based on a proper infection protection. This chapter is focused on practical means to handle and treat patients with suspect VHF or other dangerous agents to avoid spread to personnel and environment

Keywords

Viral haemorrhagic fever · VHF · Ebola · Lassa · Other VHFs · SARS · MERS Nipah · Biohazard-level 4 agents · High-risk infections · Information · Infection control · Hygiene · Disinfection · PPE · Emergency · Transport · Admittance

B. M. Andersen, *Prevention and Control of Infections in Hospitals*,
https://doi.org/10.1007/978-3-319-99921-0_88

88.1 Purpose

- Protect healthcare professionals and close contacts against infection from blood and other body fluids in suspected or documented high-risk, dangerous infectious disease [1–18].
- Prevent spread of infection by means of infection control barriers.
- Patients or personnel should not be exposed to dangerous infections which may be serious to health or life [19, 20]. It is not acceptable to place a patient with not defined disease in the same room as a patient with known high-risk disease (WHO).

88.2 Comprise

1. *Patient* without signs of infectious disease, but recently in the last 3 weeks from known epidemic area abroad where there is an outbreak of severe, highly infectious epidemic **and**
   (a) Exposed to SARS or other severe acute respiratory tract infection and been in close contact with sick people with severe acute respiratory tract infection, or
   (b) Exposed to VHF (Lassa,Ebola, etc.) and been in close contact with sick people with bleeding in the skin and high fever, or
   (c) Exposed to bird flu and been in contact with sick birds—suspected of having bird flu
2. *Patient* with signs of infectious disease, recently arrived in the last 3 weeks from a known epidemic area abroad **and**
   (a) Have symptoms of severe infection with high fever *and rash/bleeding* (VHF), or
   (b) Have severe respiratory tract infection and been in close contact with patients with severe respiratory tract infection (e.g. SARS or MERS), or
   (c) Have severe respiratory tract infection and been in direct contact with sick birds—suspected of having avian influenza
3. *Personnel and others* who have treated such patients—unprotected.
4. *Environment and equipment, etc.* which have been in contact with such patients—unprotected.

88.3 Responsibility

The hospital's management provides written plans for handling such cases and of that necessary resources are available.

The department management at the ambulance/emergency department, infectious medicine and anaesthetic and intensive care units must have procedures for the treatment of such patients and other key personnel who have undergone special training and necessary exercises.

The department management admitting and handling such patients are responsible for personal protective equipment—PPE—which is:

- Easily accessible,
- Properly packaged and checked
- That personnel are trained in use and undergo courses in donning (take on) and doffing (takeoff) PPE
- That personnel receive general training in isolation regimes (*see Chap. 19 on Isolation*)

Personnel must use the PPE in the correct situation and properly according to routines. Possibly contact an infection control personnel for advice.

Each user of the equipment must be responsible for a proper and safe use.

88.4 Practical Measures [16–18]

Patients (persons) with no symptoms of infection are usually at low risk of transmitting infection to others, but are still treated with the use of PPE because of some contagiousness which may occur during incubation phases.

Patients with infection symptoms (see above) must be considered as high-risk infectors.

88.4.1 Emergency Action—Transport of High-Risk Patient—"Ebola" Example

Emergency/ambulance personnel are often the first who meet and take care of a patient outside hospital. The patient may have known or unknown infections. Emergency personnel should be especially aware of and handle this situation.

88.4.1.1 Before You Are in Contact with the Patient: At Home, Hotel Room and Patient Room

1. Contact the doctor in charge and ask for advice (contact infection control personnel).
2. Close access to the room/ambulance; mark the door *strict isolation*, and notify others present.
3. Take on the following PPE: cap, respirator (P3 mask), goggles, phantom hood that covers the head and neck, shoe covers, waterproof gown with long sleeves or overall with a hood and double gloves. Learn the order of clothing, and control each other.
4. In agreement with the doctor in charge, enter the patient room (with barrier guidance).
5. Put a regular surgical mask or P2 mask without breathing valve on the patient—preferably let the patient do this himself.
6. If possible, the patient places himself on the transport stretcher.

7. Cover the patient's skin, sore and the entire body as much as possible during transport (e.g. bed sheet, gown, heat coat).
8. Contact the advisor in charge by phone, and ask for further assistance to which reception.
9. Avoid transport through corridors where there are other people.
10. Rooms, fixtures and everything that have been in contact with the patient are treated as infectious. The patient's equipment is left and the room is sealed until a complete disinfection is done.

88.4.1.2 If You Are Already in Direct Contact with the Patient (in the Same Room at Home, Hotel Room, Patient Room) and Detect Suspected Infection "Ebola" (Unprotected) Without PPE

PPE should be taken on before further work with the patient.

1. Do not leave the room, but walk away from the patient, and be calm and explain.
2. Hand disinfection (alcohols 70–85%) inactivates most dangerous viruses.
3. Move right outside the patient's room and do not go elsewhere.
4. New hand disinfection. Contact the doctor in charge by phone and ask for assistance.
5. Notify others present about the need for PPE and other assistance. PPE equipment should always be ready in the ambulance—minimum for two persons.
6. Put on PPE: Gown—waterproof/overall; shoe covers; cap; phantom hood; respirator, P3 mask; goggles/visor; and two pairs of gloves (disinfect hands before wearing gloves).
7. Go back to the patient.
8. Put surgical mask or P2 mask without breathing valve on the patient, or ask the patient to put a mask on themselves. Perform calm with gentle movements so that no particles are swirled up.
9. If the patient is able to it, he will put himself on the stretcher.
10. Cover the patient's skin, sore and the entire body as much as possible during transport (e.g. bed sheet, gown, etc.).
11. Contact the doctor in charge by phone and ask for further assistance to which reception.
12. Avoid transport through corridors where there are other people.
13. Rooms, fixtures and everything that have been in contact with the patient are treated as infectious. The patient's equipment is left and the room is sealed until complete disinfection is done.

88.4.1.3 PPE-Doffing (Removal of PPE) After Contact with High-Risk Patient: In Sluice or in Rooms Separate from the Patient

1. Doffing must be checked by another person wearing PPE.
2. Wash the gloves outside with chloramine 5%, chlorine bath 5%, 60 s; or hand disinfectant.

3. Remove the shoe cover—carefully put it in the waste bag—and move to "clean place".
4. Remove both gloves carefully, put directly into the waste bag, and do not touch the skin.
5. Wash your hands in new chlorine bath for 60 s or hand disinfectant for 60 s.
6. Put on new gloves before further doffing.
7. Remove carefully PPE in this order: gown, goggles/visor, phantom hood (if used), respiratory protection (P3 mask) and cap, and touch the areas that have been at least infected (usually backside of the body). Disinfect your hands with gloves between each procedure, and follow the written instructions, or see specifically under the infection protection regime—*strict isolation*. Check that used equipment does not contaminate the skin or the clothes under PPE during the doffing. Everything is placed in the waste bag (eventually separate bags for textiles, goggles etc.).
8. Finally remove the gloves and perform hand hygiene.
9. The waste bag is carefully closed and placed in a new clean waste bag that is disinfected outside with chloramine 5%.
10. Wash your hands thoroughly, possibly in a new chlorine bath afterwards.
11. Change clothing that has been used under PPE. Used textiles are treated as infectious in separate textile bag marked infectious.
12. Shower with Hibiscrub (chlorhexidine soap)—body and hair—before new clothes are taken on.
13. After the transport, exposed personnel (contact with the patient without the use of PPE) should be discontinued and followed up 21 days after exposure (VHF).

88.4.1.4 Transport Equipment (Ambulance, Stretcher, Wheelchair, etc.)

1. After use in high risk situations, disinfect the equipment with chloramine 5%, and optionally gas disinfect with hydrogen peroxide dry gas.
2. Use PPE during this procedure; dressing and undressing as outlined above.

88.4.1.5 Blood and Other Spills of Biological Material

1. Disinfect as usual with chloramine 5% or household chlorine.
2. Use PPE during this procedure, dressing and undressing as outlined above.

88.4.1.6 Note! Prevent Spread of Infection from the Patient

- Surgical mask or P2 mask without breathing valve is placed on the patient.
- Skin, sore, etc. are covered as much as possible during transport (e.g. put on bed sheet or plastic cover loose over the patient, but do not cover the head).
- Everything that has been in contact with the patient is treated as infectious. The same precautions as outlined above.
- It is possible to transport the patient in a separate plastic container (stretcher surrounded by plastic).

88.4.1.7 PPE: Equipment, Pre-packed, Expiration Date!

PPE infection box: PPE—equipment for 2–8 persons; listed on outside of the box. Complete PPE sets are in the box.

- Virus impermeable gown with long arms and tight wrists. Complete overall can be used.
- Gloves with long cuff, solid, double, pulled over wrists (Note! Make sure the gloves are ok). Record expiration date.
- Hood/cap that holds the hair in place.
- Tightly sealed mask with hepafilter (P3). Record expiration date.
- "Phantom hood" with long neck covering the head and neck.
- Protective goggles that are tight to the skin and so large that you can use your own glasses inside.
- Boots or shoe covers.
- Two waste bags that can be closed.

PPE infection box or equivalent with pre-packaged PPE sets can be stored at:

- Ambulances, external
- Intensive department's isolate
- Clinical chemical department
- Infection department
- Microbiological department
- Emergency reception
- Children's section
- Emergency room

Main storage for PPE in the hospital: Should be available on a 24-h basis, but under control and rotation/replacement of infection control personnel in cooperation with Central warehouse or other local solutions.

88.4.2 Notifications

- Outbreak of serious high-risk infectious disease—import patient.
- Outbreak of severe, uncontrollable epidemic disease.

88.4.3 Department's Notification Tasks

88.4.3.1 Who Should Notify?

- Responsible physician, doctor in charge, nurse, supervisor and ambulance service
- Microbiological department (in case of specific agent/resistance/clinical data)
- Corporate health service (suspected of serious infection transferred to staff)

- Primary health services if detected outbreaks of severe high-risk infection disease that require admission and high-risk isolation treatment at the hospital
- The Director of the National Institute of Public Health, the County Governor/County Council and the National Public Health Authority (special infections, according to the Infection Control Act, etc.)

88.4.3.2 To Whom Should It Be Notified?

- Medical officer (isolation and treatment)
- Infection control unit
- Department management
- Hospital management (in case of death, resource-intensive measures, serious contagious epidemic situation)
- Hospital emergency preparedness group (severe contagious disease, unusual disease and major epidemic outbreak)
- The company doctor (on infection transferred to staff)
- Primary health services if detected outbreaks of serious high-risk infectious disease that can lead to infection in the population
- National Institute of Public Health, the County Governor/County Council and the National Public Health Authority (special infections, according to the Infection Control Act, etc.)

88.4.4 Notification Method/Urgency

By telephone, e-mail, fax and writing immediately. The message is assessed primarily by professional responsible personnel at the relevant department by extent/severity.

88.4.5 Meeting Place for the Emergency Preparedness Group

The Director of the hospital leads the Emergency Group and decides when it is necessary to call the group to the Director's office. See Chap. 81 on the Preparedness Group.

88.4.6 Actions and Responsibilities

88.4.6.1 Increased Preparedness

The emergency preparedness group assesses the situation on a continuous basis and checks that:

- Infection isolates are available in the required amount and quality (regular air pressure control).
- A feasible plan for cohort treatment of defined infectious patients, mobilization and relocation of other patients.

- Competent personnel available for the relevant infection control work.
- Available and adequate containment equipment (respiratory protection, gown, gloves, etc.).
- Overview of defined stocks with PPE and disinfectants.
- Actual preventive vaccines are set (flu, rabies, anthrax, BCG, diphtheria, tetanus, polio, plague, etc.).
- A plan for further treatment of infected patients and exposed personnel.
- Notify relevant laboratories and X-ray departments and other departments/contacts of the patient so that they prepare measures.
- A plan for trapping up capacity.

88.4.6.2 Alarm

The Emergency Group activates current personnel to participate in the mission.

88.4.6.3 Priorities

1. High-risk isolates are staffed by infection professionals using PPE.
2. Fastest possible diagnosis/identification of microbe (clinical examination and laboratory studies, including microbiological diagnostics).
3. Quick message to exposed persons and responsible health personnel about measures necessary around exposed cases (name, address, number of persons exposed, measures).

See Chap. 82 on scenarios

88.4.7 Information Duty

The Director is responsible for external information to the Director of the National Institute of Public Health, the County Governor/County Council, the National Public Health Authority (according to Infection Control Act) and the National Health Directorate and the Ministry of Health and Care.

Note! Plan your work, and do not walk outside the area of infection with PPE on! Avoid unnecessary transport! Avoid many participants!

88.5 Background Information

VHF virus and a number of other viruses are considered to be the world's most dangerous infection agents, with very high mortality, lack of therapeutic possibilities and often absence of effective vaccines [1–16]. These viruses are identified as "biohazard-level 4" agents and are treated at the highest level of infection protection with strict isolation measures [2–8, 11, 16–18].

There is a large travel activity to epidemic and endemic areas in the world. Many travellers are becoming sick when going abroad, and some get symptoms after arrival to homeland, mostly harmless infections. A few persons may return very sick or be in incubation period of more dangerous infections, when returning home. This situation may need plans for patient treatment procedures to ensure early isolation of the most serious infectious diseases, such as VHF [1–14]. Viral diseases can have a relatively long incubation times (2–21 days). Many tropical-subtropical viral diseases are transmitted through insects and animals in certain geographical areas, with small ability to spread in most European countries. However, some serious infections may be spread regardless and are especially occurring as a nosocomial problem, like the SARS, MERS and Ebola.

At least 14 patients with Ebola disease were transported to Europe and the United States (11 patients) for hospital treatment in 2014. There was no secondary spread from VHF import cases in Europe and the United States from 1999 until the Ebola outbreak in 2014. Then there were three cases of nosocomial spread to personnel in hospitals, two in the United States and one in Spain, despite alleged use of strict containment routines. This indicates that it may be a high risk of spread of infection through intensive treatment and handling of ill persons. In most outbreaks vaccines or specific antiviral drugs are not available. Therefore, infection control must be based on knowledge, proper use of PPE and disinfectants, effective infection control plan and isolation preparedness [21].

88.5.1 Lassa Fever

Arenavirus group, known since 1969 (in Nigeria, West Africa), mortality is 27–44%. As a rule, it is small outbreaks [7]. Outbreak of Lassa fever is going on in West-Africa, Nigeria in 2018; with until now: 562 confirmed cases, 144 deaths and a case fatality of 25.6% (promed-mail 18 Nov 2018).

88.5.2 Other Haemorrhagic Viruses [16]

Bolivian haemorrhagic fever (Machupo virus); mortality 5–30%. Sabia virus is little known, but the CDC's laboratory infection experience with this virus is described. [8] Congo-Crimean haemorrhagic fever (CCHF) has been known since 1944 and was detected in Kosovo and Pakistan in 2001. Pakistan is an endemic area for CCHF, and especially butchers, farm workers and persons handling animals are prone to infection via blood [22].

88.5.3 Marburg

Filovirus, registered since 1967 (Marburg, Republic of Congo) with mortality rate 17–20%, seldom cause of disease.

88.5.4 Ebola Virus

Ebola is a long filovirus, registered 1972 with mortality rate 42–89% [1, 9, 11, 12, 16, 23–25].

Ebola virus has subtypes: Zaire, Sudan, Ivory Coast and Reston with small genomic differences and variation in mortality. Catchers may be infected by contact with sick monkeys (gorilla), bats and several other animals and "bushmeat". The antibody level is often relatively high in this population. Vaccines have been under development for over 10 years (DNA vaccine in plasmid/adenovirus modified vaccine with Ebola antigen was worked with before 2008) but again tested and some are used now. Latest outbreaks were in Uganda (2000, 2007), Gabon (2001, 2002) and Sierra Leone, Guinea and Liberia from 2014. In 2017, Ebola virus disease caused epidemic situation in the Democratic Republic of Congo (DRC) -with until now; 356 confirmed cases, 231 deaths, 39 health care workers infected, and 34 800 vaccinated. The epidemic is still going on with more than 20 new cases per 48 hours. (Promed-mail Nov 24 2018).

- *The Uganda epidemic in 2000* with Ebola virus led to 428 cases and 173 deaths—40%.
- *Sierra Leone, Guinea, the Liberia epidemic in 2014* with Ebola virus resulted in 28,429 cases, of which 11,297 died (per 9.10.2015) [26]. CDC calculated an underreporting of cases by a factor of 2.5.

A total of 876 health professionals were registered with Ebola, of which 509 died, as of July 17, 2015 (WHO). Outbreaks were caused by lack of knowledge, routines and the idea of WHO, CDC, and other organizations that the risk of transmitting infection is contact and within metre from the patient [21, 23–32].

This was also shown by the example from Norway [21, 27, 28, 32].

- In October 2014, an Ebola-infected, Norwegian physician was transferred to Norway from the Bo Ebola Clinic treatment centre in Sierra Leone, run by the Norwegian Medicines sans borders (MSB).
  - The Bo Ebola Clinic opened 19 September 2014.
  - Two weeks later, 2–4 October, four healthcare personnel at the Bo Clinic got Ebola; two died.
  - The Norwegian Ebola case was transferred to a high-level isolate in Norway and survived.
  - All four had worked together in the Bo triage area: 25–26 September.
  - Standard equipment in the Bo triage area was gloves and surgical mask, because the healthcare personnel working there should hold 1–2 m distance to the patients, according to WHO and to the Norwegian Public Health Institute.
  - "Then they could not be infected by droplets", said the Norwegian administrator of the centre.
  - "Triage was an area to talk with the patients—little PPE's was used in order to create confidence in the local population"!

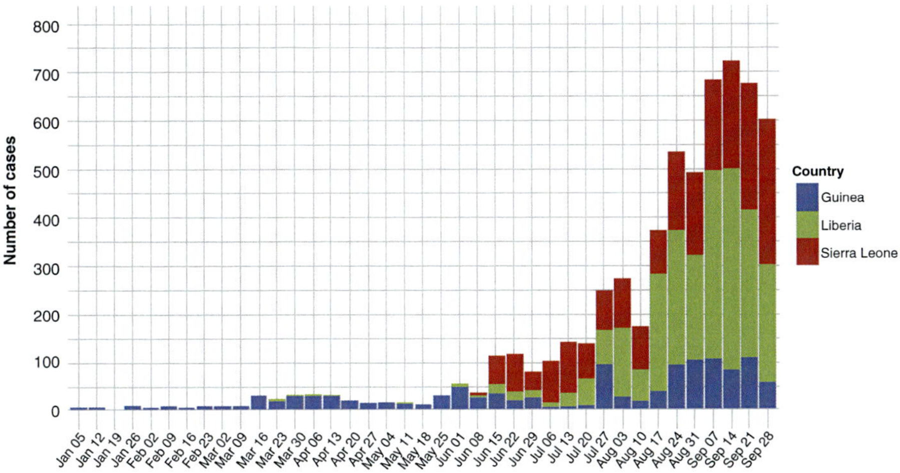

Fig. 88.1 Confirmed and probable cases of Ebola virus disease in Guinea, Liberia, Sierra Leone. Data are based on official information reported by Ministries of Health. These numbers are subject to change due to ongoing reclassification, retrospective investigation and availability of laboratory results. **Source**: WHO 2014

- In all, 21 health workers in the Medicines sans borders were Ebola-infected in October 2014, and 10 of them died. [27]
- Still, the Norwegian Institute of Public Health continued to follow the WHO's "1-m distance rule" for infection risk.

The epidemic had, in the beginning, a slow escalation that could have been controlled by the right means. From summer 2014, there was a rapid escalation with spreading to towns and cities (Fig. 88.1) [21, 28, 32]. Not before 8 August 2014, the WHO declared that the Ebola outbreak was a "public health emergency of international concern" (PHEIC) [28, 32]. The epidemic reached its peak 14 September 2014.

88.6 Lack of Infection Control Routines [21, 28, 32]

WHO, CDC and the United Kingdom established springtime 2014 guidelines for contact and droplets in a radius of 1 m from the Ebola patient [21, 28–32]. Outside the 1-m zone, personal protective equipment—PPE—was usually unnecessary, see Table 88.1. The spread of Ebola disease and death among many patients, including many healthcare professionals, was observed despite following WHO and CDC's guidelines [26, 28]. In 20 October 2014, CDC changed its routines for the use of PPE, focused more on training in donning and doffing PPE in sluices, use of head and neck coverings, use of P3 mask and observation of and check by a dedicated person that this work properly [33]. Healthcare staff underwent proper training in

Table 88.1 Recommended use of infection protection equipment; PPE (personal protective equipment) in Ebola virus guidelines from the World Health Organization (WHO), United Kingdom (UK) and Centres for Disease Control and Prevention (CDC), USA (source: Andersen BM *Hospital Health Care* 2015; March [28, 32])

Comparison of recommended PPE equipment for Ebola infection in WHO, UK and CDC guidelines [21, 28–34]				
	WHO 2014[a] September	UK 2014[b] September	CDC 2014[c] August	CDC 2014[d] October 20
Spread of Ebola infection				
Direct contact	Yes	Yes	Yes	Yes
Indirect contact	?	Yes	Yes	Yes
Airborne?	No	No	No	No
Use of PPE at				
Suspected cases of Ebola				
Eye protection	Yes	Yes	Yes	
Gown	Yes	Plastic apron	Yes	
Gloves	Yes	Yes	Yes	
Mask/surgical mask	Yes	Yes	Yes	
Respiratory protection/N95/P3 mask etc.	No	No	No	
Hair/head protection	No	No	No	
Specific shoes/shoe covers	Yes	No	No	
Confirmed cases of Ebola				
Eye protection	Yes	Yes	Yes	Yes
Gown	Yes	Yes	Yes	Yes
Gloves	Yes	Yes	Yes	Yes
Mask/surgical mask	Yes	No	Yes	No
Respiratory protection/N95/P3 mask etc.	No	Yes	No	Yes
Hair/head protection	No	No	No	Yes
Specific shoes/shoe covers	Yes	No	No	Yes
Aerosol-producing procedures				
Respiratory protection/N95/P3 mask etc.	Yes	Yes	Yes	Yes
Hair/head protection	No	No	No	Yes
Specific shoes/shoe covers	Yes	No	Yes	Yes

[a]WHO. Interim infection prevention and control guidance for care of patients with suspected or confirmed filovirus haemorrhagic fever in health-care settings, with focus on Ebola. September 2014

[b]UK, Department of Health. Management of hazard group 4 viral haemorrhagic fevers and similar human infectious diseases of high consequences. September 2014

[c]CDC. Infection prevention and control recommendations for hospitalized patients with known or suspected Ebola haemorrhagic fever in US hospitals. August 2014

[d]CDC. Guidance on personal protective equipment to be used by healthcare workers during management of patients with Ebola virus disease in US hospitals, including procedures for putting on (donning) and removal. October 20, 2014

Fig. 88.2 PPE use for Ebola virus infection. Source: http:imag.cdn2.vietnamnet.vn

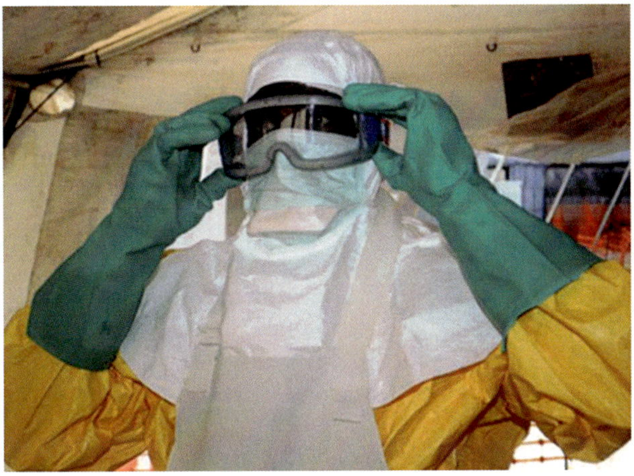

the use of PPE and other infection control measures before being sent out in the field. From January 2015, WHO also changed its schedule, but still with regular mask, with the exception of aerosol-generating procedures and still "within a meter of the patient" [34].

It is discussed whether Ebola infects via air or not; important for infection control measures [21, 28, 32]. Earlier studies have warned that air transmission cannot be excluded, as shown in animal experiments [9, 11, 16, 23–25, 35]. Based on high risk of fatal progression, preventive measures are better than belated wisdom. However, in April 2015, CDC and WHO still postulated that "Ebola is not spread through air, water or food". Since the Ebola virus may occur in large quantities in saliva and tears and mucous membranes during disease, studies generally show that drops from cough and sneezing may spread up to 9 m away [36].

Ebola virus survives a long time in biological materials such as blood and other body fluids/secretions (urine, semen, saliva), 9 weeks or more after onset of the disease and also post mortem [37]. Very long-lasting carrier status, and relapse of carrier status occurs even after the patient has been declared healthy. The virus may occasionally be detected in tissues in the body such as in the eye, lungs, testicles—with relapse of the infection observed several times, last with a Scottish nurse who became ill again, "Post-Ebola Syndrome" [26].

There is increasing scepticism regarding the management of the Ebola epidemic, also from the WHO internal evaluation group [38]. Airborne infection and re-aerosols from equipment and bedclothes and textiles cannot be ruled out, which means that personnel and others who treat such patients must use a better protection [21, 28, 32, 39–43] (Fig. 88.2).

During formation of aerosols, including production of re-aerosols, all types of viruses can become airborne. Therefore, all high-risk virus with high mortality, "biohazard-level 4" should be treated as *strict isolation*—(air, contact, blood, secretions, tissue, etc.); the most advanced infection control regime available! There is, however, a high risk of self-contamination during PPE donning and doffing, mainly because of protocol deviations, even for doffing assistants and trained observers [32, 44–46].

References

1. Arthur RR. Ebola in Africa discoveries in the past decade. Eurosurveillance. 2002;7:33–6.
2. Crowcroft NS, Morgan D, Brown D. Viral haemorrhagic fevers in Europe—effective control requires a co-ordinated response. Eurosurveillance. 2002;7:31–2.
3. Wirtz A, Niedrig M, Fock R. Management of patients with suspected viral haemorrhagic fever and other potentially lethal contagious infections in Germany. Eurosurveillance. 2002;7:33–42.
4. Hugonnet S, Saxon H, Pittet D. Management of viral haemorrhagic fevers in Switzerland. Eurosurveillance. 2002;7:42–4.
5. Crowcroft N, Brown D, Gopal R, Morgan D. Current management of patients with viral haemorrhagic fevers in the United Kingdom. Eurosurveillance. 2002;7:44–8.
6. Swan CM, van der Broek PJ, Wijands S, van Steenbergen JE. Management of viral haemorrhagic fever in the Netherlands. Eurosurveillance. 2002;7:48–50.
7. Crowcroft N. Management of Lassa fever in European countries. Eurosurveillance. 2002;7:50–2.
8. Armstrong LR, Dembry LM, Rainey PM, Russi MB, Khan AS, Fischer SH, et al. Management of a Sabia virus-infected patient in a US hospital. Infect Control Hosp Epidemiol. 1999;20:176–82.
9. Feldmann H, Slenczka W, Klenk HD. Emerging and reemerging of filoviruses. Arch Virol Suppl. 1996;11:77–100.
10. Borio L, Inglesby T, Peters CJ, Schmaljohn AL, Hughes JM, Jahrling PB. Hemorrhagic fever viruses as biological weapons. Medical and public health management. JAMA. 2002;287:2391–405.
11. Peters CJ. Marburg and Ebola—arming ourselves against the deadly filoviruses. N Engl Med. 2005;352:2571–3.
12. Outbreak of Ebola virus disease in western Uganda. MSIS report 24/2007.
13. Duh D, Saksida A, Petrovec M, et al. Viral load as predictor of Crimean-Congo Hemorrhagic fever outcome. Emerg Infect Dis. 2007;13:1769–72.
14. Gurley ES, Montgomery JM, Hossain MJ, et al. Person-to-person transmission of Nipah virus in a Bangladeshi community. Emerg Infect Dis. 2007;13:1031–7.
15. WHO. Infection prevention and control of epidemic—and pandemic-prone acute respiratory disease in healthcare. WHO/CDS/EPR/2007.6.
16. Andersen BM. Ebola, Lassa, and other haemorrhagic viruses. In: Handbook in hygiene and infection control for hospitals. Part 1. Medical microbiology. Bergen: Fagbokforlaget; 2014. p. 291–9.
17. Andersen BM. Other serious viral infections—zoonoses. In: Handbook in hygiene and infection control for hospitals. Part 1. Medical microbiology. Bergen: Fagbokforlaget; 2014. p. 278–90.
18. Andersen BM, Hochlin K, Rasch M. Viral haemorrhagic fever (VHF) and other serious viral diseases. In: Handbook in hygiene and infection control for hospitals. Ullevål University Hospital; 2008. p. 575–82.
19. Directorate of Labor Inspection. Regulations on protection against exposure to biological factors (bacteria, viruses, fungi and more) in the workplace, December 19, 1997.
20. European Parliament and Council Directive 2000/54/EC of 18 September 2000 on the protection of workers from the risks related to exposure to biological agents at work.
21. Andersen BM. Infection control is not working. Promed-mail; 14 Sept 2014.

22. Promed mail October 6, 2015. Crimean-Congo Haemorrhagic fever Pakistan.
23. Jahrling PB, Geisbert TW, Jaax NK, Hanes MA, Ksiazek TG, Peters CJ. Experimental infection of cynomolgus macaques with Ebola-Reston filoviruses from the 1989-1990 US. Epizootic. Arch Virol Suppl. 1996;11:115–34.
24. Mwanatambwe M, Ymada N, Arai S, et al. Ebola haemorrhagic fever (EHF): mechanisms of transmission and pathogenicity. J Nippon Med Sci. 2001;68:370–5.
25. Public Health Agency Canada. Ebola Virus; August 2014.
26. Promed mail October 9, 2015. Ebola update. WHO, Scottish nurse relapse, suspected, research, funding.
27. Olsen T. 21 health workers in medicines sans borders infected—10 died. Aftenposten; 10 Oct 2014.
28. Andersen BM. International infection control guidelines for Ebola. Hospital Healthcare Europe. Facilities management. www.hospitalhealthcare.com. Accessed April 2015.
29. WHO. Interim infection prevention and control guidance for care of patients with suspected or confirmed filovirus haemorrhagic fever in health-care settings, with focus on Ebola; Sept 2014.
30. CDC. Infection prevention and control recommendations for hospitalized patients with known or suspected Ebola haemorrhagic fever in US hospitals; Aug 2014.
31. UK, Department of Health. Management of hazard group 4 viral haemorrhagic fevers and similar human infectious diseases of high consequences; Sept 2014.
32. Andersen BM. Infection control guidelines that did not work against Ebola in 2014. www.webbertraining.com. Accessed 5 Oct 2017.
33. CDC. Guidance on personal protective equipment to be used by healthcare workers during management of patients with Ebola virus disease in US hospitals, including procedures for putting on (donning) and removal; 20 Oct 2014.
34. WHO. Steps to put on personal protective equipment (PPE) including gown. WHO 2015 1.
35. Weingartl HM, Embury-Hyatt C, Nfon C. Transmission or Ebola virus from pigs to non-human primates. Sci Rep. 2012;2:article number: 811.
36. Bourouiba L, Dehandschoewerker E, Bush JWM. Violent expiratory events: on coughing and sneezing. J Fluid Mech. 2014;845:537–63.
37. Prescott J, Bushmaker T, Fischer R, et al. Post-mortem stability or Ebola virus. Emerg Infect Dis. 2015;21:856–9.
38. WHO. Report of the Ebola Interim Assessment Panel, July 2015 to WHO.
39. Brousseau LM, Jones R. Commentary: health workers need optimal respiratory protection for Ebola. Cidrap.umn.edu. Accessed 17 Sept 2014.
40. Edmond MB, Diekema DJ, Perencevick EN. Ebola virus disease and the need for new personal protective equipment. JAMA. 2014;312(23):2495–6.
41. Shears P, O'Dempsey TJD. Ebola virus disease in Africa: epidemiology and nosocomial transmission. J Hosp Infect. 2015;90(1):1–9.
42. Weber D, Fischer WA, Wohl DA, Rutala WA. Protecting personnel from acquiring Ebola virus disease. Infect Control Hosp Epidemiol. 2015;36(10):1229–32.
43. Osterholm MT, Moor KA, Kelley NS, et al. Transmission of Ebola viruses: what we know and what we do not know, vol. 6. Minneapolis. mbio.asm.org: Centre for Infectious Disease Research and Policy, University of Minnesota; 2015. p. e00137-15.
44. Kwon JH, Burnham CD, Reske K, Liang SY, Hink T, Wallace MA, et al. Assessment of health-care worker protocol deviations and self-contamination during personal protective equipment donning and doffing. Infect Control Hosp Epidemiol. 2017;38:1077–83.
45. Janke C, Heim KM, Steiner F, et al. Beyond Ebola treatment units: severe infection temporary treatment units as an essential element of Ebola case management during an outbreak. BMC Infect Dis. 2017;17:124.
46. Selvaraj SA, Lee KE, Harrell M, Ivanov I, Allegranzi B. Infection rates and risk factors for infection among health workers during Ebola and Marburg virus outbreaks: a systematic review. J Infect Dis. 2018;218(Suppl 5):S679–89.

Biological Terror: Anthrax-Suspected 89

Abstract
Anthrax is still endemic or hyperendemic on all continents in the world, mainly as a zoonose among unvaccinated cattle. Natural anthrax in human is associated with contact with sick animals and animal products. The bacterium *Bacillus anthracis* is producing lethal toxins and spores that can survive in the environments for hundred years or more. Minimum infectious dose is 1–3 spores, and toxin-producing anthrax may cause cutaneous, lung or intestinal anthrax, dependent on transmission via contact, air or food. The non-cutaneous anthrax has a very high lethality. In the Middle Age epidemics of anthrax, called "Black Bane" (black poison), caused a large number of deaths among humans and animals in Europe and killed half of the sheep livestock in Europe during the 1800th century. Today, about 2000 people are infected each year, mostly cutaneous and some oropharyngeal or intestinal cases, from eating or handling infected meat. During peace time, there are few incidents of threats using bioterror weapons like anthrax. However, in autumn 2001 anthrax was spread in the United Sates by "powder letters" (US Postal Service) to congress represented with spread of aerosols through the mail distribution systems. In all 22 cases were registered; 11 lung anthrax (5 died) and 11 cutaneous anthrax (all survived), mostly postal service-associated workers, and 32,000 persons got prophylaxis with antibiotics for many weeks. In this chapter, cases with suspected anthrax—randomly or intentionally—admitted to hospitals are described according to handling, treating and infection control.

Keywords
Anthrax · *Bacillus anthracis* · "Splenic fever" · Malign pustule · Biological terror "Powder letters" · Zoonosis · Toxins · Spores · Infection control · Hygiene Isolation · Disinfection

B. M. Andersen, *Prevention and Control of Infections in Hospitals*,
https://doi.org/10.1007/978-3-319-99921-0_89

89.1 Purpose

- To describe some measures to handle persons who are suspected infected/contaminated with biological terror agents, like anthrax, when admitted to hospital [1–3].

89.2 Comprise

- All health workers handling/taking care of persons/patients and equipment associated with suspected infection/contamination with biological terror agents.

89.3 Responsibility

The hospital's management provides written plans for how to react in situations where personnel and others may be exposed to known/unknown serious communicable disease and a practical arrangement for how to handle the situation.

The *infection control officer* at the level of where the problem occurs, and at the departments/ward where the infection may spread, is responsible for following local emergency plans.

Personnel who unprotected have come in a seriously contagious situation and may have been exposed to infectious agents are responsible for contacting the nearest responsible/infectious unit for advice and of following written guideline and practical advice.

Note! No admission via main reception!

89.4 Practical Measures [4–8]

In connection with the threat of using biological weapons, the following measures should be taken internally:

- *Emergency plan: isolate capacity, transport, PPE, disinfectants, other equipment, personnel, etc.*—see emergency preparedness plan, disaster plan, hygiene instructions and infection protection.
- *Patient with symptoms possible anthrax* or similar *biological* weapon [9–11]:
  - Placed directly (not via reception!) in isolate—for airborne infections with strict isolation measures (contact, air, blood and tissue, etc.).
  - Check that ambulance personnel/porter/primary contacts are monitored for exposure to this type of infection (see emergency preparedness plan, hygiene manual, etc.).

89.4.1 Suspected Anthrax

In general, risk of spread of anthrax infection between patients is very small, regardless of type of anthrax, wounds, lung or intestinal affection. Anthrax spores live for many decades in the environment but are not defined as normal biological microbes in the environment in most countries in Europe, today [12, 13].

- *Patient with symptoms/suspicion of anthrax is* admitted directly into isolate for airborne infections (air and contact isolation) through direct external access from outside of the isolate.
- *Patient detected with suspected anthrax after admittance to hospital (inpatient, outpatient clinic)* is a seldom and unexpected discovery. In this situation infection control measures are usually not in place. This may be biological terrorism or other suspicion of anthrax infection.
  - *Example:* Random discovery of possible anthrax in wound from a patient in a four-bed room. The patient has been hospitalized for 3 days due to a deep purulent wound, fever and respiratory symptoms. A variety of contacts with personnel/visitors and a possibility that personnel, patients and visitors may have been exposed to bacteria/spores.
  - Verify the diagnosis "suspected anthrax" with clinical and microbiological findings.
  - If confirmed diagnosis, consider following measures in consultation with *infection control personnel* who have the advisory and coordinating responsibility for the infection control at the hospital.

    1. *Report and inform the manager in charge*; see reports; contact infection control personnel.
    2. *Personnel who have been in contact with the patient/equipment,* immediately wash hands. Then disinfect the hands in 5% chloramine (effect on spores). Take so on surgical mask, cap, gown and gloves prior to further care and treatment of the index patient and roommates in the same room. Be careful with bedding so that no spores/bacteria are released to the air.
    3. *The room closes,* signs are put on the door. Nobody leaves the department until registered and informed about what to do. If biological terror of anthrax is suspected, room disinfection is awaited until examinations and samples are taken from the patient's and any co-worker's equipment (possibly powder).
    4. *Patients* in the same room—roommates—of the index case are isolated in a separate room, transferred in a clean bed with surgical mask if coughing and should undergo wash/shower with Hibiscrub if possible in new room.
    5. *The index patient is isolated* (air and contact isolate). Prior to transfer to the isolate, the patient is placed in a clean bed, and a surgical mask is placed on the patient if he is coughing. The patient should undergo wash/shower with Hibiscrub if possible in the isolation unit.
    6. The bed and all of the patient's equipment are left in the first room and the room is closed.

7. *Disinfection.* Bed and entire room with equipment may be disinfected first with hydrogen peroxide gas by robot, then with 5% chloramine for at least 1 h; see point 10.
8. *The department is closed* for entry of new patients and personnel.
9. *Samples* of roommates and exposed persons; nose, throat and wounds. Notify the microbiological department.
10. *Exposure to infection—removal of possible contaminants.* Exposed persons/personnel who have been in contact with the index patient should wear a clean gown over their clothes and shoe covers and go directly to a designated wardrobe. Take off clothing and shoes carefully to avoid transmitting contaminants to the air. The used clothes are placed in an infection waste bag. Shoes are put in a separate waste bag for disinfection. Everything is treated as infectious. Shower with soap/Hibiscrub and water. Change to new clothes in a clean place in the wardrobe.
11. *Disinfection of rooms*—use P3 mask, cap, goggles, long-sleeved waterproof gown, double gloves and shoes that can be autoclaved/burned. All disposal barrier equipment is treated as infected waste that is burned - or autoclaved. Remember disinfection of fixtures and equipment. Hydrogen peroxide dry gas robot can be used first (with spore tests) in all relevant rooms before chloramine 5% disinfection with effect for at least 1 h, before ordinary cleaning.
12. Consider the need for *environment tests before* decontamination (swabbing with sterile gas moistened with sterile saline/water on suspected areas—biological terrorism?).
13. *Registration*—Personnel at the department and other personnel who have been in contact with the patient are registered (as for MRSA). Exposed persons who have been in the actual patient rooms are registered. The department's management is responsible for registration and to report to potentially exposed persons.
14. *Exposed persons* contact infectious outpatient clinic after appointment. Samples are taken from the throat, nose and wounds for cultivation. Microbiological laboratory is notified.
15. *Protection during further work at the department/ward before microbiological clarification.* Use surgical mask, cap, gown and gloves for all patient care (as in MRSA). Each patient is protected with a separate barrier.
16. *Further working situation for* exposed personnel, while the test result is not available, can work, but use masks, cap, gloves and gowns. Do not work at other departments (like MRSA).
17. *Positive tests of anthrax*—Personnel and others start treatment and possible vaccination and leave the work. Further follow-up of infection specialist.
18. *Treatment*—Upon detection of *Bacillus anthracis* in personnel and others is treatment with Ciprofloxacin 500 mg × 2 started for 60 days, alternatively doxycycline 100 mg × 2 for 42–60 days, possibly penicillin (in most cases penicillin sensitivity).

89.4.2 Information

- The Director is informed on a regular, daily basis.
- Information to cooperating and surveying health authorities, the media, etc. is due to the fact that managers, by virtue of their position, are responsible within their field of medicine cf. the hospital's procedure for statement to the press/media. The information director coordinates and facilitates this work.

89.5 Background Information

Anthrax is still endemic or hyperendemic on all continents in the world, mainly as a zoonose among unvaccinated cattle. Natural anthrax in human is associated with contact with sick animals and animal products [12]. *Bacillus anthracis* is producing lethal toxins and spores that can survive in the environments for hundred years or more. Minimum infectious dose is 1–3 spores, and toxin-producing anthrax may cause cutaneous, lung, or intestinal anthrax, dependent on transmission via contact, air or food [13]. The non-cutaneous anthrax has a very high lethality. In the Middle Age, epidemics of anthrax, called "Black Bane" (black poison), caused a large number of deaths among humans and animals in Europe and killed half of the sheep livestock in Europe during the 1800th century [12]. Today, about 2000 people are infected each year, mostly cutaneous and some oropharyngeal or intestinal cases, from eating or handling infected meat [12, 13]. During peace time, there are few incidents of threats using bioterror weapons like anthrax. However, in autumn 2001 anthrax was spread in United States by "powder letters" (US Postal Service) to congress represented with spread of aerosols through the mail distribution systems [12]. In all 22 cases were registered; 11 lung anthrax (5 died) and 11 cutaneous anthrax (all survived), mostly postal service-associated workers. Thirty-two thousand persons got prophylaxis with antibiotics for many weeks [12].

References

1. Ministry of Labour and Administration. Regulations on protection against exposure to biological factors (bacteria, viruses, fungi and more) in the workplace. FOR OSLO: 1997-12-19 nr.1322.
2. Sehulster LM, Chinn RYW, Ardunio MJ, et al. Guidelines for environmental infection control in health-care facilities. CDC MMWR. 2003;52:1–42.
3. Rutala WA, Weber DJ. Disinfection, sterilization, and control of hospital waste. In: Mandell, Douglas, and Bennets principles and practice of infectious diseases. 8th ed. vol 2. Philadelphia: Elsevier Churchill Livingstone; 2015. p. 3294–309.
4. Directorate of Labour Inspection. Regulations on protection against exposure to biological factors (bacteria, viruses, fungi and more) in the workplace; December 19, 1997.
5. European Parliament and Council Directive 2000/54/EC of 18 September 2000 on the protection of workers from the risks related to exposure to biological agents at work.
6. Emergency preparedness at Ullevål University Hospital in connection with biological weapons. http://www.ulleval sykehus.oslo.kommune.no/default.asp?page=/News&Id=23370 (25.10.2001).

7. Andersen BM. Anthrax and emergency routines at Ullevål University Hospital. Tidsskr Nor Legeforen. 2002;122:852–5.
8. Andersen BM, Lereim I. Suspicion of the use of biological weapons—for example anthrax. In: Handbook in hygiene and infection control for hospitals. Ullevål University Hospital; 2008. p. 583–5.
9. Rebman T. Chapter 120: Infectious disease disaster: bioterrorism, emerging infections, and pandemics. APIC text of infection control and epidemiology; 2014. p. 1–22.
10. English JF, Cundiff MY, Malone JD, et al. Bioterrorism readiness plan: a template for healthcare facilities. APIC, CDC. 4/13/99.
11. Rebman T, The 2008 APIC Emergency Preparedness Committee, St. Louis, Missouri. APIC State-of-the-art report: the role of the infection preventionist in emergency management. Am J Infect Control. 2009;37:271–81.
12. Andersen BM. Anthrax. Bacteria and disease. Epidemiology, infections and infection protection. Oslo: Gyldendal Akademika; 2005. p. 9–44.
13. Andersen BM. Bacillus anthracis. In: Handbook in hygiene and infection control for hospitals. Part 1. Medical microbiology. *Fagbokforlaget*; 2014. p. 148–50.

Preparedness in Connection with Biological Weapons

90

Biological sabotage-treatment of post-mail

Abstract

During autumn 2001, anthrax was spread in the United States by "powder letters" (US Postal Service) to congress represents with spread of aerosols through the mail distribution systems. As a result of this happening, a lot of fake "powder letters" and parcels were sent to—and within many countries, also in Norway. Official and large company buildings with many people present are most often the goal by this form of bioterrorism, therefore preparedness plans must be in order.

Keywords

Biological sabotage · Bioweapon · Preparedness · Infection control · Hygiene Disinfection · Infected post-mail

90.1 Purpose

Describe a scenario in the primary phase of dangerous transferable diseases, like biological sabotage of post-mail and practical measures to avoid spread of infectious agents from post-mail.

90.2 Comprise

All persons that have been in contact with contaminated post-mail and/or contaminated environment where spread of biological weapons and/or dangerous microbes are suspected.

B. M. Andersen, *Prevention and Control of Infections in Hospitals*,
https://doi.org/10.1007/978-3-319-99921-0_90

90.3 Responsibility

The hospital's management provides written plans for how to react in situations where personnel and others may be exposed to known/unknown serious communicable disease, including bioweapon, and a practical arrangement for how to handle the situation.

Infection Control Officer at the level of where the problem occurs, and at the departments/ward where the infection may spread, is responsible for following local emergency plans.

Personnel who unprotected has come in a seriously contagious situation are responsible for contacting (per telephone) the nearest responsible/infectious unit for advice and of following written guideline and practical advice.

90.4 Practical Measures for Treatment of Suspected Mail: During Threats [1]

In connection with the threat of using biological weapons, the following measures should be taken internally regarding the handling of mail/parcels:

Unopened mail: Suspicious, unknown package mail/letter from abroad with content other than regular sheets/journals and more:

- Do not open; gently put it into a yellow, transparent plastic bag.
- Throw away promotional materials unopened.
- Contact the addressee internally at the hospital.
- If unknown to the addressee, put it aside in an infection container, and contact eventually the police (to check sender, redirects, etc.)

Opened mail: If any suspicious material is found, powder and the like from an unknown addressee, it may be dangerous:

- Leave the envelope with material lying on the bench—*do not sniff/smell on the contents!*
- Wash your hands immediately, disinfect with chlorine/alcohol before doing anything else.
- Place a clean plastic bag all over the shipment.
- Report to the department management who contact the police and report to infection control personnel. The department management register persons exposed to the material (persons in the same room). The extent of measures is decided by the infection control physician.
- Exposed persons take off clothes on site. Cloths are placed in a waste bag that closes and is stored for microbiological test response. Then the hands are washed/disinfected.

- Exposed persons (in the same room) go to the nearest wardrobe, take off the rest of the clothes, put it into a new waste bag and shower. Reapply clothes and continue working as usual.
- The suspected mail will be removed by the police/healthcare staff; microscopy of powder is done, and samples are cultured at microbiological laboratory or what is determined according to plan.
- Samples of exposed persons are relevant: nose, throat, hands and any clothes if spilled outwards.
- The room closes. If the activity is to be maintained, immediately disinfect the room. Equipment that cannot be disinfected is packed into waste bags for infectious agents.
- *If positive test of the mail-parcels*: Exposed person is tested and immediately treated prophylactically. Other people who were in the room are being tested and prophylactically treated at the infectious outpatient clinic. In addition, consider vaccination of infected persons, if inhalation is not excluded.

Reference

1. Andersen BM, Lereim I. Preparedness for biological weapons. In: Handbook in hygiene and infection control for hospitals. Oslo: Ullevål University Hospital; 2008. p. 586–7.

Dangerous Infectious Agents Combined with Hazardous Chemicals

91

Abstract

In extreme situations during war and terror, and also during peacetime, there may be sudden outbreaks of unknown illness with a high lethality. In addition, there may be a larger number of healthy people who may be exposed to the harmful agent(s) and yet with no symptoms. This situation may be caused by dangerous, high-risk microbes or by dangerous chemical agents and gases or by microbes and chemicals in combination—if intended action. The exposure may happen via aerosol, dust/dirt, food or water, etc. and may involve wounds and other injuries that need treatment (injuries from explosions, bombs, etc.). Patients may be highly contaminated by infectious agents/chemicals on clothing and skin when coming for further treatment in hospitals. This chapter describes the first steps of taking care of exposed persons: how to handle, decontaminate and remove dangerous agents and give first help.

Keywords

High-risk microbes · Hazardous microbes · Hazardous chemicals Decontamination · Infection control

Intent, scope and responsibility, see serious, common contagious scenarios, Chap. 82.

91.1 Purpose

To handle persons exposed to dangerous agents like microbes and/or chemical agents without spreading the contamination.

To protect patients, personnel and others against spread of infection and contamination.

B. M. Andersen, *Prevention and Control of Infections in Hospitals*,
https://doi.org/10.1007/978-3-319-99921-0_91

91.2 Comprise

All health care workers that are handling heavily contaminated (infectious agents and/or chemicals) persons or equipment during the first steps when admitting to hospitals.

91.3 Responsibility

The hospital's management provides written plans for how to react in situations where personnel and others may be exposed to known/unknown serious communicable disease, including bio-weapon, and a practical arrangement for how to handle the situation.

Infection Control Officer at the level where the problem occurs, and at the departments/ward where the infection may spread, is responsible for following local emergency plans.

Personnel who unprotected has come in a seriously contagious situation and may have been exposed to infectious agents is responsible for contacting (per telephone) the nearest responsible/infectious unit for advice and for following written guideline and practical advice.

91.4 Practical Measures [1, 2]

Healthy people who have been exposed to the harmful agent(s) and yet with no symptoms may perform a rapid decontamination with showering, bathing, changing clothes, medical prophylaxis, etc. outside the hospitals. Here the civil defence has a high responsibility to assist the population.

91.4.1 Hazardous Microbial Contamination: With or Without Hazardous Chemicals

91.4.1.1 Preparedness

Notify the person in charge at reception, who further communicates messages according to emergency preparedness plan. Infection control personnel are contacted to protect personnel, other patients and the environment.

Decide as far as possible if the patient is highly contaminated by infectious agents on clothing and skin (aerosol, dust/dirt, water) and/or of chemically dangerous agents. In case of suspected chemical agents, diagnostic equipment is prepared for the detection of hazardous chemical agents (CAM). CAM can be used on the patient before entering the hospital.

1. *Reception* redirects transport of the suspected case to external access to the isolate for airborne infections with negative air pressure. All intensive treatment takes place at this isolate (respirator treatment and more).

2. *Isolates for airborne infections are* prepared with decontamination rooms and sluice function. The negative pressure ventilation must be checked, and there must be protective equipment for a minimum of ten persons.
3. *Consider the* need to empty the isolation unit for other patients (if there are other patients isolated).
4. *Persons in charge (two persons)* take on protective equipment: respiratory protection, cap, tight-wearing glasses, double gloves, special waterproof gown or overalls, phantom hood (with surgical cap below), shoe covers and other disposable equipment. Additionally raincoats and boots when showering the patient. Eventually fresh air systems.
5. *Assistance (one to two persons)* prepares with PPE in the same way but stays outside the isolate/in the sluice and takes care of the in-and-out delivery of equipment and contaminated waste, as well as checking the proper removal of PPE.

91.4.2 Biological Dangerous Agent: Not Chemical

1. *Patient infected with dangerous agent but not contaminated on clothing or skin is* admitted directly through external access into the isolate. Diagnostics, treatment and registration are put into effect. Continue isolation treatment for clarification/treatment effect, etc.
2. *Patient infected* via *contaminated aerosols, dust, dirt and water* (for instance, biological weapons) on clothing and skin.
   - Place the patient in airborne isolation with direct access from outside or in a preinstalled decontamination tent placed outside the isolation unit.
   - Ask the patient to close the eyes and mouth and breathe calmly through the nose. Meanwhile wash the face gently and quickly with water and hibiscrub (chlorhexidine wash) or chloramine 5% (remove infectious tissue around the nose/mouth/eyes).
   - Respiratory protection (P3 mask) should be applied to the patient before quickly and carefully (re-aerosols) taking off the clothes before showers/whole body wash with hibiscrub. Remove the mask while the patient showers and start washing/showering the head. Finally put on a new respiratory protection.
3. *After decontamination*, the patient is moved in a clean bed with new equipment and with P3 mask on a new isolate, while the first isolate may be decontaminated or clarified to the next patient.
4. *The patient is* treated and taken care of in the isolate. Continue isolation treatment for clarification/treatment effect, etc. Intensive treatment is carried out in this isolate. *Surgery*, preferably in airborne isolation, see below and separate chapter.

91.4.3 Biological Infection: Suspected Combined with Chemical Dangerous Substances

Person exposed to—or possibly contaminated by—dangerous microbes and/or hazardous chemical agents. The hazardous chemical substance may damage the skin and mucous membranes of the patient but will not cause a danger to personnel if personal protective equipment/chemical barrier equipment is used.

Use chemical protective clothing outside of PPE. Otherwise, follow treatment as above: Sect. 91.4.2, 1–4.

91.4.4 Surgical Treatment: Infectious Agent: High Risk with or Without Chemical Agent

91.4.4.1 Emergency Operation

Reception clarifies diagnostic equipment for detection of hazardous chemical agents (CAM).

Patient decontaminates as described above.

After decontamination, the patient is moved to a new bed with P3 mask to an isolate or to an operating room equipped for infectious surgery. Avoid transport through patient wards; clean the bed throughout, and place a clean sheet over the bed before transport. The decontamination room is cleaned/decontaminated.

Preparation of the operating room: Optimally, the operating room should have direct access from the outside and be a complete separate unit. The unit should have a sluice system, negative air pressure and disinfected air and waste water. If not present, consider the following solution:

1. Use the operation department's "infectious room"—preferably with negative air pressure, 15 pascal or lower. Current system today is "multiresistant tuberculosis" scheme (see separate chapter). All unnecessary equipment is removed, and all openings and valves are taped over with plastic. The ventilation is turned off. Separate air extractor aggregate disinfect air out from the room. HEPA filters are put on all technical equipment that is air-cooled. Exhaust gases and ventilation air from the patient are directed directly into the extractor unit.
2. *If there is no time or situation to prepare the operating room*, use a peripherally located operating room that is closed and sealed and the ventilation is turned off (PPE for ten people).
3. Personnel for cleaning and internal service are notified.
4. It may be appropriate with a separate transport of contaminated waste, etc.; internal service is notified.
5. Evaluate the stop of the operating program of the whole operation department, and empty the operating department for unauthorized persons.

After surgery, the patient wakes up in the operating room and is transferred into a new bed that is covered with a clean bed sheet, and use respiratory protection on the patient during transport to airborne isolate. Avoid transport through patient areas; prefer external transport to isolate.

The operation unit is decontaminated as usual after high-risk infections. Machinery and other technical equipment which inner parts cannot be heat disinfected or treated with 5% chloramine may be gas sterilized—considered by infection control personnel. Hydrogen peroxide dry gas can be used for disinfection of equipment, ducts, etc., which are hardly available with common surface disinfection. The equipment must then be started so that the gas is pulled through internal parts. Use spore control to document the effect. Gas disinfection has killing effect on most bacteria, bacterial spores and virus after approximately 3 h of disinfection (no effect on *Mycobacteria*). After gas disinfection, disinfect surfaces with 5% chloramine- for one hour.

91.4.5 Not Infectious, Only Dangerous Chemical Agent: Hospital Emergency Preparedness Plan

Chemical agent: liquid, powder and gas (respiratory system and/or the skin).

Decontamination room may be in close proximity to reception; must have direct access from outside, negative air pressure and separate exhaust duct to remove toxic gases, and should have quality bathroom, equipped with shower and wash on stretcher and with separate ventilation. Alternatively, a separate tent outside can be used. Also *a negative air pressure isolate* with separate entrance and disinfection room can be used for decontamination of chemical agents, if separate air extraction does not access other ventilation systems.

The patient is treated immediately in the decontamination room, and, if appropriate, the extent of injury and measures recorded.

After decontamination, the patient follows the usual procedures in the hospital, depending on the condition. Further treated as non-infectious.

References

1. Andersen BM, Lereim I. Contamination of dangerous contaminants/chemical substances. In: Handbook in hygiene and infection control for hospitals. Oslo: Ullevål University Hospital; 2008. p. 588–91.
2. Andersen BM. *Bacillus anthracis*. In: Bacteria and diseases. Epidemiology, infections and infection control. Oslo: Gyldendal Akademisk; 2005. p. 9–44.

Infection Control Resources 92

Abstract
Healthcare-associated infections (HAIs) constitute major additional costs for the health service and society as a whole and unnecessary suffering and death among patients. Resources put in place to combat hospital infections appear to reduce infections by 30–70% and at the same time are very profitable. In high-income countries, the prevalence of healthcare-associated infections in mixed patient populations may be 7–10%. During the last 20 years, HAIs have become more dangerous with more resistant microbes, associated with indefensible use of antibiotics. The nexus of cause and effect is the use of antibiotics like "sweets," both in human and animal medicine, combined with a great neglect of hygiene and infection control, "to treat bad hygiene and lack of infection control by bad antibiotics". Today there is a short stay in hospitals. A high burden on each patient bed; overcrowding, and on each personnel; understaffing, results in a higher risk of HAIs. By establishing at least one infection control nurse (ICN) per 250 somatic patient beds and one infection control physician (ICD) per 1000 beds, hospital infections have been reduced by one-third. However, the number of infection control personnel should be assessed by number of admissions and other activities of the hospital. Investments in infection control personnel, statistics, technical equipment, etc. for monitoring and preventing of hospital infections pays for hospitals, patients and society as a whole. It is a clear cost-benefit measure.

Keywords
Infection control · Infection control nurse (ICN) · Infection control doctor (ICD) Healthcare-associated infection (HAI) · Resources · Surveillance · Prevention Containment · Resistant microbes · Epidemics · Nosocomial infections · Hygiene nurse · Hygiene

B. M. Andersen, *Prevention and Control of Infections in Hospitals*,
https://doi.org/10.1007/978-3-319-99921-0_92

92.1 Purpose

- To protect the patient, personnel, environment, healthcare institution and the society in general, against spread of healthcare-associated infections, by the presence of competent and updated infection control personnel (ICP):
  - That are working with the hospital staff to establish relevant infection control routines, guidelines, hygienic measures, surveillances and practical solutions during outbreaks
  - Participate in planning and working with emergency measures concerning infectious outbreaks

92.2 Comprise

- All ICP responsible for the infection control work at the hospital
- All personnel and leaders working together with ICP during preventive controls, surveillances, reports, methods and emergency situations

92.3 Responsibility

The hospital's management is responsible for ensuring enough resources, including infection control personnel, for proper infection control work at the hospital and for the presence of an updated Infection Control Programme, updated internal guidelines, surveillance systems, quality of hygienic standard and for other control and prevention of infections at the hospital, according to guidelines, activity and actual laws.

The infection control management is responsible for updating and implementing the Infection Control Programme at the hospital, for surveillances, control and prevention of spread of infections and for emergency plans and guidelines concerning outbreaks of infections. Infection control reports to the hospital management: hygienic problems, outbreaks, deviations from procedures etc., that may result in infection risk for patients, personnel or others.

Department management provides implementation of routines concerning hygiene, control and prevention of infections, according to the infection control programme, and contacts infection control concerning hygienic issues, questions and information concerning infectious diseases.

Staffs follow routines concerning hygiene and infection control. Deviations from internal guidelines and procedures should be reported to the management and to infection control unit.

92.3.1 Burden of Hospital-Associated Infections

Hospital infections constitute major additional costs for the health service and society as a whole and unnecessary suffering and death among patients [1–30].

Resources put in place to combat hospital infections appear to reduce infections by 30–70% and at the same time are very profitable [1–13, 24].

92.3.1.1 Cost of Some Hospital-Associated Infections

Central line-associated bloodstream infection (CLABSI), ventilator-associated pneumonia (VAP), surgical site infection (SSI), catheter-associated urinary tract infection (CAUTI) and *Clostridium difficile* infection (CDI) are estimated to cost:

One case of	was in the USA (2013) estimated to [17]
• CLABSI	• 45,800 USD
• VAP	• 40,145 USD
• SSI	• 20,785 USD
• *C difficile*	• 11,285 USD
• CAUTI	• 900 USD

92.3.2 The Need for Infection Control Resources

Hayley et al. (1985) showed that by establishing an infection control nurse (ICN/ICP) per 250 somatic patient beds and an infection control physician (ICD) per 1000 beds, hospital infections were reduced by one-third (32%), postoperative wound infections by 20–35%, urinary tract infection by 38%, sepsis by 35%, and pneumonia by13–27% and other types by 32% [2].

Investments in personnel, statistics, technical equipment, etc., work on prevention, monitoring and follow-up of hospital infections pays for hospitals, patients and society as a whole. It is a clear cost-benefit measure [2–17].

During the last 30 years, different needs for infection control personnel have been calculated in relation to the number of somatic beds or the number of hospitalizations, see table below [2, 3, 6, 7, 12, 16, 19–31]. Number of personnel should be assessed by number of admissions and other activity of the hospital. This is important because of shorter stay, more and more patients (also risk patients) pass the hospital admission and discharge systems, and there is a higher burden on each patient bed.

Minimum requirements are [32]:

- Infection control doctor (ICD)/epidemiologist
- Infection control nurse (ICN) (hygiene nurse)
- Bioengineer, medical microbiologist and specialist in infection medicine
- Mercantile personnel for prevalence and incidence surveys, reports, routines and messages
- Data and statistics. Continuous access to microbiological findings at the hospital
- Technical equipment (instruments for detecting of microbes, dirt, particles, ventilation conditions, air pressure conditions, etc.)
- Training, knowledge and experience; hospital staff, as well as internal updating of knowledge

- Work descriptions and functions
- Mandate descriptions for infection control personnel
- Organization and position/responsibility in the hospital
- Hygiene Committee
- Antibiotics Committee, Building Committee, Purchasing Committee, etc.
- Infection control laboratory, including microbiology and study of environmental microbes [32]

In 2005, the number of infection protection personnel per 1000 beds in 12 countries in Europe are as follows [26]:

• 1.2 ICD[a]
• 3.4 ICN
• 1 computer engineer
• 1 epidemiologist
• 1 administrative/mercantile support
• 1 technique, monitoring
• SUM: At least 9.3 full-time positions per 1000 patient somatic beds.

[a]At least 6 years postgraduate training with specialty/subspecialty in infection control [26]

92.3.2.1 Infection Control Nurses (ICN): Hygiene Nurse

Needs relative to the number of somatic beds vary from one ICN per <100 patient beds to one ICN per 365 beds (see Table 92.1). The ratio of personnel to numbers of somatic patient beds depends on complexity, acute activity and patient categories.

92.3.2.2 Infection Control Physician (ICD, Infection Control Doctor)

The need of ICDs in somatic departments is calculated to one ICD per 800–1000 somatic hospital beds; see Table 92.2. In Belgium, ICD is a separate medical specialty. The Netherlands required in 2007 one medical microbiologist per 806 patient beds or one per 25,000 admissions [27].

Consensus reports for infection control generally lack specific recommendations regarding staffing of infection control nurses [3–36]. This may lead to a lack of follow-up and implementation of infection prevention [33–36].

The need for infection protection personnel and technical assistance is increasing in somatic emergency hospitals. Scheckler et al. wrote already in 1998 that “the old ratio of one ICP per 250 beds is no longer adequate”. “In most acute care hospitals today, the scope of work of ICP is much greater than that provided by the old ratio” [31]. The Delphi project from 2002 has made a graded staffing plan in relation to the hospital type and nursing home [24]. From Canada, ICP is proposed and assessed by workload in both hospitals (1:100) and nursing homes (1:250), and similar is recommended in France (1:100) [3, 25]. A recent systematic study of hospital organization, management and structure of infection protection in Europe supports this assessment [37].

Table 92.1 Needs for infection control nurse (ICN-ICP) in hospitals per number of beds in somatic hospitals

Hygiene nurse, infection control nurse (ICN), infection control personnel (ICP) in relation to somatic beds				
ICN/ICP number	Per number of patient beds	Comment	Country	References
1	250	SENIC	United States	Haley et al. [2]
1	700		Belgium	Mertens et al. [19]
1	386		United Kingdom	Emmerson et al. [12]
0.2–0.75	250		Switzerland	Pittet et al. [20]
1.5	200		United States	JCAHO [21]
1	150		United States	US Navy
1.5	200		United States	Hoffman and Grant [22]
1.1	250		Canada	Zoutman et al. [23]
1	100 first	1/250 next	United States	Klevens et al. 2002/[16]
0.8–1	100	"Delphi"	United States	O'Boyle et al. [24]
1	133	2003	Quebec, Canada	Publ. Hlth Canada [3]
1	100	2003 special	Quebec, Canada	Publ. Hlth Canada [3]
3	500		Canada	Health Canada [25]
1	150–250	LTCF	Canada	Health Canada [25]
3.4	1000		Europe 12 countries	Voss et al. [26]
1	178		Netherlands	van den Broek et al. [27]
3	1000[a]	1995–2007	Norway	Andersen et al. [28]
1	100		France	Carlet et al. [6]
1	400	"historic"	France	RAISIN [7]
1	167	average	USA NNIS	Stone et al. [29]
0.6	250	LTCF	Canada	Zoutman et al. [30]

LTCF long-term care facilities, Nursing Home, *SENIC* Great American Study, *NNIS* hospital network in the United States
[a]In addition, more than 200 psychiatric patients

92.3.3 Education and Responsibility for ICN/Hygiene Nurses [38]

In accordance with the Act on Specialist Health Care Services §§ 2-1 a, 3 -3,3-4, and Regulations on infection protection in the health service of 17 June 2005, pursuant to Law 5 August 1994 no. 55 on protection against communicable diseases §§ 4-7,7-11, the following mandate is made for ICN/hygiene nurses in Norway:

- Hygiene nurse (ICN) shall have formal education such as hygiene nursing care, administrative experience, management training, teaching competence and good written and oral ability. Experience and special education in surgery, intensive medicine or emergency medicine is the basis for further education as a hygiene nurse.

Table 92.2 Needs for infection control doctor (ICD) in hospitals per number of somatic beds or admissions

Infection control doctor (ICD) in relation to somatic beds				
ICD number	Per number of patient beds	Comment	Country	References
1	1000	SENIC	United States	Haley et al. [2]
1	1700		Belgium	Mertens et al. [19]
1.2	1000		Europe 12 countries	Voss et al. [26]
1	806	1/25,000 admissions	Netherlands	van den Broek et al. [27]
1	800		France	Carlet et al. [6]
1	800		France	RAISIN [7]
1	1000[a]	1995–2007	Norway	Andersen et al. [28]

SENIC Great American Study
[a]In addition, more than 200 psychiatric patients

- Hygiene nurse is responsible for the ongoing functions/tasks that can naturally be linked to hospital hygiene work in accordance with the hospital's infection control program.
- Examples of important tasks:
  - Advice and information on hospital hygiene work
  - Prevalence and incidence surveys, follow-up and feedback
  - Participate in infection tracing, infection monitoring and infection control measures
  - Participate in infection control procedures and guidelines
  - Work with quality assurance of sterile equipment, other equipment, textiles, cleaning, etc.
  - Teach and arrange further education of health professionals
  - Participate in development and research work
  - Provide advice, guidance and information to other hospitals and municipalities
  - Attend hygiene forums, relevant building/rebuilding committees, working environment, meetings and emergency preparedness groups
  - Attend regional and international infection control meetings

92.3.4 Responsibility, Mandate, Education and Work for Infection Control Doctor (ICD) (Hospital Hygienists) [36]

In accordance with the Act on Specialist Health Care Services §§ 2-1 a, 3 -3,3-4, and Regulations on infection protection in the health service of 17 June 2005, pursuant to Law 5 August 1994 no. 55 on protection against communicable diseases §§ 4-7,7-11, the following mandate is made for ICDs in Norway:

- ICD should be a specialist in medical microbiology or infectious medicine, and in the long term, a speciality in infection control should be established.

- ICD coordinates the infection protection work in the hospital and should in such cases be directly subject to the management at the hospital, lead the infection prevention work, and be the adviser to the hospital's management and towards the different departments at the hospital.
- ICD is the head of the department for hygiene and infection protection and organizationally associated with quality and patient safety.
- The hospital management, director of the hospital, has overall responsibility for the infection control program at the hospital, while the ICD has the medical professional responsibility for designing and maintaining the program as part of the hospital's internal control system.
- Responsibility for implementing the program lies with the line manager.
- The infection control program contains two organizational and medical professional parts that constitute measures within (a) infection monitoring and (b) infection prevention.
- The ICD/ICN should be represented in the hospital's quality committee, building committees and other committees to ensure and improve the hospital hygiene standard (e.g., new building/rebuilding, purchasing of medical equipment, practical methods and new techniques, routines, products, etc.).
- ICD shall have a *professional free and independent position* that allows for quick, effective and independent advice regarding infection prevention and infection control measures.
- Internal reporting regarding hospital infections or suspected hospital infections shall be directed to infection protection personnel and through the usual reporting obligation for deviations to quality department. This applies to all departments at the hospital, both in terms of prevalence, incidence investigations and reporting of single cases according to reporting routines included in the infection control program.
- ICD reports to the Director of the hospital, to the National Institute of Public Health and the Public Health Authority in the County for major outbreaks and particularly hazardous infections/situations. In addition, the ICD reports to the Director on deaths due to hospital infection and/or resource-intensive measures [38]. Prevalence and incidence of hospital infections are reported to the health authorities on an ongoing basis.
- ICD and ICN shall have free access to information, use and processing of, for example:
  - Microbiological results (daily, weekly and monthly annual reports, etc.)
  - Other patient data (clinical data, prevalence and incidence)
  - Consumption of antimicrobial agents (weekly reports, defined daily doses (DDD)/department)
  - Staff data, if actual for infection tracing and environmental measures
- ICD shall—in collaboration with the microbiological department—have access to the necessary laboratory capacity and technical staff in the work with infection-preventive measures and tracing of outbreaks.
- ICD and ICN shall contribute to the planning and teaching of hospital hygiene and infection control to medical students and physicians and to other healthcare personnel in the hospital hygiene.
- A hygienic forum, or similar like that, should be an advisory board headed by the ICD.

92.3.5 Organization, Management, Staffing and Part-Time Work

Infection control work depends not only on a functional infection control team but also on the organization and management of the hospital, burden on patient beds, staffing and workload [28, 37]. MRSA infections are spread by understaffed personnel in intensive care units, new-born departments and many other types of hospital departments [28, 37, 39–54].

Intensive care units An increase of MRSA cases in intensive department is most often related to increased work pressure among nurses [39–41]. Such outbreaks can be controlled by avoiding overcrowding [40]. A study demonstrated that MRSA infection increased significantly among hospitalized patients when more than seven out of eight beds were in use (87%) [41]. The intensive patient is usually critically ill. In case of high work pressure, the number of infections in such patients increases [42]. Among 1800 intensive patients, a higher staffing level was associated with over 30% reduction of the infection risk. By keeping nursing/patient ratio of more than 2.2, a reduction of infections of 27% was calculated. Too low staffing in intensive departments has been linked to 50% increase in hospital infections [43]. Overcrowding and understaffing have also been associated with blood catheter infections from central catheters and with hepatitis C transmission during dialysis [44–46].

New-born intensive units At Ullevål University Hospital, MRSA outbreaks occurred in the new-born intensive care department in 2002 [47]. This department was understaffed with many part-time employees who worked at several hospitals at the same time (especially at hospitals in Sweden). There was a chronic overcrowded unit; small patient space and isolates were missing, and patients from different parts of the ward were gathered in fewer rooms to save personnel night-time and weekends. This led to a larger spread of infection [47]. Later on, in 2010, the condition and management were unchanged at new-born, while at the same time, there was a large overcrowding, heavy under-capacity, mixing of patients from different patient rooms and at the same time spread of a serious infection with gentamicin-resistant *S. aureus* among the children [48].

A study of 3.65 million paediatric patients in California showed that resource-based nurse staffing was related to significantly reduced cases of postoperative lung complications, including pneumonia and postoperative sepsis [49].

Other departments in hospitals Overcrowding is an important factor for the transmission of MRSA and other MDRO-bacteria also within other parts of the hospital [50]. An occupancy rate above 85% of patient beds causes a rapid turnover of patients and shorter stay time per patient and is significantly associated with MRSA proliferation in Northern Ireland and in England [51–53]. A Finnish study showed that the overall risk of hospital infections increases during long working time, high levels of work pressure and poor cooperation between staff [54].

Good organization and management can reduce hospital infections [55–57].

92.4 Background Information

92.4.1 The Burden of Infections That Can Be Prevented

Infections are very common both outside and inside healthcare institutions—move between institutions and between the community and institutions, following patients, personnel, visitors and equipment. Globally, it is, for example, estimated that two out of seven people in the world have infections with *Staphylococcus aureus* each year.

Healthcare-associated infections (HAIs) constitute major additional costs for the health service and society as a whole and unnecessary suffering and death among patients [1–30]. Resources put in place to combat hospital infections appear to reduce infections by 30–70% and at the same time are very profitable [1–13, 24].

Studies have shown that in high-income countries, the prevalence of healthcare-associated infections in mixed patient populations may be 7–10% [58]. The burden is higher in the developing world. Prevalence studies show a large variation between hospitals and between countries, with a pooled prevalence of 10.1% HAI [58]. The prevalence is significantly higher in high- and then in low-quality studies, 15.5% versus 8.5%, respectively, and is very high in intensive care units, 30% or more [58].

During the last 20 years, there has been a change in HAIs towards more dangerous infections, more resistant microbes, associated with indefensible use of antibiotics. The nexus of cause and effect is the use of antibiotics like "sweets," both in human and animal medicine, combined with a great neglect of hygiene and infection control in developed countries. It is the same as "to treat bad hygiene and lack of infection control by bad antibiotics."

WHO summarizes this problem in 2014 [59]:

1. High proportions of resistance were reported in all regions to common treatments for bacteria causing infections in both healthcare settings and in the community.
2. Antibacterial resistance has a negative effect on patient outcomes and health expenditures.
3. Treatment options for common infections are running out.
4. Despite limitations, the report demonstrates worldwide magnitude of antibacterial resistance and surveillance gaps [59].

The overall economic impact of this situation is very high, with reduced consumer income, employment and savings, and increased national investment and spending in healthcare delivery [60]. The result for most developed countries is a reduced gross domestic product (GDP) by 1.4–1.6% [60].

- In the United States, 1.7–2 million healthcare-associated infections are calculated each year (population 300 million), which leads to 99,000–103,000 deaths (5.8%) and direct extra costs of 20–40 billion USD each year [1, 4, 14–16, 58].

  - A meta-analysis of costs and financial impact during the period 1986–2013 in the United States showed that hospital infections were a "major supplier" of illness and death that could be prevented [17]. Five types of hospital infections, catheter-associated sepsis (CLABSI), ventilator-associated pneumonia (VAP), postoperative wound infection (SSI), *Clostridium difficile* infections and catheter associated urinary tract infections (CAUTI), amounted to 400,000 infections and ten billion USD, annually [17].
  - CDC's annual HAI progress reported 722,000 HAIs and 75,000 deaths during stay in US acute care hospitals in 2011 [61]. One in every 25 patients caught infection in hospitals. There was a 50% decrease in CLABSI between 2008 and 2014, 17% decrease of SSI, 8% decrease of CDI, 13% decrease of MRSA bacteraemia and no change in CAUTI [61].
  - Estimated burden of *antibacterial resistance* in the United States was in 2013 more than 23,000 deaths, more than two million illnesses and overall social costs up to 20 billion USD direct and up to 35 billion indirect [59].
- In Europe (population, 500 million), HAI may cause 16 million extra days of hospital stay and 37,000 attributable deaths and and contribute to additional 110,000 annually [58]. Annual direct cost is estimated to seven billion Euro [58].
  - Estimates between 2011 and 2012 from data from 1150 hospitals in 30 European countries resulted in more than 2.5 million HAIs with estimated deaths in 90,000 people, annually [62]. One in every 20 patients caught an infection during stay in hospital. Cassini et al. estimated that around a third of infections were preventable through better hygiene, detection and improved infection control [62]. Pneumonia, SSI and urinary tract infections had the highest numbers of cases per year, while bacteraemia and pneumonia had the highest death rate [62].
  - Estimated burden of *antibacterial resistance* in Europe is 25,000 deaths per year, 2.5 million extra hospital days and approximately 1.5 billion Euro per year [60].
- In Thailand (population, 70 millions), the burden of *antibacterial resistance* results in >3.2 million extra hospital days, >38,000 deaths and >1.5 billion USD in direct and indirect costs per year [59].
- In Norway (population, five million), the four types of HAIs registered, urinary tract infection, lower respiratory tract infection, SSI and bacteraemia, may cause infections in 5–10% of admitted somatic patients [1, 18, 63, 64]. These four types amount to approximately 45,600 patients with HAIs each year [1, 63]. With five extra hospital days (900–1000 Euro/day), the four HAIs may cost at least 205 million in direct annual additional hospital expenses [1, 63].

92.4.2 The Quantitative Need for Infection Prevention Staffing

As shown in the tables above, the quantitative needs assessment is varying between countries and hospitals and may be results of knowledge, mandate, responsibility, resources, patient categories, meaningfulness and organization of infection prevention. Recently, a systematic study was done to quantify infection prevention staff and coverage needs in five states (34 hospitals, 583 ambulatory sites, 26 in-home and long-term care programs) in the United States [65]. When the need of infection control personnel was aggregated across the organization, "the comprehensive review results yielded a new benchmark of 1.0 infection prevention full-time equivalent per 69 beds if ambulatory, long-term care or home care are included" [65].

Since the patients are staying shorter and shorter time in hospitals and return back to primary healthcare or to other hospitals with infections/carrier state, they may spread infections to others that in turn are seeking medical help in the healthcare. This is to create an "evil circle" of preventable and expensive infections in the healthcare and society. The study of Bartles et al. puts focus on this problem and proposes an even more effective and comprehensive way to reduce preventable infections [65].

References

1. Andersen BM. Occurrence, costs and mortality of hospital infections. In: Handbook in hygiene and infection control for hospitals, Part 1. Norway: Fagbokforlaget; 2014. p. 26–30.
2. Haley RW, Culver DH, White JW, et al. The efficacy of infection surveillance and control programs in preventing nosocomial infections in university hospitals. Am J Epidemiol. 1985;121:182–205.
3. Public Health Agency of Canada. Essential resources for effective infection prevention and control programs: a matter of patient safety—a discussion paper (2010). Updated July 26, 2010.
4. Umscheid CA, Mitchell MD, Doshi JA, Agarwal R, Williams K, Brennan PJ. Estimating the proportion of healthcare-associated infections that are reasonable preventable and the related mortality and costs. Infect Control Hosp Epidemiol. 2011;32:101–14.
5. CDC. National and state healthcare-associated infections (HAI). Progress report; 2015.
6. Carlet JM, Astagneau P, Brun-Buisson C, et al. French national program for prevention of healthcare-related infections and antimicrobial resistance, 1992-2008. Positive trends, but perseverance needed. Infect Control Hosp Epidemiol. 2009;30:737–45.
7. RAISIN-working group. "RAISIN" - a national program for early warning, investigation and surveillance of healthcare-related infection in France. Euro Surveill. 2009;14. pii: 19408.
8. Pronovost PJ, Goeschel CA, Colantuoni E, et al. Sustained reductions in catheter-related bloodstream infections in Michigan intensive care units: observation study. BMJ. 2010;340:309.
9. Rioux C, Grandbastien B, Astagneau P. Impact of a six-year control program on surgical site infections in France: results of the INCISO surveillance. J Hosp Infect. 2007;66:217–23.
10. Astagneau P, L'Hériteau F, Daniel F, Parneix P, et al. Reducing surgical site infection incidence through a network: results from the French ISO-RAISIN surveillance system. J Hosp Infect. 2009;72:127–34.
11. Coignard B. Raisin. National NI prevalence surveys results, 2001-2006. http://www.invs.sante.fr/raisin.
12. Emmerson AM, Enstone JE, Griffin M, Kelsey MC, Smyth ET. The second national prevalence survey of infection in hospitals - overview of the results. J Hosp Infect. 1996;32:175–90.
13. Pittet D, Harbarth S, Ruef C, et al. Prevalence and risk factors for nosocomial infections in four university hospitals in Switzerland. Infect Control Hosp Epidemiol. 1999;20:37–42.
14. Leape LL, Brennan TA, Laird N, et al. The nature of adverse events in hospitalized patients: results of Harvard Medical Practice Study II. N Engl J Med. 1991;324:377–84.

15. Scott DR, CDC. The direct medical costs of healthcare-associated infections in US hospitals and the benefits of prevention. CDC.Gov., 1 September 2012.
16. Klevens RM, Edwards JR, Richards CL Jr, et al. Estimating healthcare-associated infections and deaths in US hospitals, 2002. Public Health Rep. 2007;1222:160–6.
17. Zimlichman E, Henderson D, Tamir O, et al. Healthcare-associated infections: a meta-analysis of costs and financial impact on the US health care system FREE. JAMA Intern Med. 2013;173:2039–46.
18. National Public Health Institute. Prevalence of healthcare-associated infections and antibiotic use (PIAH); 2014.
19. Mertens R, Jans B, Kurz X. A computerized national network of nosocomial infection surveillance in Belgium. Infect Control Hosp Epidemiol. 1994;15:171–9.
20. Pittet D, Francioli P, von Overbeck J, Raeber PA, Reuf C, Widmer AF. Infection control in Switzerland. Infect Control Hosp Epidemiol. 1995;16:49–56.
21. The Joint Commission on Accreditation of healthcare Organizations. JCAHO 1997 accreditation manual for hospitals. Oakbrook Terrace; 1996.
22. Hoffman J, Grant L. National Nosocomial Infection NNIS system. Infect Control Hosp Epidemiol. 1997;18:475–8.
23. Zoutman DE, Ford BD, Bryce E, et al. The state of infection surveillance and control in Canada acute care hospitals. Am J Infect Control. 2003;31:266–73.
24. O'Boyle C, Jackson M, Henly SJ. Staffing requirements for infection control programs in US health care facilities: Delphi project. Am J Infect Control. 2002;30:321–33.
25. Health Canada. Development of a resource model for infection prevention and control programs in acute, long term, and home care settings; conference proceedings of the Infection Prevention and Control Alliance. Am J Infect Control. 2004;32:2–6.
26. Voss A and A Panel of ESGNI Members. The training in hospital infection control. Clin Microbiol Infect. 2005;11:33–5.
27. van den Broek PJ, Kluytmans JAJW, Ummels LC, Voss A, Vanderbroucke-Grauls CMJE. How many infection control staff do we need in hospitals? J Hosp Infect. 2007;65:108–11.
28. Andersen BM, Rasch M, Hochlin K, Tollefsen T, Sandvik L. Hospital-acquired infections before and after healthcare reorganization in a tertiary university hospital in Norway. J Public Health. 2009;7:1–7.
29. Stone PW, Dick A, Pogorzelska M, et al. Staffing and structure of infection prevention and control programs. Am J Infect Control. 2009;37:351–7.
30. Zoutman DE, Ford BD, Gauthier J. A cross-Canada survey of infection prevention and control in long-term care facilities. Am J Infect Control. 2009;37:358–63.
31. Scheckler WE, Brimhall D, Buck AS, et al. Requirements for infrastructure and essential activities in infection control and epidemiology in hospitals: a consensus panel report. Infect Control Hosp Epidemiol. 1998;19:114–24.
32. Voss A. Guidelines: how to develop, read and apply. Training course in hospital epidemiology, 7–10 Nov 2001 Brugge. SHEA/CDC/ESCMID.
33. Friedman C, Barnette M, Buck AS, et al. Requirements for infrastructure and essential activities in infection control and epidemiology in out-of- hospital setting: a consensus panel report. Infect Control Hosp Epidemiol. 1999;20:695–705.
34. Murphy D, Carrico R, Warye K. Building the infectious prevention system of tomorrow: proceedings of the 2007 APIC futures summit. Am J Infect Control. 2008;36:232–40.
35. WHO. Core components for infection prevention and control programs. Geneva: WHO; 2008.
36. Hale R, Powell T, Drey NS, Gould DJ. Working practices and success of infection prevention and control teams: a scoping study. J Hosp Infect. 2015;89:77–81.
37. Zingg W, Holmes A, Dettenkofer M, et al. Hospital organization, management, and structure for prevention of health-care-associated infection: a systematic review and expert consensus. Lancet Infect Dis. 2015;15:212–24.
38. Infection Control Program. Ullevål University Hospital, Oslo, 2006–2011.
39. Vicca AF. Nursing staff workload as a determinant of methicillin-resistant *Staphylococcus aureus* spread in an adult intensive therapy unit. J Hosp Infect. 1999;43:109–13.

40. Blatnik J, Lesnicar G. Propagation of methicillin-resistant *Staphylococcus aureus* due to the overloading of medical nurses in intensive care units. J Hosp Infect. 2006;63:162–6.
41. Howie AJ, Ridley SA. Bed occupancy and incidence of methicillin-resistant *Staphylococcus aureus* infection in an intensive care unit. Anaesthesia. 2008;63:1070–3.
42. Hugonnet S, Chevrolet JC, Pittet D. The effect of workload on infection risk in critically ill patients. Crit Care Med. 2007;35:76–81.
43. Hugonnet S, Villaveces A, Pittet D. Nurse staffing level and nosocomial infections: empirical evaluation of the case crossover and case-time control design. Am J Epidemiol. 2007;165:1321–7.
44. Fridkin SK, Pear SM, Williamson TH, Galgiani JN, Jarvis WR. The role of understaffing in central venous catheter-associated bloodstream infections. Infect Control Hosp Epidemiol. 1996;17:150–8.
45. Alonso-Echanove J, Edwards JR, Richards MJ, et al. Effect of nurse staffing and antimicrobial-impregnated central venous catheters on the risk of bloodstream infections in intensive care units. Infect Control Hosp Epidemiol. 2003;24:916–25.
46. Petrosillo N, Gilli P, Serraino D, et al. Prevalence of infected patients and understaffing have a role in hepatitis C virus transmission in dialysis. Am J Kidney Dis. 2001;37:1004–10.
47. Andersen BM, Lindemann R, Bergh K, Nesheim BI, Syversen G, Solheim N, Laugerud F. Spread of methicillin-resistant *Staphylococcus aureus* in a neonatal intensive unit associated with understaffing, overcrowding and mixing of patients. J Hosp Infect. 2002;1: 1–7.
48. Grub C, Holberg-Petersen M, Medbø S, Andersen BM, Syversen G, Melby KK. A multi-drug resistant, methicillin-susceptible strain of *Staphylococcus aureus* from a neonatal intensive care unit in Oslo, Norway. Scand J Infect Dis. 2010;42:148–51.
49. Mark BA, Harless DW, Berman WF. Nurse staffing and adverse events in hospitalized children. Policy Polit Nurs Pract. 2007;8:83–92.
50. Borg MA. Bed occupancy and overcrowding as determinant factors in the incidence of MRSA infections within general ward settings. J Hosp Infect. 2003;54:316–8.
51. Cunningham JB, Kernohan WG, Rush T. Bed occupancy, turnover interval and MRSA rates in Northern Ireland. Br J Nurs. 2006;15:324–8.
52. Cunningham JB, Kernohan WG, Rush T. Bed occupancy, turnover interval and MRSA rates in English hospitals. Br J Nurs. 2006;15:656–60.
53. Cunningham JB, Kernohan WG, Sowney R. Bed occupancy and turnover interval as determinant factors in MRSA infections in acute settings in Northern Ireland: 1 April 2001 to 31 March 2003. J Hosp Infect. 2005;61:189–93.
54. Virtanen M, Kurvinen T, Terho K, et al. Work hours, work stress, and collaboration among ward staff in relation to the risk of hospital-associated infection among patients. Med Care. 2009;47:310–8.
55. McAlearney AS, Hefner J, Robbins J, Garman AN. The role of leadership in eliminating healthcare-related infections: a qualitative study of eight hospitals. Adv Health Care Manag. 2013;14:69–94. Cunningham.
56. Saint S, Kowalski CP, Banaszak-Holl J, Forman J, Damschroder L, Krein SL. The importance of leadership in preventing healthcare-related infection: results of a multisite qualitative study. Infect Control Hosp Epidemiol. 2010;31:901–7.
57. B B, Harris AD, Richards CL, et al. Does health care role and experience influence perception of safety culture related to preventing infections. Am J Infect Control. 2013;41:638–41.
58. WHO Patient Safety, Allegranzi B, et al. Report of the burden of endemic healthcare-associated infections worldwide. Geneva: WHO; 2011.
59. WHO. Antimicrobial resistance. Global report on surveillance 2014. Geneva: WHO; 2014.
60. Roberts R, Hota B, Ahmad I, Scott R, Foster SD, Abbasi F, et al. Hospital and societal costs of antimicrobial-resistant infections in a Chicago teaching hospital: implications for antibiotic stewardship. Clin Infect Dis. 2009;49:1147–84.
61. CDC. HAI Data and statistics. Healthcare-associated infections in the United States, 2006-2016: a story of progress. CDC; 2016.

62. Cassini A, Plachouras D, Eckmanns T, et al. Burden of six healthcare-associated infections on European population health: estimating incidence-based disability-adjusted life years through a population prevalence-based modelling study. PLoS Med. 2016;13(10):e1002150.
63. Andersen BM. Economic consequences of hospital infections in a 1,000 bed university hospital in Norway. Infect Control Hosp Epidemiol. 1998;19:805–7.
64. National Public Health Institution. Infections. Oslo; 2017.
65. Bartles R, Dickson A, Oluwatomiwa B. A systematic approach to quantify infection prevention staffing and coverage needs. Am J Infect Control. 2018;46:487–91.

Definitions

Infection: Invasion or presence of microbes that damage the tissue or tissue function—with or without symptoms. The infection may be acute with symptoms or chronic with or without symptoms.

- *Colonization* is when microbes are present without damaging tissues or functions.
- *Infection carriers*: Persons who are carriers of potentially infectious microbes without being clinically ill (colonized or symptomless infection).
- *Hospital-associated infection* is infection—due to treatment or stay at a hospital—and not present or in the incubation phase upon admission. Usually, hospital infection is registered:
  - Up to 30 days after discharge from the hospital
  - By implanted prosthesis/foreign body up to 1 year
- *Nosocomial* ("house common") *infection*: Hospital-associated infection and divided into 12 disease groups developed by the Centers for Disease Control and Prevention, CDC, Atlanta, USA, 1988 and later revisions [1–4]. The following are listed:
  1. Urinary tract infections (symptomatic)
  2. Upper and lower respiratory tract infection
  3. Gastroenteritis
  4. Surgical site infections: superficial and deep
  5. Infection in burns, other skin and soft tissue infection
  6. Intra-abdominal infection
  7. Osteomyelitis
  8. Septicaemia (bacteraemia)
  9. Meningitis
  10. Infection associated with intravascular tracheal intubation/canula equipment
  11. Infection in new-borns within 4 weeks, staphylococci
  12. Infections not covered by the points above

  Many nosocomial infections are easily spread between patients, personnel and the environment in the "common house".
- *HAI* healthcare-associated infections are associated with infections encountered in treatment and stay in the health service, hospitals, nursing homes, home care facilities, outpatient clinics, medical centres, etc.

B. M. Andersen, *Prevention and Control of Infections in Hospitals*,
https://doi.org/10.1007/978-3-319-99921-0

- *CLABSI* Central line-associated bloodstream infection
- *SSI* Surgical site infection
- *VAP* Ventilator-associated pneumonia
- *UTI* Urinary tract infection
- *CAUTI* Catheter-associated urinary tract infection
- *PIVC* Peripheral intravenous catheter
- *CVC* Central intravascular catheter
- *HD* Haemodialysis
- *PD* Peritoneal dialysis
- *Point Prevalence*: point registration of a given indicator, for example, number of patients with hospital infection at a predetermined time and date, expressed as percentage of the total number of patients in attendance [4]. The prevalence of hospital infections may be somewhat higher than the incidence. At the completion of point prevalence only four times a year, the result will be approximately results in the case of incidence. Short stay at the hospital.
- *Incidence*: continuous registration over time intervals, for example, the number of patients with hospital infections within 3 months expressed as percentage of the total number of patients in the same period of time.
- *Infection control* program: a program that includes all necessary measures to prevent and counter hospital infections and for the management and follow-up of outbreaks of such infections [1–4]. It shall contain necessary measures for (a) infection monitoring, (b) infection prevention, (c) measures for control of outbreaks, and (d) emergency preparedness for serious/extensive infection.
- *Municipal infection control unit*: healthcare unit designated by the municipality to provide infection control assistance to healthcare institutions at municipal level. The unit may be located in hospitals and staffed with infection control nurses and infection control doctor (specialist in medical microbiology or infectious medicine).
- *Infection control* is a second-line special function associated with hospitals/healthcare enterprises.
- *Medical microbiology*: the teaching of micro (small) organisms that can cause disease in humans.
- *Bacteria* are prokaryotic cells without core membranes, with many mitochondria, active mitosis systems and contain both DNA and RNA.
- *Viruses* are not living organisms, actively infectious nucleic acids, either DNA or RNA.
- *Prions* are not living, do not have DNA or RNA and are actively infectious protein molecules.
- *Medical parasitology*: the teaching of protozoans (single-celled organisms) and helminths/worms (multicellular organisms) that affect human beings. A parasite lives on another living creature.
- *Fungi* are yeast and a variety of other fungi, occasionally associated with allergies and serious infections, especially in patients with a defect of normal immune system.

- *Infections* are microorganisms such as bacteria, viruses, fungi, parasites and prions that can cause disease or unfortunate carrier status in humans.
- *The source of infection* is usually a patient, convalescent or healthy carrier but may also be infected animals (*Salmonella*, *E coli*, *Listeria*, *Brucella*, etc.), fish, insects or contaminated food, water and environment.
- *Infection transmission* can occur directly and indirectly by contact, blood and secretions/excretions, stab injuries, and via air, drops of varying size, droplets (aerosols) and skin and dust particles. Infection can also be transmitted via infected food and water.
  - *Contact contamination*: when the infectious agent is deposited on or in the environment around the patient (e.g., diarrhoea) and includes all direct contact with the infected patient or indirect contact, with equipment and fixtures in the patient's room (via hands, equipment, clothes, etc.)
  - *Airborne/droplet contamination (including contact)*: when contaminant spread into the air as drops of different size and weight or as small, droplet nuclei (dried drops, <5 μm). Also contagious (bacteria, viruses, etc.) skin or dust particles can float in the air for hours around the patient and partially fall down on the surfaces and furniture of the room. *Note! Droplet contamination* is airborne and must be treated as such. Some may separate drop from airborne contamination, which does not occur in real life.
  - *Re-aerosolization*: when contaminants present in the environment are blown up in the air by shaking/blowing, for instance, during bed making, rapid door movements or with heavy air stream in the room.
  - *Blood-borne infection*: certain types of infections that can be introduced directly through the skin or through damaged mucous membranes. This can happen in case of stab or sharp injury, sexual contact, infection from mother to child during childbirth, intravascular drug use, direct contact with open wounds (if you have open wounds or eczema) and rarely by contaminated transfusions or contaminated medical equipment.
- *Droplet nuclei* are microscopic particles less than 5 μm that are residues of dried drops, for example, produced when a person coughs, sneezes, cries, sings or "speaks loudly". Droplets are floating in the air for many hours to days and can follow air currents out of the patient's room and via air vents.
- *Epidemiologically important microbes*: (a) easily transmissible - infectious, (b) make outbreak of infections, (c) may cause serious disease, (d) can contribute to treatment problems, (e) are often long-term survivors in the environment, (f) are often affected by and selected by antimicrobial consumption; type and amount, and (g) usually robust against heat and chemicals.
  - Bacteria: MRSA, VRE, and ESBL-, CRE-, CP- and NDM-1 producing Gram-negative rod bacteria, *Clostridium difficile*, other MDROs, *Klebsiella* sp., *Enterobacter* sp., *Serratia* sp., *Pseudomonas aeruginosa*, *Acinetobacter species*, *Burkholderia cepacia*, *Stenotrophomonas maltophilia*, *Listeria monocytogenes*, *Legionella* sp., *Mycobacterium tuberculosis* and other mycobacteria, etc.

  - Virus: influenza virus, parainfluenza virus, avian influenza virus group, respiratory syncytial virus (RSV), metapneumovirus, enterovirus group, adenovirus group, norovirus, rotavirus, sapovirus, hemorrhagic virus, and coronavirus such as SARS and MERS.
  - Fungi: *Aspergillus* and others that specifically infect immunosuppressed.
  - Parasites: *Giardia* and other parasites that are contaminating drinking water.
- *Virulence* is the ability of microbes to cause disease when the infection is deposited at an appropriate recipient site (receptor, for example, lung tissue) in a person susceptible to infection (not immune). Virulence is usually related to low dose of the agent and long-term survival in the environment. Particularly low infection doses are well known for lung tuberculosis (one bacterium), EHEC (about 10 bacteria), shigella (about 100 bacteria) and norovirus (about 10 virus particles).
- *Resistant*: a bacterium may be resistant (survive), for example, to penicillin. This treatment has no effect on the bacterium (survives) or on the infection (ongoing).
- *Sensitive*: a bacterium may be sensitive to penicillin, and this treatment causes the bacteria to be killed and the infection disappears.
- *ESBL*: "extended spectrum beta-lactamases". Bacteria that produce special enzymes that make them particularly resistant to all beta-lactam antibiotics such as penicillin, cephalosporins and eventually carbapenems.
- *MDROs*: multidrug-resistant organisms – microbes that are resistant to many antimicrobial medicaments.
- *MDR*: "multidrug-resistant" resistance to many types of antibiotics.
- *MRSA*: meticillin-resistant *Staphylococcus aureus.*
- *VRSA:* vancomycin-resistant *Staphylococcus aureus.*
- *VRE:* vancomycin-resistant enterococci.
- *CP*: carbapenem resistant to imipenem, meropenem, etc. by producing special enzymes that breaks down carbapenem antibiotics, among others.
- *CRE*: carbapenem-resistant *Enterobacteriaceae.*
- *NDM-1:* New Delhi metallo-beta-lactamase 1, a resistance gene that can be transmitted between gram-negative rod bacteria and elicit complete antibiotic resistance.
- *CD*: *Clostridium difficile*—gram-positive spore-forming bacterium that provides diarrhoea—selected by antibiotics that inhibit other intestinal flora. High carrier rate without symptoms—easily transmitted—nosocomial outbreaks.
- *CDI*: *Clostridium difficile* infection.
- *SARS*: Severe acquired respiratory syndrome. Epidemic and "pandemic" coronavirus, transmitted from animals, in 2003, started in China, Guangdong, and ended after approximately 6 months. Since then, no outbreaks have occurred. Nosocomial outbreaks are very important and easily transmitted to staff.
- *MERS*: Middle East respiratory syndrome coronavirus. Epidemic coronavirus, probably transmitted from animals and bats, started in the middle of spring 2012. Nosocomial outbreaks are very important and may be transmitted to staff.
- *CJD*: Creutzfeldt-Jakob disease. Prion disease with variants "mad cow disease".

- *CDC*: Centres for Disease Control and Prevention. State Centre in the United States for the prevention and control of infections.
- *ICN/ICP*: infection control nurse/infection control personnel and hygiene nurse.
- *ICD*: infection control doctor and infection control physician.
- *PPE*: personal protective equipment, respiratory equipment such as gloves, surgical mask, cap, gown, etc.
- *HEPA filter*: high-efficiency particulate air filter. The filter removes 99.97% of all particles larger than equal to 0.3 μm at a defined air flow. There are a number of virus particles less than 0.3 μm, but these are still caught in the filter.
  - HEPA filter is used for respiratory protection—like P3 masks and portable respiratory systems, as protection against infectious agents.
  - Used to shield patients who are highly immunosuppressed (air overpressure with HEPA filters on the inlet air).
  - Use on air outlets/recirculation from isolates for infectious disease to catch adverse contaminants.
  - Used as LAF (laminar air flow) ceilings or other types of filters in the operating room to get clean enough air into the room and to the surgical site.

References

1. Garner JS, Jarvis WR, Emori TG, Horan TC, Hughes JM. CDC definitions for nosocomial infections, 1988. Am J Infect Control. 1988;16:128–40.
2. Haley RW, Culver DH, White JW, et al. The efficacy of infection surveillance and control programs in preventing nosocomial infections in university hospitals. Am J Epidemiol. 1985;121:182–205.
3. Horan TC, Andrus M, Dudeck M. CDC/NHSN surveillance definition of health care-associated infection and criteria for specific types of infections in the acute care setting. Am J Infect Control. 2008;36:309–32.
4. Andersen BM, Hochlin K, Rasch M. Prevalence studies. In: Handbook in hygiene and infection control for hospitals; 2008. p. 671–8.